Putting Prevention into Practice

Problem Solving in Clinical Prevention

EDITED BY

RICHARD K. RIEGELMAN, M.D., Ph.D.
Professor of Health Care Sciences and Medicine, George Washington
University School of Medicine and Health Sciences; Attending
Physician, George Washington University Hospital, Washington

GAIL J. POVAR, M.D., M.P.H.
Associate Professor of Health Care Sciences and Medicine, George
Washington University School of Medicine and Health Sciences;
Attending Physician, George Washington University Hospital,
Washington

LITTLE, BROWN AND COMPANY
BOSTON/TORONTO

Contents

Preface

Our system's philosophy might be condensed in the motto as "Millions for cure and not a penny for prevention."

W. Hutchinson [1], 1886

"The physician's function is fast becoming social and preventive; rather than individual and curative" [2]. So wrote Abraham Flexner in his 1910 report on medical education. In 1932, the Committee on the Cost of Medical Care again forecast a future in which medical practice would be increasingly concerned with prevention [3]. Most recently, the Report on the General Professional Education of the Physician (GPEP report) strongly endorsed an emphasis in medical education on "promoting health and preventing diseases" [4].

Despite such assertions, teaching prevention has remained very much in the background. Barker and Jonas report that "Some 40 years of effort . . . to teach prevention as an integral part of clinical medicine . . . have met with limited success" [5]. Yet, the emphasis in medicine has changed markedly in the last few years. The public and the profession are paying increasing attention to health promotion and disease detection. Reports of preventive strategies are as likely as "rescue" techniques to capture a newspaper's front page. Such a social and medical evolution mandates a new focus. Skills essential to the practice of prevention are no longer peripheral to either medical practice or to mainstream medical education. Our goal in producing this text is to facilitate the integration of clinical preventive medicine into the medical curriculum.

To accomplish this goal, we have tried to define the critical skills that lie at the convergence of three related disciplines: clinical preventive medicine, primary care, and medical decision making. Clinical epidemiology, decision analysis, cost-effectiveness analysis, and health policy evaluation represent essential skills for the intelligent interpretation of proposed preventive interventions. With such training, the physician's endorsement of preventive strategies is enhanced. Lewis has written, ". . . the primary role of the physician is to legitimize and emphasize the value of certain preventive practices . . ." [6]. We believe that the doctor who most fully appreciates the foundation of well-constructed preventive policies is their most effective advocate.

To accomplish this role, physicians need to be able to think through the official recommendations. They must be prepared to read between the lines. Ultimately, they must be equipped to choose to adopt, to question, or even to reject such recommendations. To teach these skills, we have attempted, in the words of the GPEP report, to ". . . offer educational experiences that require students to be active, independent learners and problem solvers, rather than passive recipients of information" [4].

We have been guided by the assumption that the specific issues in prevention will continue to change dramatically. What is necessary are the skills to approach *new data* and *new problems* in a flexible, analytic fashion. Thus, our text is not a compendium of information, attempting to cover the range and breadth of topics in clinical prevention. Rather, we have selected representative problems that will guide the student or clinician in the development and application of fundamental assessment skills. The cases are familiar territory—cholesterol, breast cancer, rabies, atrial fibrillation. The approach, we believe, is new.

Putting Prevention into Practice: Problem Solving in Clinical Prevention is written by and for clinicians. The book offers a range of clinical issues and preventive medicine approaches. The authors' unique interests, backgrounds, and philosophies are evident in the individual cases. The cases, however, share common characteristics. Each presents a clinical scenario, characterizes the clinical issues, walks the reader through the available data, reviews the unanswered questions, and returns to the individual patient. Above all, the cases are designed to be clinically relevant and intellectually stimulating. We hope you will agree!

R. K. R.
G. J. P.

References

1. Hutchinson W. Health insurance, or our financial relation to the public. JAMA 1886;7:477–481.
2. Flexner A. Medical education in the United States and Canada. A report to the Carnegie Foundation for the Advancement of Teaching, Bulletin No. 4. Boston: Updyke, 1910.
3. Committee on the Cost of Medical Care. Medical care for the American people. Final report of the Committee on the Costs of Medical Care. Chicago: University of Chicago Press, 1932.
4. Muller S (Chairman). Physicians for the twenty-first century. Report of the Project Panel on the General Professional Education of the Physician and College Preparation for Medicine. J Med Educ, November 1984;59:2.
5. Barker WH, Jonas S. The teaching of preventive medicine in American medical schools, 1940–1980. Prev Med 1981;10:674–688.
6. Lewis CE. Teaching medical students about disease prevention and health promotion. Public Health Rep 1982;97:210.

Contributing Authors

EVE BARGMANN, M.D.
Assistant Professor of Health Care Sciences and Medicine, George Washington University School of Medicine and Health Sciences; Attending Physician, George Washington University Hospital, Washington

HOWARD J. BENNETT, M.D.
Associate Professor of Health Care Sciences and Child Health and Development, George Washington University School of Medicine and Health Sciences; Attending Pediatrician, Children's Hospital National Medical Center, Washington

BENJAMIN C. BLATT, M.D.
Associate Professor of Health Care Sciences and Medicine, George Washington University School of Medicine and Health Sciences; Attending Physician, George Washington University Hospital, Washington

RISA BETH BURNS, M.D.
Assistant Professor of Emergency Medicine, George Washington University School of Medicine and Health Sciences; formerly, Resident, Department of Health Care Sciences, George Washington University School of Medicine and Health Sciences, Washington

JAMES F. CAWLEY, M.P.H., PA-C.
Associate Professor of Health Care Sciences and Associate Director, Master of Public Health Program, George Washington University School of Medicine and Health Sciences, Washington

LAWRENCE J. D'ANGELO, M.D., M.P.H.
Associate Professor of Child Health and Development and Medicine, George Washington University School of Medicine and Health Sciences; Chairman, Department of Adolescent and Young Adult Medicine, Children's Hospital National Medical Center, Washington

KATHLEEN K. DAVIS, M.D.
Assistant Clinical Professor of Health Care Sciences and Medicine, George Washington University School of Medicine and Health Sciences; Attending Physician, George Washington University Hospital, Washington

GENE A. H. KALLENBERG, M.D.
Assistant Professor of Health Care Sciences and Medicine, George Washington University School of Medicine and Health Sciences; Attending Physician, George Washington University Hospital, Washington

MARIANA KASTRINAKIS, M.D.
Assistant Professor of Medicine and Child Health and Development, George Washington University School of Medicine and Health Sciences; Attending Physician, George Washington University Hospital, Washington

LILA T. McCONNELL, M.D.
Assistant Professor of Health Care Sciences, Division of Geriatric Medicine, George Washington University School of Medicine and Health Sciences; Attending Physician, George Washington University Hospital, Washington

ROBERT J. MELFI, M.D.
Fellow in Endocrinology, George Washington University School of Medicine and Health Sciences; formerly, Resident, Department of Health Care Sciences, George Washington University School of Medicine and Health Sciences, Washington

L. GREGORY PAWLSON M.D., M.P.H.
Acting Chairman and Professor of Health Care Sciences, Medicine, and Health Services Administration, George Washington University School of Medicine and Health Sciences; Attending Physician in Geriatric Medicine, George Washington University Hospital, Washington

GAIL J. POVAR, M.D., M.P.H.
Associate Professor of Health Care Sciences and Medicine, George Washington University School of Medicine and Health Sciences; Attending Physician, George Washington University Hospital, Washington

RICHARD K. RIEGELMAN, M.D. Ph.D.
Professor of Health Care Sciences and Medicine, George Washington University School of Medicine and Health Sciences; Attending Physician, George Washington University Hospital, Washington

TERESA M. SCHAER, M.D.
Chief Geriatrician, St. Peter's Hospital, New Brunswick; formerly, Geriatric Fellow, Department of Health Care Sciences, George Washington University School of Medicine and Health Sciences, Washington

WALTER A. STEIN, M.A., PA-C.
Assistant Professor of Health Care Sciences and Director, Physician Assistant Program, George Washington University School of Medicine and Health Sciences, Washington

ALAN W. STONE, M.D.
Associate Professor of Health Care Sciences and Medicine, George Washington University School of Medicine and Health Sciences; Attending Physician, George Washington University Hospital, Washington

TEEKIE WAGNER, M.D., M.P.H.
Assistant Professor of Health Care Sciences and Child Health and Development, George Washington University School of Medicine and Health Sciences; Attending Pediatrician, Children's Hospital National Medical Center, Washington

ROBERT E. WALKER, M.D.
Pulmonary Fellow, Hospital of the University of Pennsylvania, Philadelphia; formerly, Resident, Department of Health Care Sciences, George Washington University School of Medicine and Health Sciences, Washington

MARK I. WEISSMAN, M.D.
Assistant Professor of Health Care Sciences and Child Health and Development, George Washington University School of Medicine and Health Sciences; Attending Pediatrician, Children's Hospital National Medical Center, Washington

Putting Prevention into Practice

Problem Solving in Clinical Prevention

Introduction

PART ONE

Reading Between the Lines of the Official Recommendations

CHAPTER ONE

RICHARD K. RIEGELMAN
GAIL J. POVAR

Yesterday's panacea becomes today's placebo. Today's cure may be tomorrow's carcinogen. In every direction we look, change and uncertainty surround the practice of medicine. How can clinicians cope?

One might be tempted to adhere to the tried and true, resisting change at every turn. At the other extreme is the tendency to adopt the conclusions of the latest study or the newest official recommendations, equating what is new with what is good. In *Putting Prevention into Practice*, we present a third alternative: to accept uncertainty and change as a permanent condition and learn to read between the lines of the official recommendations.

The goal of *Putting Prevention into Practice* is to help you think through the problems of clinical preventive medicine. We will approach this important task by providing you with the background and practice to (1) characterize the problem, and (2) evaluate the solutions. Equipped with these skills, you will be prepared to read between the lines of the official recommendations.

Before forging ahead, let us take a look at a relatively straightforward situation you may confront in clinical preventive medicine. What questions occur to you as you read through the case? What answers can you offer? See how far you get in thinking through the questions.

Reye's syndrome is a rare, life-threatening disease of children, characterized by vomiting, hepatic abnormalities, and mental changes that may progress to coma and death. Reye's syndrome usually follows viral infections, especially influenza and chickenpox. The treatment of Reye's syndrome, once diagnosed, is largely supportive, with no known cure available. Recently, the use of aspirin but not acetaminophen has been suggested as a contributory cause of Reye's syndrome.

One of your patients brings in a bottle of children's aspirin and reads you the official recommendations, which state:

Children and teenagers should not use this medicine for chickenpox or flu symptoms before a doctor is consulted about Reye's syndrome, a rare but serious disease.

This recommendation sounds simple enough, but let's delve a little deeper. Take a minute to list the questions you would want answered before you accept the recommendation.

You might have asked the following questions:

1. What data is needed to establish that aspirin is a contributory cause of Reye's syndrome?
2. What are the risks and benefits of using aspirin versus the alternatives?
3. When in the natural history of the disease is the intervention occurring?
4. Who is the target of the intervention?
5. How is the recommendation being implemented?
6. What intervention options have been rejected and why?

Did you ask other questions as well? These are the kinds of questions this book will teach you to ask and to answer. For a preview of the completed process for this case, turn to the final chapter. We will arrive at the analyses demonstrated in the last chapter by focusing on the development of our two important skills, characterizing the problem and evaluating the solution.

Characterizing the Problem

Problem solving in clinical prevention requires us to answer the following questions:

What causes the disease? We will review the methods and criteria used to establish the contributory causes of a disease and identify who is at risk.

How can we detect the presence of the disease? We will review the methods used to assess screening tests for early intervention.

Evaluating the Solutions

To evaluate the solutions, we must address the following questions:

What are the benefits, risks, and costs of potential interventions? We will review the methods of risk-benefit analysis, decision analysis, and cost-effectiveness analysis to help answer this question.

When in the natural history could we intervene? We may choose among primary prevention (intervention before the disease develops), secondary prevention (intervention during the asymptomatic stage of disease), or tertiary prevention (intervention after the appearance of clinical disease).

Who could be the target for the intervention? We may direct intervention to the individual, the group at risk, the population at large, including individuals not at risk.

What strategies for preventive intervention are available to us? We may choose from three basic strategies that differ in the degree of external force and individual decision making required. These strategies include information, motivation, and obligation.

Finally, how should we choose among the options?

Applying These Skills

Having developed the ability to characterize problems and evaluate solutions, you will undoubtedly want to apply what you have learned. Thus, the heart of this book consists of 14 cases that will help you learn problem solving in clinical prevention. The cases are divided into primary, secondary, and tertiary prevention. Each case challenges you to characterize the problem, evaluate the solutions, and apply them to individual patients. The busy clinician will not always be able to take such an in-depth approach. However, having worked through these cases, you will be prepared to ask the right questions when problem solving in clinical prevention. To help you, we will provide a checklist of appropriate questions in the final chapter.

The approach we recommend in *Putting Prevention into Practice* will not provide you with all the answers or even the right answer. It will, however, serve as a framework for organizing your thoughts as you raise issues and seek the best solution. Despite so much uncertainty in medicine, thinking through problems in an organized manner should enable you to make well-informed decisions and to act wisely.

Characterizing the Problem

PART TWO

Rates, Risk Factors, and Causation

CHAPTER TWO

RICHARD K. RIEGELMAN

Measurements of the rates of disease are tools for analysis that are basic to defining the natural history of a disease, identifying who is at risk for contracting a disease, and evaluating the cause of a disease. In this chapter, we will demonstrate, using the relationship between cigarettes and lung cancer, how rates of disease can be used to accomplish each of these purposes.*

Rates of Disease

TYPES OF RATES

There are three basic types of rates that characterize the risk of disease: incidence rates, prevalence rates, and case-fatality rates.† Let us look at how these three basic types of rates are defined and interpreted.

Incidence rates are used to estimate the probability of developing a disease.‡ They are defined as follows:

$$\text{Incidence rate} = \frac{\text{no. of individuals who develop the disease over a period of time}}{\text{total person-years at risk}}$$

Incidence rates are the basic measure of risk for developing a disease over a period of time. However, limitations of available data frequently require that we use mortality or death rates to assess the risk of disease. Mortality rates aim to approximate the risk of dying from a disease. Over

---

*In this book we will use the term *rate* as synonymous with a proportion. Biostatisticians, at times, further distinguish between a rate and a proportion. To be called a rate, a measure must also contain a unit of time in the denominator.

†Rates are, strictly speaking, only an approximation of risk. Mathematical expressions of risk include the number of individuals who could develop the disease in the denominator. Since this rarely is known and changes from day to day, we approximate those at risk by using an estimate of the number of individuals in a population at one point in time.

‡Biostatisticians and epidemiologists often distinguish between cumulative incidence and incidence rates. Cumulative incidence contains in the denominator the number of individuals in the population at the beginning of the time period. Strictly speaking, the cumulative incidence is synonymous with risk.

9

an extended period of time, mortality is related to incidence rates as follows:

Mortality rates = incidence rate × case-fatality rate

Case-fatality rates estimate the probability of dying from a disease once it develops. They reflect the number of individuals who die divided by the number of individuals who develop the disease. Case-fatality rates, unlike incidence rates, are affected by the success of medical intervention designed to cure disease or prolong life despite the presence of disease. Thus, one must be careful not to equate mortality rates with risk of developing the disease.

In addition to incidence rates and case-fatality rates, we need to use *prevalence rates,* to provide a comprehensive picture of the risk of disease. Prevalence rates estimate the probability of having a disease at a point in time. The numerator in prevalence rates represents the number of people in a population who have the disease at a point in time, whereas in incidence rates the numerator is the number of people who acquire or develop the disease over a period of time. Prevalence rates are defined as follows:

$$\text{Prevalence rate} = \frac{\text{no. of individuals who have the disease at a point in time}}{\text{no. of individuals who are in the population at risk at the same point in time}}$$

Clinically, prevalence rates are a starting point for the diagnosis of disease, since they estimate the risk or probability that an individual in a population has the disease. For rare disease, prevalence rates are related to incidence rates approximately as follows:

Prevalence rate of a disease

= incidence rate of the disease × average duration of the disease

Taken together, the incidence, case-fatality, and prevalence rates reflect the risk at three key points in the natural history of a disease. Thus, in clinical medicine, we need to define these rates if we are to define the natural history of the disease.* This may be depicted as follows:

Development of disease	Diagnosis of disease	Outcome of disease
Incidence rate	Prevalence rate	Case-fatality rate

Now let us look at the case of lung cancer and cigarette smoking to illustrate some of the concepts just described.

LUNG CANCER AND CIGARETTES.   In the United States, lung cancer accounts for more deaths than any other cancer. There are four major types of lung or bronchogenic cancer: epidermoid (also called squamous cell), adenocarcinoma, large cell, and small cell carcinoma. Epidermoid carcinoma is the most common. All four types have a poor prognosis. The 2-year case-fatality rate is approximately 90 percent.

_____ STUDY QUESTION 2-1

Dependable incidence rates for lung cancer are not available. Mortality rates have generally been substituted. From what you know about the case-fatality rates, is it reasonable to use mortality rates as an estimate of incidence rates?

Risk Factors

Incidence rates provide a useful figure for assessing the factors that contribute to disease occurrence. By comparing incidence rates between

---

*Incidence, prevalence, and case-fatality rates share the common feature that their denominators are all estimates of the number of individuals at risk of experiencing the event included in the numerator. Rates always have numerators that reflect the number of diseases or events, whereas the denominators reflect the number of individuals in the population at risk for the same disease or event. Rates are thus an approximation of risk. In contrast, ratios do not require that the numerator be related to the denominator. Therefore, ratios are not an estimate of risk.

Mortality ratios are the most frequently used ratios. Mortality rates are defined as follows:

$$\text{Mortality ratio} = \frac{\text{no. of individuals dying from a disease}}{\text{no. of individuals dying from all diseases}}$$

Mortality ratios are a useful means of determining which are the most important causes of death at particular ages, but they do not tell us about the risk of death.

populations or by observing changes in incidence rates over time, we frequently can suspect the existence of factors associated with disease in groups.

Let us imagine that we have observed a difference in the incidence of a disease between two populations or have observed a change in the incidence of the disease over time. What are the possible reasons for differences or changes in the incidence of the disease?

Differences in incidence rates between populations or changes in the same population over time may be artifactual or real. *Artifactual changes* may be the result of

1. Differences or changes in the definition of the disease.
2. Differences or changes in efforts to search for the disease.
3. Differences or changes in the technology available for detecting the disease.

When these artifactual causes do not explain the differences in rates that we have observed, then we can conclude by elimination, that the changes are real. *Real changes* (1) may be explained by differences or changes in the characteristics of the population at risk or (2) may reflect actual increases in the incidence rate of disease for similar individuals.

Differences or changes in the characteristics of the population at risk may involve variations in the age, sex, or racial distribution of the population. Such variations produce real difference in the risk of certain diseases for the population as a whole. This does not necessarily mean, however, that individuals of the same age, sex, or race have different levels of risk.

Because age is such an important determinant of the risk of disease, rates of disease frequently take into account the age distribution of a population, using age standardization.* Standardization helps us obtain a fairer comparison of the risk of disease for individuals of the same age in different populations or at different times. Age standardization using the direct method compares two populations, asking: How many events, such as death, would have occurred in population 1 if it had the age distribution of population 2. Often, the data from a population is standardized using the indirect method. This method compares the observed

---

*Standardization can be performed for any characteristic that may affect the risk of disease, if one has data on the frequency of the characteristic for subgroups of the population.

number of events, such as death, in a population to the number that would have been expected in the general population. The indirect method can produce a ratio known as the standardized mortality ratio.

$$\text{Standardized mortality ratio} = \frac{\text{observed no. of deaths}}{\text{expected no. of deaths}}$$

Real increases in the incidence rate of disease for similar individuals may be owing to

1. New or increased frequency of risk factors for disease that herald further increases in the disease over time.
2. Cyclical or epidemic fluctuations in the incidence of disease that produce temporary increases in the risk of disease. These increases may be self-limited, and subsequent decreases in the incidence of the disease may occur.
3. Increases reflecting special susceptibility of a subgroup or cohort of the population that produce real but temporary increases in the incidence of disease owing to their so-called cohort effect.

Thus, real increases in incidence rates of disease may have a variety of implications for the future incidence rates of disease.

_____ STUDY QUESTION 2-2
Figure 2-1 summarizes the changes that have occurred in the age-standardized mortality from lung cancer in the United States in recent years. (a) Do you think these are real or artifactual changes? (b) Can you hypothesize an explanation for these changes? (c) What are the limitations of these trends in predicting the future risk of dying from lung cancer?

The rates of a disease help us characterize the risk posed by the disease among groups of individuals. Changes or differences in rates among groups may suggest factors associated with the disease. These group associations or ecological associations, however, do not establish the existence of a risk factor. *Risk factors are characteristics of individuals that are associated with the development of disease in the same individual.* To be a risk factor, a characteristic must be more commonly associated with individuals who develop a disease than with those who do not develop the disease. Association simply implies that the factor and the disease occur together more frequently than expected by chance alone. A risk

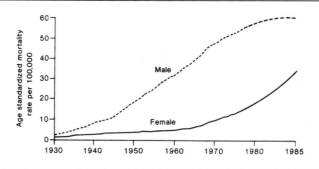

Fig. 2-1. Age-standardized mortality rates for lung cancer among white men and women in the United States for selected years from 1930 to 1985. Rates are standardized on the United States population of 1940. (Based on data supplied by the American Cancer Society.)

factor may be unalterable, such as age, sex, or race, or potentially alterable, such as cholesterol level, hypertension, or cigarette smoking.

To define the risk factors for a disease, we need to do more than observe changes or differences in rates among groups or populations. We need to compare individuals with the disease to those without the disease. Much of clinical research on the etiology of disease is devoted to studies that retrospectively or prospectively compare individuals with and without a disease to determine the risk factors associated with that disease. Let us briefly look at the measures used to describe and measure risk factors.

RELATIVE RISK
Relative risk is a fundamental measure of the importance of a risk factor. Relative risk tells us the probability of the disease if the risk factor is present compared to the probability of disease if the risk factor is absent. Relative risk is defined as follows:

$$\text{Relative risk} = \frac{\text{probability of developing the disease if the factor is present}}{\text{probability of developing the disease if the factor is absent}}$$

A relative risk of 1 indicates that there is no association between the factor and the disease. A relative risk of less than 1 suggests that the factor is associated with *less* disease, whereas a relative risk of more than 1 indicates that the factor is associated with *more* disease. There is no upper limit to the size of the relative risk, but the lower limit is zero. The higher the relative risk, the stronger the association between the risk factor and the disease.*

Notice that relative risk does not tell us the actual magnitude of the risk. It tells us the relative probability of disease if the risk factor is present, compared to the probability of disease if the risk factor is absent. This distinction has important clinical implications. For example, let us imagine a relative risk of 10 in these two clinical situations:

The incidence of disease for those without the risk factor is 1 per 100.

The incidence of disease for those without the risk factor is 1 per 10,000.

The implication of a relative risk of 10 in these two situations is very different. In the first situation, the probability of disease if the risk factor is present is increased 10-fold from approximately 1 per 100 to 1 in 10. In the second situation, if the risk factor is present, the probability of disease increases from approximately 1 per 10,000 to 1 per 1000. Despite the same relative risk, the absolute risks for those with the risk factor are strikingly different. The difference depends on the underlying incidence rate of the disease for those without the risk factor. Thus, to characterize the absolute risk of developing disease, one needs to know the incidence of disease for those without the risk factor as well as the relative risk resulting from a given risk factor.

Risk factors frequently operate together to increase the probability of developing a particular disease. The presence of two or more risk factors may produce independent effects that add one to another, or they may produce effects that cause the risk to multiply.

LUNG CANCER AND CIGARETTES.   Classic data on the risk of lung cancer was collected by the American Cancer Society in the 1950s. Almost 190,000 American men aged 50 to 60 years were followed for 44 months to assess the relationship between cigarette smoking and lung cancer. Figure 2-2 shows the data com-

---

*In retrospective or case-control studies, the odds ratio is used as an approximation of relative risk. Ninety-five-percent confidence limits can be calculated and often appear in parentheses after the relative risk. If the range of the 95-percent confidence limits does not include an odds ratio or relative risk of 1, then the relative risk or odds ratio is statistically significant at the $p < .05$ level.

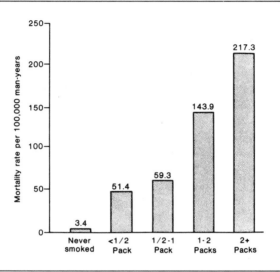

Fig. 2-2. Age-adjusted death rates from malignant neoplasm of lung (exclusive of adenocarcinoma) by amount of cigarette smoking at beginning of prospective study in 1952. (Adapted from EC Hammond and D Horn. Smoking and death rates: report on 44 months of follow-up of 187,783 men. JAMA 1958;166:1159, 1294.)

paring the mortality from lung cancer and the quantity of cigarette smoking. The relative risk for those who smoked less than one-half pack per day compared to those who never smoked is calculated as follows:

$$\text{Relative risk} = \frac{51.4}{3.4} = 15.1$$

_____ STUDY QUESTION 2-3

Calculate the relative risk of cigarette smoking at each of the other levels compared to those who never smoked.

LUNG CANCER AND CIGARETTES.   The risk of cigarette smoking often interacts with other risk factors. For instance, cigarette smoking, hypertension, and cholesterol are approximately additive risk factors for coronary artery disease. The effect of cigarettes may also be multiplicative. The presence of cigarette smoking in the context of asbestos exposure multiplies the risk of lung cancer as compared to the risk from asbestos exposure alone.

_____ STUDY QUESTION 2-4
Assume that an individual has a relative risk of 2 for coronary artery disease
from cigarettes, 2 from hypertension, and 3 from cholesterol. What is this individual's approximate overall relative risk compared to a comparable individual
without any of these risk factors?

_____ STUDY QUESTION 2-5
Assume that an individual exposed to asbestos has a relative risk of lung cancer
of 5. Assume that the same individual's relative risk of lung cancer owing to
smoking is 10. What is this person's overall relative risk of lung cancer compared
to the average individual for whom asbestos exposure or cigarettes are not a risk
factor?

ATTRIBUTABLE RISK
Incidence rates and relative risks are the fundamental measures that,
when used together, define the clinical probability of disease for individuals. However, if one is interested in the potential consequences of reduction or elimination of the risk factor one also needs to consider additional concepts known as attributable risk and population attributable
risk. Attributable risk and population attributable risk are also referred
to as attributable fraction (exposed) and attributable fraction (population), respectively. Some authors also refer to them as attributable risk
percentage and population attributable risk.

Attributable risk and population attributable risk are related concepts
that address somewhat different questions. Attributable risk addresses
the question: What proportion of the disease *among those with the risk
factor* is associated with or potentially attributable to the risk factor? Attributable risk thus measures the potential clinical impact for those with
the risk factor. In a particular study, the attributable risk is expressed by
the following formula:

$$\text{Attributable risk} = \frac{\begin{array}{c}\text{incidence of the disease}\\ \text{among those with}\\ \text{the risk factor}\end{array} - \begin{array}{c}\text{incidence of the disease}\\ \text{among those without}\\ \text{the risk factor}\end{array}}{\begin{array}{c}\text{incidence of the disease among those}\\ \text{with the risk factor}\end{array}}$$

Relative risk can be converted to attributable risk using the following
formula:

$$\text{Attributable risk} = \frac{\text{relative risk} - 1}{\text{relative risk}}$$

This conversion formula holds true when the relative risk is greater than 1. When the factor under study is protective and therefore has a relative risk less than 1, the attributable risk equals $(1 - \text{relative risk}) \times 100$. The following table demonstrates the relationship between relative risk and attributable risk.

Relative Risk	Attributable Risk (%)
1	0
2	50
4	75
10	90
20	95
100	99

Notice that even a small relative risk of 2 means that 50 percent of the cases of disease among those with the risk factor is potentially attributable to the risk factor. A risk factor with a relative risk of 10 may explain a large proportion of the cases of disease among those with the risk factor.

The closer the attributable risk is to 100 percent, the more strongly the disease is associated with or potentially attributable to the risk factor. If a cause and effect relationship exists, the attributable risk tells one the maximum percentage reduction in disease one could expect among those with the risk factor if the effects of the risk factor were totally and immediately eliminated.

A second form of attributable risk is known as population attributable risk. Population attributable risk asks about the potential community impact of the risk factor as opposed to the impact on those with the risk factor. Since communities are usually composed of individuals with and individuals without a risk factor, population attributable risk takes into account the proportion of a population that has the risk factor. Thus, population attributable risk addresses the question: How much of the disease in a community is potentially attributable to the risk factor? Population attributable risk is related to the relative risk (RR) and the proportion of the population with the risk factor (b) by the following formula:

$$\text{Population attributable risk} = \frac{(b)\,(RR - 1)}{(b)\,(RR - 1) + 1}$$

Table 2-1. Relationship among population attributable risk (PAR), relative risk (RR), and proportion of the population with the risk factor (b)

RR	b (%)	PAR (approximate %)
2	1	1
4	1	3
10	1	8
20	1	16
2	10	9
4	10	23
10	10	46
20	10	65
2	50	33
4	50	60
10	50	82
20	50	90
2	100	50
4	100	75
10	100	90
20	100	95

   The relationship among relative risk, proportion of the population with the risk factor, and population attributable risk is summarized in Table 2-1. Notice that if the risk factor is uncommon (1 percent, for instance), the relative risk must be substantial before the population attributable risk starts to increase. On the other hand, if the risk factor is common (50 percent, for instance), even a small relative risk means that the potential community impact will be substantial. When the prevalence of the risk factor is 100 percent (i.e., everyone has the risk factor), note that the population attributable risk equals the attributable risk.

   The concept of population attributable risk, like attributable risk, does not guarantee that reductions in disease will result from altering the risk factor. Rather, those concepts tell us the maximum that can be expected if a cause and effect relationship exists. We will discuss what we mean by a cause and effect relationship, but let us first return to our examination of cigarettes and lung cancer.

—————————————————————————— STUDY QUESTION 2-6

Let us assume that for the average cigarette smoker the relative risk for lung cancer is 20. What is the attributable risk for lung cancer among smokers?

—————————————————————————— STUDY QUESTION 2-7

Let us assume that 50 percent of a population smokes cigarettes and that the average relative risk of lung cancer for smokers is 20. What is the population attributable risk of lung cancer from cigarette smoking?

—————————————————————————— STUDY QUESTION 2-8

What are the implications when a disease such as lung cancer has a high incidence and the attributable risk and the population attributable risk are both high?

Causation

The concept of risk factors for disease must be distinguished from the concept of causation. To be a cause of disease or, more strictly speaking, a *contributory cause,* a factor must fulfill all the following criteria:

1. The cause is associated with the disease (the effect).
2. The cause precedes the disease (the effect).
3. Altering the cause alters the disease (the effect).

The term *risk factor* can be used whenever the first criterion of causation—association—is fulfilled. We will use the term *risk factor* in this way. Others use this term only after the second criterion is also fulfilled. To be a risk factor, however, a characteristic does not need to satisfy the third criterion of causation. Factors such as age, sex, race, or socioeconomic status can be risk factors without fulfilling the third criterion of contributory cause. Such risk factors may be useful for identifying individuals who are at increased risk of developing a disease. However, to answer the question of why certain individuals are at risk, we must ultimately look beyond risk factors to contributory cause.

ESTABLISHING THE FORMAL CRITERIA
FOR CONTRIBUTORY CAUSE

The criteria for contributory cause can be established based on data from the three basic types of clinical studies: retrospective (case-control), prospective (cohort), and experimental (controlled clinical trials).

Retrospective studies begin after the development of the disease and look back in time to assess the presence or absence of risk factors. They are capable of establishing the existence of an association between a risk factor and a disease. Remember, though, that an association is only the first of three criteria needed to establish contributory cause. The fact that such studies begin after the development of disease makes it more difficult for them to establish that the risk factor precedes the disease. It is always possible that the disease occurs first and brings about the development of the risk factor. Also because they begin after the development of disease, retrospective studies are prone to a series of biases that may call into question the existence of a true association. For instance, it has been shown that the incidence of lung cancer is very high among those who recently stopped smoking cigarettes. Ceasing to smoke cigarettes, however, may be a response to, rather than the cause of, the lung cancer. Retrospective studies may also produce false associations, in part owing to their dependence on recall and reporting. Recall errors tend to occur when the study patients, who are aware of the existence of disease, more thoroughly search their memories for commonly occurring, subjectively recalled events. Reporting error may occur when those with the disease are put under increased pressure to report confidential information.

Prospective or cohort studies begin before the development of disease. They assess the future occurrence of disease among groups with and without the risk factor under study. Prospective studies are capable of establishing an association. In addition, when doubt exists, prospective studies are more useful than retrospective studies in assuring that the cause precedes the effect. Prospective studies are also less prone to biases owing to recall and reporting. However, both prospective and retrospective studies may produce spurious or false associations as a result of the methods used to select study and control groups. Selection bias occurs whenever study or control group patients are different from all those who could have been selected and this difference affects the outcome (subsequent disease or prior characteristic) being measured.

The third basic type of study is the *experimental study*, usually referred to as controlled clinical trials. This design is theoretically capable of meeting all three criteria of contributory cause. What distinguishes controlled clinical trials of preventive therapy is that individuals are randomized to receive or not to receive a therapy designed to alter a risk factor for disease.* Randomization implies that individuals have a known probability of being assigned to a treatment group or a control group. It does not imply that the individuals are randomly selected or selected by chance from a large population. The randomization process does not assure that the study and control groups will be identical. By chance alone, one group may contain individuals who have a worse outlook or prognosis. Factors that differ between groups and that appear to affect outcome are known as *confounding variables*.

All three types of studies must take into account confounding variables. Confounding variables can be recognized and prevented at the beginning of studies by the process of pairing or matching, or they may be taken into account or controlled for after the data has been collected using statistical techniques such as regression analysis.

When properly performed, controlled clinical trials enable the investigator to assess the association between the risk factor and the disease; to assure that the risk factor occurs prior to the development of the disease; and to determine whether altering the risk factor results in an altered incidence of the disease. If all three of these criteria are fulfilled, then the risk factor under study can be said to be contributory cause of the disease.

Note that a contributory cause is not necessarily the most immediate biologic explanation for the effect. Some epidemiologists distinguish between direct and indirect contributory causes. A direct contributory cause is the most immediate known biologic link between the cause and the effect. The following may be direct and indirect contributory causes:

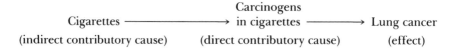

The performance of controlled clinical trials often is not possible. Once a strong association between a risk factor and a disease has been established, randomization may be considered unethical by doctors or patients. Difficulty in obtaining the necessary numbers or administrative

---

*Blinding of investigators and patients is frequently performed as part of controlled clinical trials, in an effort to eliminate bias and control for the placebo effect. However, blinding often is unsuccessful or impractical, and so it is highly desirable but not required for all controlled clinical trials.

logistics may also preclude a controlled clinical trial. When it is not practical or ethical to use a controlled clinical trial to assess whether altering the cause alters the effect, natural experiments may be adequate substitutes. Natural experiments take place when changes in the frequency of risk factors occur in a population without intervention by an investigator. When carefully observed, natural experiments may help establish that altering the cause alters the effect.

ESTABLISHING ANCILLARY CRITERIA FOR CONTRIBUTORY CAUSE
At times, we wish to make judgments about the existence of cause and effect relationships when the formal criteria of contributory cause cannot be fulfilled. In these situations, additional circumstantial evidence often is used as supportive evidence for the existence of a contributory cause. Ancillary criteria that support the existence of a contributory cause include

The strength of the association between the risk factor and the disease as measured, for example, by the size of the relative risk.

The consistency of the association from one study population to another.

The biologic plausibility of the relationship as deduced from clinical or basic scientific data.

The existence of a dose-response relationship implying that greater exposure to the risk factor is associated with a greater incidence of disease.

Data supporting each of these criteria help bolster the argument that a risk factor is actually a contributory cause. Nonetheless, the criteria do not prove the existence of a contributory cause. In addition, none of these four criteria for establishing contributory cause are essential. A risk factor with a modest but real association may be a contributory cause. Consistency is not essential since it is possible for a risk factor to operate in one population but not another because of the existence or absence of other prerequisite conditions. Biologic plausibility assumes we understand the relevant biologic processes. Finally, a dose-response relationship, though common in medicine, is not required for a cause and effect relationship: Even small exposures may produce dramatic effects, and high doses (such as radiation to the thyroid) may cause less cancer risk than low-dose exposures. Therefore, one cannot exclude the possibility that a risk factor is a contributory cause if these ancillary criteria remain unfulfilled.

Contributory causes must be distinguished from necessary and sufficient causes of disease. *Necessary cause* implies that a risk factor is required for the development of a disease. *Sufficient cause* implies that a risk factor is sufficient to produce the disease by itself if present. Necessary and sufficient causes of disease are very rare in clinical medicine.

LUNG CANCER AND CIGARETTES.   The data suggesting an association between cigarettes and lung cancer goes back to the 1940s when case-control studies demonstrated an increased risk of lung cancer among those who smoked cigarettes. The results of a series of prospective studies performed in the 1950s are shown in Table 2-2.

_____ STUDY QUESTION 2-9
Which criteria of contributory cause are established by this data?

_____ STUDY QUESTION 2-10
What supporting criteria for contributory cause are established by this data?

_____ STUDY QUESTION 2-11
Controlled clinical trials are the optimal means of establishing whether altering the cause alters the disease. Do you think it would be feasible or ethical to perform a controlled clinical trial for cigarettes and lung cancer?

LUNG CANCER AND CIGARETTES.   To assess whether altering the cause alters the disease, data from natural experiments have been used. In natural experiments of cigarettes and lung cancer, the risk for smokers has been compared to the risk for exsmokers. This relationship is summarized in Figure 2-3.

_____ STUDY QUESTION 2-12
Does this data satisfy the third criterion of the definition of contributory cause?

Data supporting the biologic plausibility of the relationship between cigarettes and lung cancer have included the following:

Widespread histologic changes believed to be precursors of lung cancer are seen at autopsy much more frequently among smokers than nonsmokers.
Animal experiments have demonstrated the presence of cancer initiators and promotors in cigarette smoke.

_____ STUDY QUESTION 2-13
Does this type of evidence establish the biologic plausibility of cigarettes as a contributory cause of lung cancer?

Table 2-2. Results from three prospective studies of lung
cancer mortality ratios for current smokers of cigarettes*

Subject characteristics	Prospective study		
	Doll and Hill (1956)	Hammond and Horn (1958)	Dorn (1958)
Types of subjects	British doctors	Men from 9 U.S. states	U.S. veterans
No. of subjects	34,000	188,000	248,000
Age range (years)	35–75	30–69	30–75
Months followed	120	44	78
Mortality ratios			
Nonsmokers	1.0	1.0	1.0
Smokers (cigarettes/day)			
< 10	4.4	5.8	5.2
10–20	10.8	7.8	9.4
21–39	43.7	13.9	18.1
≥ 40		21.7	23.3

*Excludes persons who smoked pipes or cigars in addition to cigarettes.
Source: Adapted from Smoking and Health Report of the Advisory Committee to the
Surgeon General of the Public Health Service, U.S. Department of Health, Education
and Welfare (USPHS publication no. 1103). Washington, D.C.: U.S. Government
Printing Office. 1964:83, 164.

_____ STUDY QUESTION 2-14
Lung cancer does occur among nonsmokers, and many smokers, even after
long-term exposure, do not develop lung cancer. How do these facts affect your
assessment of a causal relationship between cigarette smoking and lung cancer?

Summary
The concepts of incidence rates, prevalence rates, and case-fatality rates
are our fundamental tools for measuring the risk of disease for groups
of people. When we attempt to define the factors associated with disease
in individuals, we use the concept of risk factors. The relative risk measures the strength of a risk factor. It compares the probability or rate of
disease when the risk factor is present and when it is absent. Relative risk

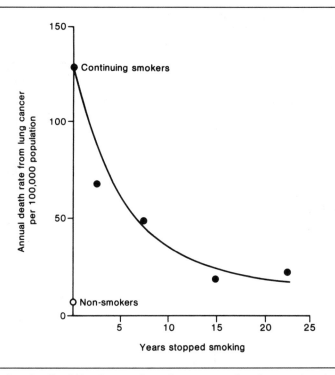

Fig. 2-3. Standardized death rates from lung cancer for cigarette smokers, exsmokers, and nonsmokers. (Adapted from R Doll, AB Hill: Br Med J 1964;1:1399, 1460.)

multiplied by the incidence rate when the risk factor is absent is used to assess the magnitude of the absolute risk.

Attributable risk asks the question: What percentage of the risk among those with the risk factor is potentially attributable to the risk factor? Population attributable risk asks a somewhat different question: What percentage of the risk of disease among a population is potentially attributable to the risk factor? Population attributable risk thus takes into account the fact that in a group or population only a proportion of the population possesses the risk factor.

Establishing contributory cause requires demonstration of an association between the risk factor and the disease. It also requires that the risk factor come before the disease. Finally, it requires that an alteration of the cause will alter the disease. When doubt remains regarding contributory cause, the strength, consistency, and biologic plausibility of the association and the existence of a dose-response relationship all provide supportive evidence. However, these ancillary criteria alone do not establish contributory cause.

The analytic tools for defining the natural history of a disease, identifying who is at risk for contracting a disease, and evaluating the cause of a disease are summarized in the following chart:

Rates	*Risk Factors*	*Causation*
Incidence rate	Relative risk	Association
Prevalence rate	Absolute risk	Prior association
Case-fatality rate	Attributable risk	Contributory cause
	Population attributable risk	Necessary and sufficient cause

Screening for Disease Control CHAPTER THREE

RICHARD K. RIEGELMAN
ALAN W. STONE
GENE A. H. KALLENBERG

Screening for disease control is the testing of asymptomatic individuals to detect the presence of risk factors for disease or a disease itself. (The term *screening* is also applied in other situations. For instance, screening may imply testing of symptomatic individuals as part of their diagnostic evaluation. Alternatively, clinicians may order a screen when they suspect a specific disease such as drug overdose in order to identify the drug or drugs taken. These uses of the term *screening* will not be used in this book.) Screening for disease control may benefit patients if (1) it enables clinicians to diagnosis a disease at an asymptomatic or preclinical phase, *and* (2) treatment at this earlier stage in the natural history of the disease leads to a longer life or reduced morbidity for those individuals who are detected by screening.

Figure 3-1 illustrates the intended benefits of screening for disease control. When screening is done at the individual level by a clinician as part of clinical care, the term *casefinding* is often applied.

Screening for disease control may be performed once, or it may be performed at intervals as part of an ongoing screening program. The results of an initial screening and a repeat screening of the same population may identify different types of cases of disease. Initial and repeat screening usually detect disease that has been present for different lengths of time.

The first time a group of individuals is screened, the cases will include a small group of individuals with disease that has recently developed; but mostly they will consist of individuals with disease that has been in the asymptomatic preclinical phase for a lengthier period of time. Together, these two types of individuals make up the cases of disease at one point in time. Thus, the cases of disease detected on initial screening approximate the *prevalence rate* of disease.

When repeating the screening process in the same population, one detects primarily those who have developed the disease in the interval between screenings. These are the individuals who have developed new disease. Thus, on repeat screening, the rate of disease detected approximates the *incidence rate*.

Prevalence cases are more numerous than incidence cases as long as we are screening for a chronic disease with a long average duration. Thus, more cases will usually be detected on initial screening than on subsequent repeat screening of the same population. It is possible, how-

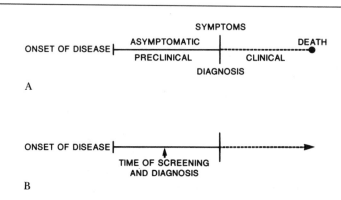

Fig. 3-1. Intended impact of screening. *A.* Natural history of a disease without screening. *B.* Natural history of a disease detected by screening and successfully treated.

ever, that by detecting cases of newly developed disease, repeat screenings may detect cases that are more responsive to treatment.

Screening for disease control takes time, costs money, and carries potential dangers, especially for those without disease who may be thought to have disease on the basis of a false positive screening test. Therefore, before advocating screening for disease control among large numbers of individuals, it is important to establish a set of criteria for a successful screening program. A screening program for a particular disease or risk factor can then be judged against these criteria. In general, the criteria address the basic questions of screening:

1. Is the morbidity or mortality associated with the disease so great that a successful screening program can be expected to benefit a substantial population?
2. Are there risk factors whose identification facilitates prevention or early detection?
3. Does early detection improve outcome?
4. Is there a testing approach that is both feasible and acceptable?

Let us define specifically what we mean by these questions and take a look at the implications of the criteria they establish. As we examine each criterion, we will see how it applies to the issue of screening for high blood pressure.

Criterion 1. Is the Morbidity or Mortality Associated with the Disease So Great that a Successful Screening Program Can Be Expected to Benefit a Substantial Population?

Screening is only worthwhile if the risk factor or disease has been shown to be a frequent contributory cause of such adverse outcomes as death or disability. Thus, before considering screening for a disease, it is important to establish that the disease is an important cause of death or disability in the population to be screened. Some diseases, such as colonic cancer, may satisfy this criterion by their severity and the frequency with which they cause death in the general population. Other diseases, such as Down's syndrome in infants delivered by women over age 35 or syphilis in homosexuals, may satisfy the criterion by the frequency of the disease in a particular risk group.

_____ STUDY QUESTION 3-1
Does hypertension satisfy criterion 1?

Criterion 2. Are There Risk Factors Whose Identification Facilitates Prevention or Early Detection?

Specifically, this question seeks to determine whether risk factors can be identified before the development of clinical disease that (1) can serve to identify high-risk groups to facilitate early detection of disease, or (2) can be modified to prevent the appearance of clinical disease. Risk factor detection may serve two possible functions in screening. A risk factor that is present prior to the development of disease can help identify a group of individuals who are at increased risk of subsequent disease. If it is possible to modify the risk factor and subsequently reduce the probability of developing disease, this is ideal. Even when a risk factor cannot be modified, the identification of a risk factor can be valuable by helping to focus the subsequent search for early diseases on a group of individuals with a high probability of developing the disease.

SCREENING FOR HIGH BLOOD PRESSURE.   High blood pressure is a risk factor for vascular disease, and modification of high blood pressure has been shown to reduce the risk of subsequent disease. In the Hypertension Detection and Follow-up Program after the screening of 150,000 individuals, 10,940 men and women 30 to 69 years old with diastolic blood pressures of 90 mm Hg or higher were followed. These individuals were randomized to "stepped-care" vigorous antihypertension management or referred to their usual source of care. The stepped-care group had a greater decrease in diastolic blood pressure which, for those with initial diastolic blood pressure in the 90– to 104–mm Hg range, resulted in a 23 percent reduction in mortality compared to the referred care group [1].

———————————————————————————— STUDY QUESTION 3-2
Does hypertension satisfy criterion 2?

Criterion 3. Does Early Detection Improve Outcome?

Does treatment begun during the asymptomatic preclinical phase result in a better outcome compared to treatment that awaits the appearance of symptoms? Before justifying screening, one should ideally establish that early diagnosis of disease through screening produces a better outcome than diagnosis and treatment once clinical disease has begun.

The benefit of a screening program is often measured by the case-fatality rate observed in a screened population compared to the case-fatality rate in an unscreened population. In other words, at a point in time after the time of screening, we need to determine the frequency of adverse outcomes among those who are screened compared to those who are not screened. The following is the definition of *case-fatality rate* often used in screening:

$$\text{Case-fatality rate} = \frac{\text{no. of deaths among the cases}}{(\text{no. of cases}) (\text{average person-years of cases observed})}$$

Note that this standard method of assessing a screening program does not take into account any adverse effects of the screening program for those who are free of disease. In addition, it does not take into account the number of individuals who must be screened to detect a case of disease. Consequently, this method of assessing effectiveness tells us only about the benefits gained and nothing about the adverse effects or costs.

There are two effects of screening itself that may create biases which cause us to overestimate the benefits of screening as measured by the

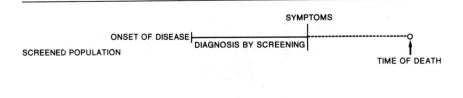

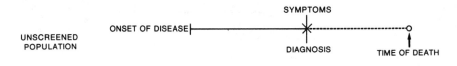

Fig. 3-2. Lead-time bias.

reduction in case-fatality rates. These biases have been called lead-time bias and length bias.

LEAD-TIME BIAS

Gaining lead time is the goal of screening. That is, by screening, we aim to diagnosis the disease at an earlier point in time. Early diagnosis, however, may or may not translate into improved prognosis. If early detection does not allow us to intervene successfully to alter the natural history of the disease, then we have gained lead time but have not increased the life span of those screened. This is lead-time bias. The case-fatality rate is artificially reduced, without actually extending the life span of those individuals whose disease is detected early (Fig. 3-2). Those diagnosed by screening may live for a longer time after diagnosis even if their *total* life span is not extended as measured from the true onset of disease [2].

Lead-time bias is most likely to occur when the period of observation is fairly limited after detection of the disease. With longer-term continued observation, the effect of lead-time bias on the case-fatality rate will diminish. Hence, it is possible to assess whether lead-time bias makes a major contribution to the reduced case-fatality rate by determining whether the case-fatality rate for those cases detected by screening remains lower than for cases detected without screening after longer-term observation.

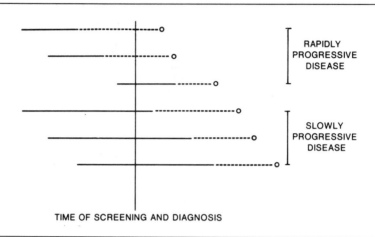

TIME OF SCREENING AND DIAGNOSIS

Fig. 3-3. Length bias. *Solid line* = preclinical phase; *dashed line* = clinical phase; *circle* = death. (Adapted from AS Morrison. Screening in Chronic Disease. New York: Oxford University Press, 1985, p. 66.)

LENGTH BIAS

Length bias is a second form of bias that can artificially reduce the apparent case-fatality rate among those screened [2]. Length bias occurs when there are two varieties of the disease that can be detected by screening, one with a short preclinical phase and the other with a longer preclinical phase. Often, a short preclinical phase will mean a rapidly progressive disease with a short clinical phase as well. The prognosis in individuals affected by such a disease may be poor even if the disease is detected early. In contrast, a disease with a longer preclinical phase often has a longer clinical phase as well. The prognosis in individuals affected by such a disease may be reasonably good even if the disease is detected after symptoms occur.

Screening identifies individuals who are in the asymptomatic preclinical phase. Because individuals with slowly progressive disease spend more time in the preclinical phase, they are more likely to be detected by a one-time screening effort. Figure 3-3 illustrates why this is so. Notice that in this example screening detects all three slowly progressive cases while they are in the asymptomatic preclinical phase. In contrast, screening only detects one of the three rapidly progressive cases while in the asymptomatic preclinical phase. This tendency for screening to detect slowly progressive disease with a better prognosis can lead to a length bias.

Because of their longer preclinical and clinical phases, cases of slowly progressive disease, which are disproportionately detected by screening, may appear to do better even in the absence of effective treatment. The disproportionate number of slowly progressive cases may make it seem that the case-fatality rate for screened cases is better than for unscreened cases even when screening has not actually increased longevity. This is what is meant by *length bias*.*

At times, screening may disproportionately detect individuals with rapidly progressive disease and produce a reverse length bias that underestimates the effects of screening. There is a suggestion that this may occur in screening for bladder cancer using cytology.

OTHER SCREENING BIASES

In addition to lead-time and length biases, two other biases may be produced by the characteristics of the population being screened and the tests being used. *Patient self-selection bias* occurs if the patient population that is screened is biologically or behaviorally different from the unscreened population in ways that affect the outcome of their disease. For instance, it is possible that those who are healthier will self-select themselves as volunteers for screening. These healthy volunteers may have a better-than-average prognosis even if they do develop the disease. This type of bias can be largely eliminated only by conducting controlled clinical trials among groups of patients for whom the screening program is proposed.

Another type of bias can occur if the tests used for screening and subsequent diagnosis produce false positive diagnoses. This *overdiagnosis bias* produces "pseudodisease"—that is, some individuals labeled as hav-

---

*Length bias is usually greatest for those cases that are detected at an initial screening examination, because initial screening samples individuals who have had asymptomatic disease for shorter and for longer periods of time. The cases of disease detected at subsequent screening examinations usually are of more recent onset. Therefore, it is possible to assess the effect of length bias also by determining the case-fatality rates for cases detected by repeat screening relatively soon after the initial screen. If those cases detected at repeat screening have a case-fatality rate that approximates the rate of those detected without screening, then length bias may have produced the apparent benefit of screening. However, if those detected by the repeat screening have a lower case-fatality rate than those who are not screened, then the improvement probably is not explained by length bias.

ing disease are truly free of disease. These people have an especially good prognosis, which thereby reduces the case-fatality rate of the cases detected by screening. Overdiagnosis bias can occur in any type of study. It can be reduced or eliminated only by employing accurate testing methods for definitive diagnosis and by "blinding" the diagnostician in a controlled trial.

RANDOMIZED CONTROLLED CLINICAL TRIALS TO ELIMINATE SCREENING BIASES

One way to minimize the problem of lead-time bias, length bias, and self-selection bias is to perform a randomized controlled clinical trial with prolonged follow-up among those with a modifiable risk factor. Such a study would randomize individuals to either an immediate treatment group or a group that receives treatment only after symptoms appear. If it is feasible and ethical to use this method, the effects of lead-time and length bias will be reduced by allowing one to assess the mortality rates of study and control group patients from the time of their entry into the study. Thus, one can assess the efficacy of early treatment directly by determining whether the early treatment group has a lower mortality rate compared to the late treatment group.

Note that a controlled clinical trial will not automatically circumvent the problems of lead-time and length biases if case-fatality rates are used as the outcome measure. A controlled clinical trial of screening, however, does allow an investigator to use mortality rates as the outcome measure in both the study and control group. Mortality rates are for the entire group, as opposed to case-fatality rates, which are for those individuals who develop the disease. Mortality rates include in the denominator all individuals in the study or control group, not just those who have the disease being studied. If mortality rates or disease-specific mortality rates are compared between study and control groups randomized to receive or not receive treatment and long-term follow-up is undertaken, the effects of lead-time and length bias can be removed. Mortality rates are not generally used to assess a screening program in the absence of a controlled clinical trial. Despite the advantages of using mortality rates, the difficulty of following all screened individuals makes the use of mortality rates impractical in most situations other than controlled clinical trials.

SCREENING FOR HIGH BLOOD PRESSURE.   A randomized controlled clinical trial with prolonged follow-up among those with a modifiable risk factor is not usu-

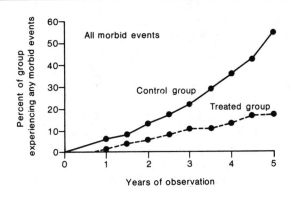

Fig. 3-4. Estimated cumulative incidence of all morbid events in patients with diastolic blood pressure averaging 90 to 114 mm Hg, and percent effectiveness of treatment in the Veterans Administration trial. (Adapted from The VA Cooperative Group on Antihypertensive Agents. JAMA 1970;213:1143–1151.)

ally performed, because once a risk factor or condition is designated as a disease, it is not considered ethical or feasible to withhold treatment until symptoms appear. An exception, however, was the Veterans Administration's study [3], which randomized individuals with diastolic blood pressures greater than 90 mm Hg to study and control groups. The follow-up data from these studies demonstrated that treatment of patients with diastolic blood pressure of 95 mm Hg or greater resulted in lower mortality and morbidity than that for individuals whose treatment was delayed until symptoms appear (Fig. 3-4).

_____ STUDY QUESTION 3-3

Does hypertension satisfy criterion 3?

Criterion 4. Is There a Testing Approach that Is Both Feasible and Acceptable?

More specifically, is there a testing approach that (1) makes it feasible to effectively detect or rule out disease at the asymptomatic preclinical stage, and (2) is satisfactory in terms of patient safety, acceptability, and affordability? In assessing a test, we need to define a group of individuals who are unequivocally free of the disease. This is done by applying a "gold standard" test. A gold standard test may be a biopsy, an angiogram, an autopsy, or any other test or combination of tests that can be agreed on as the best available means of defining the presence or absence of the disease.

If no unequivocal method is available for diagnosing early disease, equivocal cases are not usually included in assessing the utility of the test in question. Because of this tendency to consider only the clear-cut cases, the utility of a test for detecting or ruling out mild uncomplicated disease cases that are sought by screening may be overestimated.

In assessing a test's diagnostic discrimination, we compare the results obtained using the gold standard with the results obtained using the test being studied. All individuals, whether they are positive or negative by the gold standard, are independently classified as negative or positive according to the test being studied. The possible results are as follows:

	Gold standard positive	Gold standard negative
Positive test	a = true positives	b = false positives
Negative test	c = false negatives	d = true negatives

This procedure allows us to calculate a series of measurements that quantitate the information obtained from the test relative to the gold standard.

SENSITIVITY AND SPECIFICITY

The most commonly used measures of a test's informative value are sensitivity and specificity. These measures have been adopted because they reflect the information obtained from the test and do not depend on the prevalence of the disease or the characteristics of the particular population being studied. (Sensitivity and specificity may, however, depend on the stage of disease development.) These measures tell us about the inherent properties of the test independent of other information obtained from the patient.

Sensitivity is the proportion of those with disease, as defined by the gold standard, who are correctly categorized by the test. One might remember sensitivity as "positive in disease (PID)." Thus

$$\text{Sensitivity} = \frac{\text{true positives}}{\text{true positives} + \text{false negatives}} = \frac{a}{a + c}$$

Specificity is the proportion of those without disease, as defined by the gold standard, who are correctly categorized by the test. One might remember specificity as "negative in health (NIH)." Thus

$$\text{Specificity} = \frac{\text{true negatives}}{\text{true negatives} + \text{false positives}} = \frac{d}{b + d}$$

Sensitivity and specificity both can vary from 0 to 100 percent. A 100 percent sensitive and 100 percent specific test is one that agrees completely with the gold standard.

It is impossible to do better than the gold standard. When the test and the gold standard disagree, the gold standard is taken as correct. Thus, if a new test is actually better than the gold standard, it will not initially be possible to appreciate the utility of this test by sensitivity and specificity measures, since any discrepancy will be decided in favor of the gold standard.

PREDICTIVE VALUE OF A TEST
It is important to remember that sensitivity and specificity are measures of the test that do not take into account the clinical setting or situation in which the test is used. To assess how well a test performs in a particular clinical situation, we also need to take into account the probability of the disease before the test is performed. In screening, this pretest probability of disease represents the prevalence of disease among the population of individuals being screened. If a general population is being screened, then the pretest probability equals the prevalence of the disease in the general population. If a group of individuals is being screened because of the presence of a known risk factor for disease, then pretest probability is the prevalence of disease for those with the risk factor. This same principle is used for diagnosis in the presence of symptoms. For instance, if a patient is tested after an extensive clinical assessment or other laboratory testing, then pretest probability represents the clinician's best guess at the probability of the disease before performing the test.

The predictive value of a positive test and the predictive value of a negative test take into account the pretest probability of disease as well as the sensitivity and specificity of the test. Thus, they address the clinician's question: What is the meaning of a positive test or a negative test in a particular clinical situation?

The predictive value of a positive test tells us the proportion of those with a positive test who have the disease, taking into account the pretest probability of the disease. Thus

$$\text{Predictive value of a positive test} = \frac{\text{true positives}}{\text{true positives + false positives}} = \frac{a}{a + b}$$

Conversely, predictive value of a negative test tells us the proportion of those with a negative test who have the disease, taking into account the pretest probability of the disease. Thus

$$\text{Predictive value of a negative test} = \frac{\text{false negatives}}{\text{false negatives + true negatives}} = \frac{c}{c + d}$$

Predictive value of a negative test can be and is often defined as the proportion of those with a negative test who *do not have* the disease. When defined this way, predictive value of a negative tests tells us the probability that the disease is not present. Thus

$$\text{Predictive value of a negative test} = \frac{\text{true negatives}}{\text{false negatives + true negatives}} = \frac{d}{c + d}$$

This definition of predictive value of a negative test is the compliment of the previous definition. Thus if the probability that the disease is present equals 3 percent, the probability that it is not present equals 97 percent.

When using a test for screening, it is important to remember that the probability of disease before performing the test often is very low. Imagine, for instance, that we performed a screening test on a population whose prevalence of a disease is 1 per 100 or 10 per 1000 as determined by a gold standard. This situation may be represented as follows:

	Gold standard positive	*Gold standard negative*
Positive test	True positives	False positives
Negative test	False negatives	True negatives
	10	990

3. SCREENING FOR DISEASE CONTROL 41

Now let us imagine that we obtained a screening test with 90 percent
sensitivity and 90 percent specificity on each member of this population.
Let us look at the results we would obtain.

Since the sensitivity of the test is 90 percent, 9 of the 10 individuals
with the disease, as defined by the gold standard, will be correctly identified. Since the specificity of the test is 90 percent, 891 of the 990 individuals without the disease, as defined by the gold standard, will be correctly identified. These numbers may be tabulated as follows:

	Gold standard positive	*Gold standard negative*
Positive test	9	99
Negative test	1	891
	10	990

Notice from the chart that the vast majority (99 of 108) of positive
tests are actually false positives. From this chart it is possible to calculate
the predictive value of a positive test and the predictive value of a negative test.

$$\text{Predictive value of a positive test} = \frac{9}{9 + 99} = \frac{9}{108} = 8.3\%$$

$$\text{Predictive value of a negative test} = \frac{1}{1 + 891} = \frac{1}{892} = 0.1\%$$

This tells us that if the probability of disease before the test is 1 percent,
then the probability after obtaining a positive test is 8.3 percent. After
obtaining a negative test, the probability is 0.1 percent. The meaning
that can be derived from these figures is that screening tests in general
may effectively rule out disease, but they are not capable of definitively
diagnosing disease. Rather, screening usually identifies a group of individuals who need more accurate testing.

INCREASING PREDICTIVE VALUE OF A TEST
Most screening tests result in a high percentage of false positives. This
is an intrinsic problem with screening. It can be minimized by identifying and screening high-risk groups. High-risk groups are composed of

individuals with one or more risk factors for disease that increase the prevalence of the disease in the high-risk population and, hence, its pre-test probability. Thus, screening high-risk populations increases the predictive value of a positive test for any particular level of test sensitivity and specificity.

Another strategy for increasing the predictive value of a screening test is to use the result of initial screening tests as a basis for deciding on the frequency of subsequent screening. Papanicolaou smear results, initial cholesterol levels, or blood pressure levels may be used to classify individuals as low-risk or high-risk, as a basis for determining the frequency of or need for further follow-up testing.

MULTIPLE TESTS IN SCREENING FOR DISEASE
It is generally necessary to employ more than one test to diagnose the disease for which screening is being conducted. Tests may be ordered in sequence or simultaneously to reach a diagnostic decision. The use of *sequential testing* may lead to a diagnosis using the following strategy:

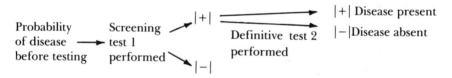

In using this strategy, the probability of disease after the results of screening test 1 are positive becomes the probability of disease before performing definitive test 2. Test 2 is then used to separate test 1's true positives from its false positives. This strategy works better than the simultaneous strategy when the available tests have a high enough sensitivity to detect a large proportion of those with the disease. In this situation, the sequential strategy allows one to reduce the number of false positives. This occurs even though each test may not in and of itself be able to correctly identify a high proportion of those who are disease-free. To be successful, tests 1 and 2 must give independent results. If both tests give false positives in the same type of clinical situation, then little is gained by using the tests in sequence.*

*In sequential testing the results are the same if test 2 is used first. The choice of which test to use in a sequential testing strategy is determined by considerations of costs, safety, and patient acceptance.

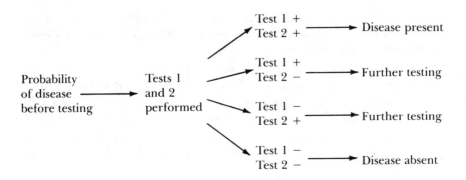

Simultaneous testing works better than sequential testing when neither test 1 nor test 2 alone is sensitive enough to detect the vast majority of those with disease. By combining tests with low sensitivity, it sometimes is possible to improve the detection rate. To use this strategy successfully, tests 1 and 2 need to detect different types or stages of disease. If both fail to detect early disease, for instance, little may be gained by using the two tests simultaneously.

To satisfy the final criterion, screening must be practical as well as satisfactory in terms of safety, patient acceptability, and affordability. In making this assessment, one must look not only at the initial screening test but also at the tests required to rule out disease among the many false positive individuals. If dangerous or expensive testing is required to rule out or diagnose the disease, the screening strategy may not be safe, acceptable, or affordable even if it is effective in achieving its other aims.

_____ STUDY QUESTION 3-4

Does hypertension satisfy criterion 4?

Summary
Screening for disease control can be an important method for reducing the mortality and morbidity caused by a disease. However, because of the time, the risks, and the costs of screening one should determine whether a particular screening strategy adequately satisfies a series of screening criteria that ask:

Criterion 1. Does the disease cause a substantial morbidity and/or mortality leading to a substantial impact on society as a whole or an identifiable sub-group of individuals in society?

Criterion 2. Are there risk factors that can be identified before the development of clinical disease which (1) can be modified to prevent the appearance of clinical disease; or (2) can serve to identify high risk groups to facilitate the early detection of disease?

Criterion 3. Does treatment begun during the asymptomatic preclinical phase result in a better outcome than treatment that awaits the appearance of symptoms?

Criterion 4. Is there a test or approach that (1) makes it feasible to effectively detect or rule out disease at the asymptomatic preclinical stage; and (2) is acceptable in terms of safety, patient acceptability and affordability?

References

1. Hypertension Detection and Follow-up Program Cooperative Group. Five year findings of the Hypertension Detection and Follow-up Program. JAMA 1979;242:2562–2577.
2. Morrison AS. Screening in Chronic Disease. New York: Oxford University Press, 1985.
3. Veterans Administration Cooperative Group on Antihypertensive Agents. Effects of treatment on morbidity in hypertension. II. Results in patients with diastolic blood pressure averaging 90 through 114 mmHg. JAMA 1970;213;1143–1152.

Evaluating the Solutions

PART THREE

Risks, Benefits, and Costs

CHAPTER FOUR

RICHARD K. RIEGELMAN
L. GREGORY PAWLSON

The job of deciding what to do is among the hardest tasks facing the medical profession in general and the individual clinician in particular. Traditionally, the decision has rested on comparison of the benefits derived from an intervention and the risks of that intervention. We will begin this chapter by looking at this process of comparing benefits or efficacy to risk or safety.

In recent years, clinicians are increasingly being asked to go beyond a comparison of the risks and the benefits of a particular intervention; they are being asked to compare two or more options to determine the best choice. In the second part of this chapter, we will introduce principles of decision analysis that are used to help us compare the options.

Finally, with the increasing emphasis on the costs of medical care, medical professionals are being asked to take explicitly into account the financial implications of their recommendations. The tools of cost-effectiveness analysis are becoming more widely used to help us quantitate the financial impact of alternative interventions. We will review the principles of cost-effectiveness analysis and look at the underlying assumptions and implications.

Let us begin by taking a look at the process of assessing the efficacy and safety of a preventive intervention.

Efficacy of Intervention

Controlled clinical trials increasingly represent the gold standard for judging the *efficacy* of preventive therapy. Such trials have several advantages in assessing how well a therapy works under ideal experimental conditions—that is, in demonstrating *efficacy*. First, randomization of individuals to study and control treatment groups helps ensure that similar types of patients receive the study treatment and the control treatment. Randomization implies that all individuals included in a study have a known probability of being assigned to a particular study or control group. Second, ideally, the blinding process helps eliminate patient or physician bias in the assessment of outcome. This is especially important when subjective outcomes are being assessed. Finally, careful follow-up in well-performed controlled clinical trials helps ensure that patients with poor outcomes are not selectively lost to follow-up.

The efficacy of treatment can be judged using a variety of study designs. The Canadian Preventive Medicine Task Force [1] and more recently, the United States Preventive Medicine Task Force [2] have ranked these studies, identifying three grades of evidence:

Grade I   Evidence obtained from at least one properly randomized controlled trial

Grade II-1   Evidence obtained from well-designed controlled trials without randomization

Grade II-2   Evidence obtained from well-designed cohort or case-control analytic studies, preferably from more than one center or research group

Grade II-3   Evidence obtained from multiple time-series studies, with or without intervention or dramatic results in uncontrolled experiments

Grade III   Opinions of respected authorities, based on clinical experience, descriptive studies, or reports of expert committees

EFFICACY VERSUS EFFECTIVENESS
Efficacy as established by controlled clinical trials should be distinguished from effectiveness. Effectiveness asks how well the therapy works under the usual conditions of clinical care as opposed to the ideal conditions of controlled clinical trials. Controlled clinical trials that establish the efficacy of a therapy cannot assure its effectiveness for the following reasons.

In a controlled clinical trial, patients are randomized to study and control groups, but they are not randomly selected for inclusion in the study. Although randomization is the hallmark of a controlled clinical trial, random *selection* is generally *not* a characteristic of controlled clinical trials. Random selection would imply that individuals are selected for an investigation by a chance process designed to choose patients representative of all those who might eventually utilize the therapy. Controlled clinical trials, on the other hand, usually select patients who meet predetermined entry criteria designed to produce a homogeneous group of patients. Thus, patients who participate in controlled clinical trials are not usually representative of all patients likely to receive the therapy. As a result, those individuals who receive the therapy in clinical practice may be less compliant, take multiple other potentially interactive medications, or be at greater risk of side effects. Alternatively, the individual clinician or the medical system may have limited expertise in using the therapy or dealing with the side effects. Therefore, it is often difficult to generalize the findings of controlled clinical trials to clinical practice.

PROBLEMS USING CONTROLLED CLINICAL TRIALS TO EVALUATE EFFICACY AND EFFECTIVENESS OF PREVENTIVE INTERVENTIONS
For many preventive treatments, it is difficult or expensive to perform controlled clinical trials. Logistic problems arise because large numbers of individuals need to be followed for long periods of time if we are to study the effects of a preventive therapy. For instance, if we hope to demonstrate the statistical significance of a true 25-percent reduction from a control group's death rate of 5 percent, we need to follow a total of approximately 10,000 individuals. Similarly, if we wish to demonstrate the statistical significance of a true 25-percent reduction from a control group's death rate of 2 percent, we need to follow a total of more than 20,000 individuals. If we perform controlled clinical trials on smaller groups of individuals, we may fail to demonstrate a statistically significant difference, even when the therapy actually produces clinically important effects.

The probability of failing to demonstrate a statistically significant difference when the therapy actually has a clinically important effect is called type II or beta error. Many small controlled clinical trials of preventive therapy are limited by their large type II errors.*

In addition to limitations imposed by sample size, one must recognize the difficulty in predicting the social impact when preventive interventions are applied to large numbers of individuals. For instance, widespread use of antibiotic prophylaxis for urinary tract infections could result in drug resistance. Alternatively, the initial success of a treatment for a venereal disease may lower social inhibitions, leading to an eventual increase in the incidence of the disease itself. To be specific, the knowl-

---

*The sample size required to ensure that a statistically significant difference can be demonstrated if there is a real difference between treatments depends on:

1. The size of the type I or alpha error that one is willing to tolerate. This is the probability of demonstrating a statistically significant difference if no true difference between treatment exists. It is conventionally set, as in our examples, at 5 percent or p = .05.
2. The size of the type II or beta error that one is willing to tolerate. This is usually set at 10 to 20 percent. In our examples we assume 20 percent.
3. The size of the true difference that we want to be able to demonstrate as statistically significant between the results of the study and control treatments.

edge that gonorrhea is treatable might reduce an individual's fear of contracting gonorrhea. This, in turn, may diminish a person's efforts to avoid contact with gonorrhea. These secondary or dynamic effects cannot be easily predicted based on one point in time or static results of a controlled clinical trial.

The difficulties inherent in extrapolating from efficacy, as demonstrated by a controlled clinical trial, to effectiveness, as defined in practice, are not meant to depreciate the importance of controlled clinical trials. Their introduction into clinical medicine has been a major advance leading to a systematic and scientific approach to evaluating therapies. However, one must be mindful of the limitations of controlled clinical trials for assessing the benefits of large-scale preventive measures.

_____ STUDY QUESTION 4-1
Imagine that a new drug called alcoholex, for alcoholism prevention, was investigated in a double-blind randomized clinical trial among prison inmates who agreed to participate immediately prior to parole. All eligible study subjects were without evidence of liver disease on biopsy. Over a 5-year period, the 1000 study group individuals taking alcoholex experienced a 1-percent incidence of alcohol-induced liver disease, compared to a 10-percent incidence of alcohol-induced liver disease among the 1000 individuals randomized to the placebo control group. Alcoholex reduced both the frequency of alcohol intake and the incidence of liver disease. The results were statistically significant. What does this study tell you about the efficacy of alcoholex? What does the study tell you about the effectiveness of alcoholex?

RISKS AND SAFETY OF INTERVENTIONS
Since the days of the thalidomide tragedy, many American physicians have come to believe that safety of therapy is the exclusive responsibility of the Food and Drug Administration (FDA). FDA approval is often equated with safety or at least with clearly defined and well-understood risks. Unfortunately, safety of therapy is even more difficult to assess than efficacy. This is especially true for rare but serious side effects. The crux of the problem is that large numbers of individuals must be exposed to the treatment before rare but serious side effects are likely to be observed.

The numbers required to ensure a 95-percent probability of observing at least one episode of a rare side effect are summarized in the "rule of three." According to the rule of three, to have a 95-percent chance of observing at least 1 case of penicillin anaphylaxis, which occurs in about 1 patient in 10,000, we need to treat 30,000 individuals. If we wish to be 95-percent certain we will observe at least 1 case of aplastic anemia from chloramphenicol, which occurs about 1 time in 50,000 cases, we would need to treat 150,000 patients with chloramphenicol. In general terms, the rule of three states that to be 95-percent certain that we will observe at least 1 case of the side effect, we need to treat 3 times the number of individuals in the denominator of the incidence rate.*

These numbers explain why controlled clinical trials cannot be expected to detect many rare but important side effects. To detect such events, we often rely on animal testing. High doses of the drug in question are usually administered to a variety of animal species on the assumption that toxic, teratogenic, and carcinogenic effects of the drug will be observed in at least one of the animal species tested. This approach has been helpful but has not entirely solved the problem. Interspecies differences have often made extrapolation to human beings difficult.

Long-term consequences of widely applied preventive treatments may be even more difficult to detect. Diethylstilbestrol (DES) was used for many years to prevent spontaneous abortions. It took decades before investigators noted a greatly increased incidence of vaginal carcinoma among teenaged girls whose mothers had taken DES.

It is only under conditions of widespread use in clinical practice that we are likely to observe these rare but serious side effects. The FDA relies heavily on reports received from the observant practicing physician. Alert clinicians and clinical investigators remain the mainstay of our current surveillance efforts.

_____ STUDY QUESTION 4-2
If alcoholex caused 1 case of bladder cancer per 3000 individuals who used the drug for 5 years, would you expect to observe a case of bladder cancer in the previously described study of alcoholex?

*The rule of three assumes that there is no background incidence of the side effect. If this side effect occurs in the absence of the medication, the numbers required to assess the side effect are even larger.

Selecting Between Therapies: Decision Analysis
Decision analysis is a method for directly comparing alternative treatments by taking into account the risks and benefits of each treatment. Decision analysis allows us to assess the alternative treatments to determine which one is likely to produce a favorable outcome under specified conditions. There are five basic steps necessary for performing decision analysis.

STEP 1. SELECTING INTERVENTIONS AND IDENTIFYING
POTENTIAL OUTCOMES
The interventions to be compared must be selected and their types of potential outcomes specified. These are then displayed in a diagram called a decision tree. For example, an intervention might have at least five potential outcomes:

1. Death owing to a complication of the preventive intervention
2. Survival of the complication of the preventive intervention with no subsequent disease
3. Survival of the complication of the preventive intervention but disease develops
4. No complications of the preventive intervention with no subsequent disease
5. No complication of the preventive intervention but disease develops

The curative approach, in which one awaits disease and treats it if it occurs, has at least four potential outcomes:

1. No disease develops
2. Disease develops with subsequent death
3. Disease develops with subsequent disability
4. Disease develops with subsequent cure

STEP 2. CONSTRUCTING A DECISION TREE FOR POTENTIAL
OUTCOMES
These potential outcomes can be diagrammed in a decision tree (Fig. 4-1). Note that even more potential outcomes are possible. For instance, if an individual develops the disease despite the therapy, he or she may die, have permanent disability, or be cured. The individual might also develop side effects of the treatment. Frequently, it is possible to com-

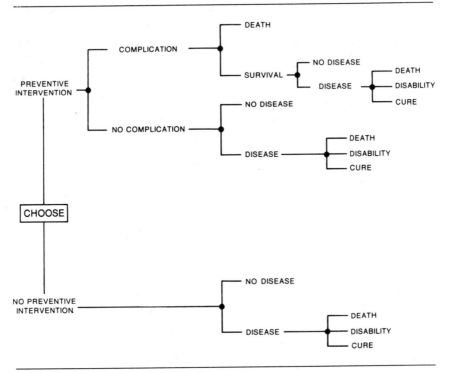

Fig. 4-1. Decision tree for potential outcomes of the curative approach.

bine or eliminate potential but rare outcomes from the decision tree to make decision analysis easier.

In their simplest form, decision trees are made up of choice or decision nodes (represented by boxes), chance nodes (represented by circles), and branches (represented by straight lines). *Choice or decision nodes* represent choices that are under the control of the decision maker.* *Chance nodes* are points at which events not directly under the decision maker's control occur or do not occur. Each *branch* of the tree represents a state or condition in which a patient can exist at a given time. The

---

*We use the term *decision maker* because decision analysis can be done from a variety of points of view, such as that of the patient, the clinician, or society.

terminal or end branch indicates an end point or outcome. The decision tree is constructed so as to represent, to the degree possible, the outcomes of decisions or choices in the time or temporal sequence in which they are likely to occur.

_____ STUDY QUESTION 4-3
Construct a decision tree comparing the option to use alcoholex in patients with medical complications of alcoholism and the option to use standard medical treatment of the complications of alcoholism.

STEP 3. ESTIMATING THE PROBABILITY OF OCCURRENCE OF POTENTIAL OUTCOMES

Having defined the potential end points or outcomes for each intervention, it is necessary to estimate the probability that each of these outcomes will occur. These outcome probabilities should add up to 100 percent for each of the decision choices being considered. Probability percentages can be obtained from estimates in the research literature, expert opinion, or estimates based on educated guesses if no other method is available. For example, one might estimate that the choice to use the curative approach will result in the following probabilities for potential outcomes.

No disease	40%
Disease with subsequent death	10%
Disease with subsequent disability	20%
Disease with subsequent cure	30%

STEP 4. ESTIMATING THE UTILITY OF EACH OUTCOME

If there are multiple possible outcomes, in addition to estimating the probability that an outcome will occur, it is necessary to estimate the utility of each outcome. Note that utility measures are not usually needed when the only options are death and cure. In this case, one would choose the decision that resulted in fewer deaths.

The term *utility* refers to the relative worth of life in the outcome state. Thus, one must determine how the decision maker feels about the relative worth of such potential outcomes as death from side effects of the preventive intervention, disease despite preventive intervention, and morbidity after developing the disease. Assessing these utilities is a very difficult part of decision analysis. We will examine how this can be done in subsequent chapters. In general, one attempts to score each of the outcomes on an interval scale of 0 to 100, where 100 equals the absence of disease and 0 equals death.*

STEP 5. COMPARING TREATMENT OPTIONS

Once steps 1 through 4 of the decision analysis process are completed, it is then possible to combine the estimated probabilities of the outcomes and their utilities for each potential intervention in order to compare the treatment options. This is done as follows:

1. Multiply the probability of a particular outcome times the utility of that outcome. This produces a utility weighted for the probability that it will occur, and it is called a weighted utility.
2. Add all of the weighted utilities for a given intervention option to yield the overall weighted utility of that intervention.
3. Directly compare the overall weighted utility of each intervention option to the overall weighted utility of other options.

For example, imagine that our decision maker ranked the utility of the four potential outcomes of the curative approach to alcohol abuse on a scale of 0 to 100, as follows:

No disease	100
Disease with subsequent death	0
Disease with subsequent disability	50
Disease with subsequent cure	80

To develop a weighted utility of the curative approach, one would multiply the probabilities and the utility value, as follows:

No disease	$100 \times 0.4 = 40$
Disease with subsequent death	$0 \times 0.1 = 0$
Disease with subsequent disability	$50 \times 0.2 = 10$
Disease with subsequent cure	$80 \times 0.3 = 24$

*As can be seen from our original decision tree (Fig. 4-1), death may occur in more than one way and may have different utilities depending on how and when it occurs. In addition, it is possible for certain outcomes to be worse than death. Decision analysis can, in theory, take these views into account by the way in which the scale is constructed. It is also possible to measure outcome in terms of cost or to make use of life expectancy measure.

Thus, the overall results of the curative approach add up to 74. This has meaning only in comparison to the overall results of the other option or options under consideration. The option with the greatest weighted utility is the one that is favored.

_____ STUDY QUESTION 4-4
Use the following probabilities and utilities to calculate an overall weighted utility for the use of alcoholex.

	Probability (%)	Utility
Death from complications of alcoholex	1	0
Survival of complication of alcoholex with no subsequent disease	2	90
Survival of complication of alcoholex but subsequent disease develops	3	50
No complications of alcoholex and no subsequent disease	85	100
No complications of alcoholex but subsequent disease develops	9	60

Therapeutic decision analysis produces an overall weighted utility for a particular intervention that takes into account the probability and the utility of each potential outcome. The overall results of decision analysis are dependent on how well the probability assigned to each outcome reflects the true probability of experiencing that particular outcome. The usefulness of the results also depends on how well the assigned utilities reflect the decision maker's true preferences.

SENSITIVITY ANALYSIS
When the weighted overall utility values between two approaches are nearly equal, small differences in probability or utility values can alter which treatment choice is most desirable. It is possible to assess how changes in utilities or changes in probabilities affect the results of a decision analysis by performing what is known as a sensitivity analysis. In a sensitivity analysis, one or more of the probabilities of an outcome or the utilities of an outcome are altered to determine how sensitive the conclusions are to these changes. For instance, if one does not know the likelihood of a particular side effect of a preventive intervention, one might start by using a best-guess estimate. Then, it would be helpful to determine how the results are affected by a smaller and larger probability of the adverse outcome.

_____ STUDY QUESTION 4-5

Do a simple sensitivity analysis by assuming that the curative approach will produce the following, more favorable outcome than originally estimated.

No disease	70%
Disease with subsequent death	5%
Disease with subsequent disability	10%
Disease with subsequent cure	15%

Assume that everything else in your decision analysis remains the same. What can you conclude from this sensitivity analysis?

USES AND LIMITATIONS OF DECISION ANALYSIS

Decision analysis attempts to measure and compare the risks and benefits given a particular set of probabilities of occurrence of potential outcomes. It also lets us take into account the preference or utilities for each potential outcome as viewed by a particular decision maker.

Most decision analyses, however, do not take into account all the variables that go into clinical decision making. For instance, decision analysis may not take into account the timing or circumstances of particular outcomes. In decision analysis, immediate death from surgical procedures is often valued as equivalent to later death from complications of treatment, whereas in clinical practice, patients may place greater worth on time in the immediate future. In addition, decision analysis usually assumes that the decision maker is risk-neutral: A risk-neutral decision maker would regard two weighted utilities of 50 as interchangeable. A risk-neutral decision maker would thus regard a choice leading to a 50-percent probability of cure plus a 50 percent probability of death as equal to a choice leading to a 100-percent probability of remaining at a utility level of 50. Many decision makers, however, are risk-aversive. Risk-aversive decision makers prefer to avoid risk of the unknown. Thus, they may choose their current partially effective therapy rather than a new therapy that holds greater potential for cure but also carries a greater risk of adverse effects.

By requiring us to be explicit about our reasoning, decision analysis can help us define the assumptions underlying medical recommendations. It can also help us identify the areas where data are lacking or where disagreement exists between individuals who favor conflicting decisions. In fact, it may help us to detect the source of disagreement and to determine the nature of the debate. Decision analysis does not make decisions. It can, however, help us to appreciate the basis for our decisions, including both the facts and the values at work. We will employ formal decision analyses in the cases that look at anticoagulation for atrial fibrillation and amniocentesis, which appear in later chapters.

Cost-Effectiveness Analysis

Decision analysis helps us balance the risks (safety) and benefits (effectiveness) of an intervention and to include in our assessment individual, institutional, or social values. Benefits, however, may or may not be worth the financial costs.*

Cost considerations have assumed increasing importance in deciding among health care options. As part of this trend, formal cost-effectiveness analysis now frequently influences such decisions. Therefore, it is important that medical professionals understand the principles of cost-effectiveness analysis so that we may appreciate its usefulness and limitations.

INFORMATION PROVIDED BY COST-EFFECTIVENESS ANALYSIS

Cost-effectiveness analysis is a method of estimating the financial cost of obtaining a desired health outcome, whether it be lives saved, disability prevented, diagnoses made, or any other desired health-related effects. It does not require us to assign a dollar amount to the worth or utility of that outcome. In other words, cost-effectiveness analysis may tell us the financial cost of saving a year of life, but it does not require us to agree on what that year of life is worth.†

When used to assess a particular health procedure or program, a cost-effectiveness analysis will generate an outcome expressed as cost per unit. This may be cost per year of life saved, cost per quality-adjusted year of life saved, cost per year of morbidity prevented, or the like. The

---

*In theory, it is possible to include financial costs among utilities assigned to a therapeutic outcome. More commonly, financial costs are considered separately as part of cost effectiveness analysis.

†In contrast to cost-effectiveness analysis, cost-benefit analysis measures all outcomes in financial terms. This allows one to compare the economic efficiency of efforts that produce different types of end results. When comparing health care strategies, for instance, cost-benefit analysis would allow direct comparison of an approach aimed at reducing mortality with an approach aimed at reducing morbidity. It also allows comparison of health benefits with nonhealth benefits such as increased production of other goods or services.

cost figures generated by a cost-effectiveness analysis do not tell us whether the result obtained is worth the cost.

COST SAVING VERSUS COST EFFECTIVENESS

At times, the financial outlays will actually be reduced by the intervention without sacrificing quality. In these rare instances, the intervention can be called *cost saving*, a special unequivocal type of cost effectiveness. More often, however, the intervention will increase costs in return for additional effectiveness in achieving a specified goal. In these circumstances, one must ask: Is the additional cost justified by the additional benefit? If the additional gain is worth the price, then the intervention can be called cost effective. An intervention can also be considered cost effective if it produces less benefit but at a substantially reduced cost. Thus, an intervention may be considered cost effective if a large reduction in cost is determined to be worth a small reduction in benefit. When looked at individually, either or both of these types of intervention—that with additional costs and additional benefits and that with reduced costs and reduced benefits—may be considered worth the price and thus cost effective. When compared to each other, however, one type may be judged *more* cost effective than the other.

Thus, the term *cost effectiveness* can be very confusing. It can refer to situations in which money is actually saved, but more often it refers to situations in which the change in benefit is worth the cost. When two or more interventions are compared, no matter how well each approach does in its own right, only one strategy will be designated as the most cost effective. Thus one must distinguish three important terms:

Cost saving refers to the situation in which an intervention actually reduces the total financial cost without reducing the benefit.

Cost effective refers to the situation in which an additional option is considered and the increased costs are considered to be worth the additional benefits or the reduced benefits are considered to be worth the substantial reduction in cost.

Most cost effective refers to the situation in which two or more options are compared and one is found to require the least cost to achieve a particular benefit.

In performing a cost-effectiveness analysis, one must begin by deciding which questions to ask and, thus, which options to consider. For example, it is possible to view the problem of cost effectiveness in renal disease in terms of (1) finding the most cost-effective means of dialysis, or (2) finding the most cost effective means of increasing the life span of renal failure patients, or (3) finding the most cost-effective means of reducing the morbidity and mortality from renal disease. For the first alternative, one would merely compare the various methods of dialysis to determine which is cheaper. For the second, one might compare the most cost effective form of renal dialysis with transplantation. For the third alternative, one might want to include as an option efforts to reduce or eliminate preventable forms of end-stage renal disease.

_____ STUDY QUESTION 4-6
Assume that the following approaches to controlling alcoholism are available:

1. Preventive intervention prior to the occurrence of medical or social consequences
2. Treatments after the detection of early medical or social consequences
3. Treatments after the appearance of life-threatening consequences

Which of these options would you study to address the following questions?

a. What is the most cost effective means of treating patients who are ill from alcohol-induced hepatic cirrhosis?
b. What is the most cost effective means of preventing death from alcohol-induced hepatic cirrhosis in the population?
c. What is the most cost effective means of preventing deaths in patients with early alcohol-induced liver disease?

CALCULATING COSTS
Having framed the questions, cost-effectiveness analysis requires that we calculate the costs. Even when adequate cost data are available, we are required to ask which costs to include and how to calculate them.

Selecting Costs for Considerations
Which costs should be considered depends largely on the perspective of the analysis. Individuals making decisions about their own care may only be interested in their out-of-pocket personal expenses. Costs to an insurance company or to society in general may not concern them. Simi-

larly, from the point of view of an insurance company or a health insurance system such as Medicare, the only costs that are relevant are those that are paid by the insurer. From a social perspective, many different financial outlays may matter, including such items as current and future medical and nonmedical expenditures.

Thus, when evaluating the costs of a preventive intervention, the costs to consider may vary enormously depending on who you are and what perspective you take. An insurance company may have to pay for the current costs of prevention, but often there is no guarantee that reductions in future health care expenditures will accrue to the same company. Thus, insurers may count as the costs the total current outlays without considering the future saving. In contrast, Medicare, a compulsory long-term insurance plan can theoretically capture some of the future reductions in health care costs. A social perspective on the costs of prevention is the broadest perspective and the one advocated by many experts in cost-effectiveness analysis. The social perspective counts all benefits regardless of who receives them, and it counts all costs regardless of who pays the bills.

Discounting
In addition to deciding which costs to apply to a cost-effectiveness analysis, one must take into account the times at which the costs and the benefits occur. This is achieved by *discounting*. Costs are discounted because economists assume that funds not spent currently can be invested in an alternative productive use that will generate a rate of return exceeding the inflation rate. This financial return might then be used to pay for future costs. Thus, economists discount costs that occur in the future.

The discount rate to use is a subject of controversy among health economists. It depends primarily on the predictions about the future return available in the economy in general. Some economists argue that a lower-than-market rate should be used for social programs that carry potential long-term benefits for future generations.

Positive outcomes that occur in the future are also discounted. Failure to discount future positive outcomes while discounting costs would result in a paradoxical situation in which it is always better to put off implementing an intervention because next year's costs will be lower but next year's benefits will be the same.

Discounting frequently is done when considering the cost of preventive programs and when comparing preventive and curative approaches. Individuals and insurance companies, for instance, may take into account the current costs of prevention while discounting the utility or worth of reduced mortality and morbidity that occurs many years later.

THE COST-EFFECTIVENESS RATIO

Cost-effectiveness analyses are usually presented as a ratio of net costs to net benefits. To understand what is meant by this ratio, let us imagine that we wished to determine the cost effectiveness of the introduction of an alcoholex prevention program into the current health care system. To calculate the cost-effectiveness ratio of such a preventive intervention, we need to estimate at least the following costs:

Cost of the alcoholex program (Cp)

Cost, if any, of treating the side effects of the alcoholex program (Cse)

Cost of treating alcohol-caused disease if the alcohol abuse program is not implemented (Ct)

Thus, the net cost of the alcoholex program equals (Cp + Cse) − Ct.*
We also need to estimate at least the following gains and losses, taking into account the effects of adjusting for quality of life:

Years of quality-adjusted life gained from reduced mortality by those enrolled in the alcoholex program (Eli)

Years of quality-adjusted life gained as a result of reduced morbidity among those enrolled in the alcoholex program, taking into account the quality-adjusted utility of life (Em)

Years of quality-adjusted life lost owing to the mortality and morbidity from the alcoholex program itself (Ese)

Thus, the net effectiveness of treatment can be expressed as (Eli + Em) − Ese.*
The cost effectiveness of a treatment is then usually expressed by combining the net cost and net effectiveness into a ratio, expressed as follows:

*The net cost and net effectiveness of treatment incorporate the effects of discounting for future costs and future benefits.

$$\text{Cost effectiveness ratio} = \frac{\text{net costs}}{\text{net effectiveness}} = \frac{(Cp + Cse) - Ct}{(Eli + Em) - Ese}$$

_____ STUDY QUESTION 4-7

Assume that the costs for an alcoholex program for 10,000 alcoholics without severe medical consequences of alcohol are:

Cp = $3,700,000
Cse = $100,000
Ct = $800,000

Assume that the effectiveness of the alcoholex program in terms of quality-adjusted years of life saved is:

Eli = 250
Em = 150
Ese = 100

What is the cost-effectiveness ratio? What is the cost-effectiveness ratio telling you?

The cost-effectiveness ratio is a useful measure of costs and benefits if a single new or additional intervention such as an alcohol abuse program is being considered. Further, it may permit comparison of two new types of interventions. This can be done if the effectiveness is measured in the same units, such as years of life saved, and if the interventions save the same number of years of life. When a curative and preventive program can be equally effective in eliminating deaths or chronic disability, then the cost-effectiveness ratio will allow us to identify the less expensive approach.

THE INCREMENTAL COST-EFFECTIVENESS RATIO

In many circumstances, one program option may be useful for a small number or special type of individual whereas another may be more applicable to larger groups or different types of individuals. In this situation, the cost-effectiveness ratio used alone may be misleading. Let us imagine, for illustration purposes, two programs, A and B.

	Program A	*Program B*
Net cost	$1,000,000	$3,000,000
Net effectiveness (years of disease-free life saved)	200	300
Cost-effectiveness ratio (dollars per year of disease-free life saved) =	$5000	$10,000

If we compare only the overall average cost-effectiveness ratio, program A looks more cost effective since each year of life saved costs $5000 in program A and $10,000 in program B. However, notice that program B, despite its higher average cost, saves more total years of life. The cost of these additional years of life saved can be calculated using the *incremental* cost-effectiveness ratio for program B compared to program A. The incremental cost-effectiveness ratio equals the cost per year of life saved for the additional or incremental years of life saved.

Incremental cost-effectiveness
    ratio of program B

$$= \frac{\text{cost of program B} - \text{cost of program A}}{\begin{array}{cc}\text{no. of years of} & \text{no. of years of}\\ \text{disease-free life} \quad - \quad \text{disease-free life}\\ \text{saved by program B} & \text{saved by program A}\end{array}} = \frac{\$2,000,000}{100}$$

In this example, the incremental cost-effectiveness ratio is $20,000 per year of life saved. This additional cost is higher than the average cost, but it may still be worth paying in order to save the additional years of life.

_____ STUDY QUESTION 4-8
Imagine that program A is an alcoholism treatment program aimed at those with alcohol-induced liver disease. Program B is an alcoholex program aimed at alcoholics without known liver disease. Given the costs and effectiveness numbers listed above, which of the following options would you choose? Justify your answer.

1. Program A
2. Program B
3. Both programs A and B
4. Neither program A nor B

References
1. Periodic Health Examination Monograph. Canadian Government Publishing Center, 1980.
2. LaForce FM, US Preventive Services Task Force. Immunizations, immunoprophylaxis, and chemoprophylaxis to prevent selected infections. JAMA 1987;256:2464–2470.

Tools for Implementation

CHAPTER FIVE

GAIL J. POVAR
RICHARD K. RIEGELMAN

Once we have acquired the tools for analysis, we are confronted with a critical question: What strategies are available to us and how should we choose a method for intervention? In selecting from among the available tools for implementation, we will address three basic considerations:

1. When in the natural history of a disease should we intervene?
2. Who should be the target of the intervention?
3. How should we implement the intervention?

When in the Natural History of a Disease Should We Intervene?

The natural history of a particular disease in an individual has three phases: predisease (no disease present), asymptomatic disease (no apparent symptoms but disease can be diagnosed), and clinical disease (symptoms apparent and disease diagnosed). Intervention during these three phases corresponds to three basic preventive options; primary, secondary, and tertiary prevention.

PRIMARY PREVENTION

Primary prevention is aimed at the individual who has not yet developed the disease (predisease). Intervention at this stage is intended to change conditions that put the individual at risk for the disease, so that he or she does not develop it. Thus, primary prevention occurs before disease and is the purest form of prevention. Using primary prevention, we may (1) attack the basic cause of the disease, (2) alter the environment to keep the cause away from humans, or (3) strengthen resistance to the disease. Examples from this book are modifying cholesterol levels to prevent myocardial infarction, regulating acceptable asbestos exposure levels for factory workers, and vaccinating children against chickenpox.

SECONDARY PREVENTION

The focus of secondary prevention is the individual in whom the disease has started but symptoms have not appeared. In secondary prevention, we treat early to prevent the disease's symptoms and complications. Using secondary prevention, we may (1) intervene after exposure to the disease, (2) detect and treat early disease before it becomes symptomatic, or (3) prevent the spread of disease by treating contacts. For example, we can treat individuals who have received high-risk bites with postexposure rabies vaccine to prevent the development of rabies, screen for breast cancer to treat early for cure, require premarital screening for syphilis to prevent congenital disease, and treat those exposed to tuberculosis, regardless of their purified protein derivative status.

TERTIARY PREVENTION
Tertiary prevention is aimed at individuals in whom the disease has become symptomatic. Most of clinical medicine is aimed at cure or control of clinical disease and can thus be considered tertiary prevention. In tertiary prevention, we treat the disease to (1) cure it or reverse its clinical manifestations, (2) control disease progression to avoid complications, (3) control the spread of disease to others, or (4) anticipate and modify the impact of clinical disease. At this level of preventive intervention we may, for example, treat recurrent herpes simplex with acyclovir or use anticoagulation to prevent embolic stroke in patients with atrial fibrillation.

At Whom Should the Intervention Be Aimed?
In addition to deciding when in the course of a disease intervention is most appropriate, one must also decide for whom the intervention is intended. Three basic social levels are possible: the individual, the group at risk, or the general population, including groups not at risk.

Preventive interventions directed at the individual level imply that decisions are being made one patient at a time. The doctor-patient encounter is the usual forum for prevention at this level. Individual intervention may include individual patient education, vaccination, case finding of early disease, or individual efforts to cure or prevent disease complications.

Preventive strategies directed to the group at risk mean that organized institutional or social interventions are being aimed at groups of individuals who are at increased risk of disease. Interventions in the group at risk may include intervention in high-risk occupational settings or organized social efforts to treat disease or prevent spread.

Preventive strategies directed at the general population target or affect a larger group of individuals than those at increased risk of disease. These strategies may include mass education, environmental modification, mass vaccination, or mass screening of an entire population.

A particular intervention can target more than one social level, depending on its intent. A doctor advising a 50-year-old woman to take calcium pills each day to lessen her chances of developing osteoporosis is practicing primary prevention at the individual level. When the doctor lectures to a senior citizens' group, giving the same advice, he or she then is practicing primary prevention to groups at risk. If the physician now offers the advice on a nationwide television program, recommending that everyone increase their calcium intake to prevent osteoporosis, he or she is practicing primary prevention at the population level.

_____ STUDY QUESTION 5-1

Imagine that all of the following options for dealing with acquired immunodeficiency syndrome (AIDS) were available. Classify each of these options according to the level of prevention employed (when) and the social level at which the intervention is aimed (who).

1. Individual "safe sex" education
2. Mass media information on "safe sex"
3. Vaccination of high-risk groups who are HIV-negative to reduce the risk of developing AIDS
4. Reversal of the clinical manifestations of AIDS through drug treatment
5. Case finding of HIV antibody–positive cases by individual physician to provide early treatment to prevent AIDS
6. Case-initiated follow-up of AIDS patients' sexual contacts so that contacts can be treated, regardless of HIV status, to prevent AIDS
7. Mass screening of all high school seniors to identify HIV antibody–positive cases and treat them to prevent AIDS and HIV spread
8. Organized screening of all transfusion recipients for HIV antibody–positive individuals so that they may be treated to prevent AIDS
9. Quarantining of AIDS patients to prevent any contact between them and other members of society

Deciding When to Intervene and Who to Target

Ultimately, we must select a preventive approach that occurs at the appropriate time and affects the right people. Primary prevention strategies have the advantage that they reduce our disease burden by blocking its very appearance. In addition, we would like to target for intervention precisely those at risk and alter their lives alone, but we must take into account a number of factors that limit our ability to design such optimal solutions.

LACK OF KNOWLEDGE

In many instances, the epidemiologic data establishing the contributory cause of a disease are lacking. For example, while we can address cigarette smoking confidently in our efforts to reduce the incidence of lung cancer, we have no similar model for colonic cancer prevention at this time. Consequently, our earliest intervention option is at the secondary level. Alternatively, we may be able to identify a risk factor or contributory cause, such as age as a risk factor for breast cancer, but have no primary intervention.

The lack of an available intervention can temper our zeal to screen for disease. If early detection does not lead to effective treatment, then screening makes little sense. There currently is no impetus to develop a screening test for multiple sclerosis as no evidence exists that preemptive therapy for mild symptoms alters the course of disease. One waits until the symptoms, by their severity, mandate intervention.

LACK OF ACCEPTABLE TREATMENT

At times, we have the knowledge to identify both a risk factor and an intervention of at least theoretical benefit. For instance, we have identified elevated cholesterol levels as a risk factor for coronary artery disease, and resins such as cholestyramine have demonstrated efficacy in the experimental situation. In the population at large, however, the side effects of cholestyramine, the bother of taking it, and so forth may substantially reduce the potential gains. Thus, a preventive strategy that is worthwhile in an idealized setting may have a more limited application to the risk group at large. Such limitations have fueled the search for a more tolerable primary intervention.

RISKS AND BENEFITS

The choice of level of intervention and target groups often results in an implied risk-benefit analysis. When an intervention, such as anticoagulation, carries substantial risk, we tend to prefer case-by-case application rather than to generalize the measure to an entire group at risk. Public service announcements suggesting that all cardiac patients ask their physicians about warfarin therapy are difficult to envision. Instead, decisions regarding the appropriateness of the therapy and the risk-benefit analyses involved occur between patients and their physicians. Thus, much, if not most, tertiary intervention takes place at the individual clinical level rather than at the public level.

COSTS

The costs associated with differing strategies will also affect our choice of when to intervene and whom to target. For instance, primary strategies (e.g., stopping cigarette smoking) may be attractive in part because they cost the health care system less than tertiary strategies (e.g., interventions aimed at limiting metastasis in patients with lung cancer). Similarly, cost considerations dictate that we direct our screening strategies at specific risk groups (e.g., persons older than 40 for colonic cancer) although we might detect a few more cases with a broader target group (e.g., if flexible sigmoidoscopies were performed on everyone older than 30).

How Should We Implement the Intervention?

The methods for implementing preventive interventions can be classified as (1) information (permissive), (2) motivation (persuasive), or (3) obligation (coercive). All three methods of implementation can be applied to any of the three target groups (Table 5-1).

INFORMATION

Information strategies vary not only by the methods used to achieve change but in the degree of external pressure each method requires. This group of strategies, as the name implies, seeks to provide the target group with data necessary to make an informed decision. The way information is provided is not necessarily psychologically neutral. For example, advertisements package information to maximize its impact and persuasiveness. As a general rule, however, such educational approaches do not use specific behavioral incentives or disincentives beyond the content of the informational message itself. Madison Avenue can only twist one's arm figuratively, not literally. Thus, the informational approach leaves the target population free to accept or reject the implications of the information. Individuals are free to change their behavior or ignore the message. Hence, information strategies are considered permissive.

MOTIVATION

The second class of implementation methods, motivation, goes beyond provision of information to employ incentives or disincentives designed to motivate change in behavior. It is a persuasive approach. Often, the

Table 5-1. Intervention implementation methods applied to each target group

Target group	Information	Motivation	Obligation
Individual	Individual receives information and initiates a preventive behavior.	Doctor tells patient to do or not to do something. Doctor suggests incentive or di incentive options.	Doctor threatens not to care for patient if . . . ; risk of legal penalty for noncompliance.
Group at risk	Make information directed at those at risk available in public areas on widespread basis.	Limit insurance by increasing premiums for risk group. Decrease access to the behavior or its paraphernalia.	Employ restrictive or punitive measures for high-risk behavior.
General population	Educate whole public (not only those at risk).	Create incentives for population as a whole to reduce risk factor. Encourage a group to work to reduce presence of risk factor in their midst.	Require whole population to participate in a risk-reduction program (e.g., fluoridation programs).

motivators are independent of the information. For instance, consider the lollipop from the pediatrician who has just administered an immunization. The child may see the lollipop as a peace offering. The pediatrician, however, might be reinforcing the child's coming to the office, so that the child will show up for the next immunization even if he or she dreads the shot itself. The information, in this case, is the need for the immunization; the motivator is the lollipop. Clearly, the lollipop strategy may fail and the child may balk at subsequent visits to the doctor. The lollipop might be persuasive most of the time, but it lacks the power to force the terrified child into the physician's office. Therefore, the subject of a motivational strategy still has choice.

OBLIGATION

Sometimes, we employ disincentives or incentives so powerful that, in theory at least, the target population can no longer choose not to engage in the behavioral change desired. We oblige or require compliance. The method is coercive. Such strategies typically employ disincentives to noncompliance that would seriously threaten one's physical or social well-being. We need only remind ourselves of the threat of a spanking as a child or of the $30 parking ticket as an adult to understand obligatory strategies. The required vaccination, without which a child may not attend public school, is an example of this kind of preventive intervention. It is important to emphasize that the obligatory approach no longer leaves the individual truly free to choose not to adopt the intended behavior.

_____ STUDY QUESTION 5-2

Consider the problem of cigarette smoking. For each cell in Table 5-1, design an intervention implementation to address this problem.

As we moved through Table 5-1, the options in some of the cells may have made us uncomfortable. Certain approaches seem either too lenient on the one hand or too draconian on the other. In fact, the three methods of intervention implementation—information, motivation, and obligation—incorporate degrees of external force or individual self-determination that may seem appropriate in some situations and in others may not. To choose among the strategic options, we must know what is at stake. Let's examine some of the advantages and disadvantages of each method.

ADVANTAGES AND DISADVANTAGES
OF EACH IMPLEMENTATION METHOD

Information

As was noted earlier, the first method of implementing an intervention relies exclusively on the provision of information to the target population. The recipients of that information may ignore it altogether, attend to it but choose not to act in accordance with it, or choose to change their behavior. The freedom to walk away from the intervention is presumed. Hence, the cigarette smoker, having read the message on the pack, is free to decide that the warning either does not apply to him or her, does not concern him or her, or at least, is insufficiently fearsome to motivate him or her to stop smoking. Preventive medicine strategies that rely solely on freedom of choice recognize that the freedom to choose change is also the freedom to refuse change. These strategies *hope* to change behavior by appealing to logic, yet the respect for individual choice, so important in our society, takes precedence over the desire to change the behavior that endangers individual health. Furthermore, the preservation of the freedom to do as one wishes is, in the informational approach, placed above the achievement of benefits to society (such as reduction of productivity losses associated with cigarette smoking). It would be wonderful if this method were successful. Unfortunately, informing people of the risks they face is often ineffective for inducing change. Many people have stopped smoking in response to the barrage of information regarding the risk of cancer, emphysema, and so forth, but many have not. When we select a strategy based on information alone, we often implicitly accept a substantial failure rate to preserve our social values of freedom of choice.

Motivation

Sometimes the failure rate of the informational approach is unacceptable. Our concern for the health of our patients or the public persuades us that a more activist intervention is warranted. It is then that we move from simply informing people to more aggressively persuading them to alter their behavior. Such efforts call for the use of the motivational methods. As noted earlier, these approaches employ behavioral incentives or disincentives that exceed information itself. The incentives or disincentives can be resisted, providing they are not coercive in nature [1]. (If they *were* coercive, the techniques would be considered an obligatory strategy.) Hence, motivating techniques still preserve freedom of choice, but they intentionally reward the desired behavior and discourage the alternative. The individual, then, must actively resist this preventive method.

The motivational method has its drawbacks. Practically speaking, it may be difficult to identify behavioral modification techniques that on the one hand promise to be effective while on the other hand steer clear of coercion. Also, campaigns that work hard at changing behavior but still claim to leave the choice with the individual set up the potential for blaming the victim: That is, if the person at risk fails to respond to the incentives or disincentives in his or her path, we may see that person as stubborn, irresponsible, or stupid. When we use either information or motivation to change behavior, we may underestimate the countervailing influences. The more convinced we are of the importance of the behavioral change, the more likely we are to see those who resist as deserving of the consequences.

Again, cigarette smoking provides a good example. The glamour of cigarette smoking as portrayed in ad campaigns, and the desire for peer group acceptance may render the teenager unable to resist smoking. Once addicted, he or she may need powerful incentives indeed to overcome the craving for cigarettes. For these reasons, some authors have been concerned that we may turn inappropriately against the smokers, noting that their apparent refusal to change is a justification for us to wash our hands of responsibility for their care [2, 3].

Alternatively, the pleasure of smoking in the present may be valued more highly by some people than the health benefits that may be obtained in the future by quitting. Motivational strategies implicitly recognize the right of the individual to choose, in effect, the "wrong" answer. We may find ourselves blaming those who persist in the behavior even though we meant to leave them a choice [2, 4]. When we believe the problem is important enough to try an active intervention such as motivation but still leave open the door for freedom of choice, we may set the stage for this sort of conflict.

Obligation

There are times when it seems clear to us that no refusal to change is tolerable. It is then that we turn to the method of obligation to achieve prevention. We use obligatory methods when we wish to make a clear statement that the health of the individual is a community concern that exceeds concern for the individual's freedom of choice [5]. At such times, we may regard the achievement or maintenance of health as more important than individual freedom [6]. This may be especially true when we seek to protect not only those engaging in the behavior that puts them at risk but also those who are put at risk by the behavior of others. When we require immunizations, we are concerned not only that the individual be protected from disease but that the community be protected from disease introduced by that individual. When we insist on pollution control in cars, it is for the benefit of all who breathe, not only for drivers on the road. Child restraint laws reflect our belief that the vulnerable must be protected when they are unable to protect themselves.

Like informational and motivational strategies, strategies that create an obligation to comply are also associated with difficulties. Freedoms may be lost beyond those that are immediately apparent (e.g., the freedom to pollute, to go without seatbelts, or to drink and drive). To enforce such obligations, the state might have to imperil privacy: Stopping cars at random to perform breathalyzer tests *requires* an invasion of privacy. A hypothetical law requiring safe sex (or no sex at all) by HIV carriers would truly bring "Big Brother" into the bedroom.

The decision to use an obligatory strategy requires us to look closely at who is at risk for the illness and who is required to alter their behavior. Our society has a long history of obligating individuals to abstain from harming others. Murder is illegal. State health departments often have the authority to control the activities of people carrying certain infections, such as keeping *Salmonella* carriers out of the food preparation business. More recently, certain industries (e.g., asbestos and chemical manufacturers) have been regulated in an effort to protect workers from undue harm. Yet one could question the morality of limiting profits or limiting numbers of jobs to achieve such protections.

The greatest ethical discomfort seems to be reserved for those situations in which we wish to obligate someone to do something for his or her benefit alone. It seems difficult to justify required exercise programs for 40-year-old men or to mandate monthly breast examinations for women older than 30. Limiting an individual's freedom "in his or her best interest" is more likely, in our society, to be viewed as intolerable meddling than as good preventive medicine policy.

Clearly, obligatory techniques may violate important political and moral values in an effort to enhance another value—health [7]. In addition, they are exceedingly difficult to enforce effectively, and if enforcement is inadequate, respect for the law generally may be undermined. We might consider the alcohol prohibition era to understand better the consequences of a legal remedy that is difficult to administer consistently.

Because they override powerful values of individual freedom and privacy, and because they are costly to enforce, obligatory methods of implementing intervention place a strong burden of proof on those who advocate their use. The risk to individuals and society must be substantial, and the likelihood of achieving compliance must be realizable. Such constraints mean that the method of obligation to achieve prevention is usually reserved as a last resort to be employed only after information and motivation have failed and the threat to the public health is indeed great. Table 5-2 summarizes the advantages and disadvantages of the three implementation methods we have discussed.

Table 5-2. Advantages and disadvantages of each implementation method

	Information	Motivation	Obligation
Advantages	Preserves freedom of choice. Often least expensive option.	Preserves some freedom of choice. More interventionist, therefore expresses more concern for the health consequences. May be more effective than information alone.	Most likely to achieve compliance if well enforced.
Disadvantages	Often ineffective. May appear to be disinterested in real behavior change.	Sets up possible victim blaming. Can be very labor intensive. Must tread line between ineffectiveness and efficacy achieved by coercion.	Often requires infringing on important moral or political values. Often very expensive to enforce properly. If inadequate enforcement, undermines respect for obligation.

STUDY QUESTION 5-3

Return to the intervention implementation strategies you identified for cigarette smoking (Study Question 5-2). How do the advantages and disadvantages of the general implementation methods just discussed apply to your strategies?

Summary

The choice of a preventive tool inevitably involves not one but a series of decisions. First, we must identify when in the natural history of the disease we should intervene. Then, we must decide who should be the target of our intervention. Finally, we must decide how to intervene. Having identified options for intervention and the advantages and disadvantages of each option, we need an approach to choosing between the options: (1) Are voluntary methods likely to be effective or are incentives or requirements needed? (2) How important is the problem with which we are dealing? Is it important enough to restrict an individual's freedom of choice? (3) What are the financial costs of the strategy? In light of the disease consequence, can we afford the preventive strategy? Are we willing to alter our priorities in order to afford it? (4) Can we accept the social consequences of implementing the preventive strategy? Can we accept the consequences of not doing so?

Now that we are equipped with the tools for characterizing the problem and evaluating the solutions, let us proceed to our case studies. These are designed to provide in-depth examples of problem solving in clinical prevention.

References

1. Faden R, Faden A. The ethics of health education as public health policy. Health Educ Monogr 1987;6:180–197.
2. Crawford, R. You are dangerous to your health: the ideology and politics of victim blaming. Int J Health Serv 1977;7:663–680.
3. Divorkin G. Voluntary health risks and public policy. Hastings Cent Rep 1981;11:26–31.
4. Meenan R. Improving the public's health—some further reflections. N Engl J Med 1976;294:45–46.
5. Beauchamp D. Community: the neglected tradition of public health. Hastings Cent Rep 1986;15:28–36.
6. Moreno J, Bayer R. The limits of the ledger in public health promotion. Hastings Cent Rep 1986;15:37–41.
7. Leichter H. Public policy and the British experience. Hastings Cent Rep 1981;11:32–39.

Primary Prevention

PART FOUR

Risk Factor Intervention

Cholesterol and Heart Disease

RISA BETH BURNS
ROBERT E. WALKER

CASE A.   Mr. L. is a 55-year-old white businessman who comes to see you for the first time complaining of chronic lower back pain. He has enjoyed excellent health since childhood, has never been hospitalized, and takes a multiple vitamin daily but no other medications. His family history is remarkable for his father who died at age 58 of "heart trouble" and a 52-year-old brother with chest pains. Mr. L. smokes one-half pack of cigarettes per day and does not engage in regular exercise. Physical examination reveals a blood pressure of 145/92, weight of 200 lb (which is 30 percent greater than his ideal weight), and normal cardiac and musculoskeletal examinations. After examining him, you emphasize the relationship between weight and back symptoms, instruct him in an exercise routine, and obtain your routine health maintenance laboratory tests. Everything comes back within normal limits except for a serum cholesterol value of 255 mg per deciliter. Repeat testing shows a fasting cholesterol level of 250 and a triglyceride level of 100.

What will you tell Mr. L. about his cholesterol level, and what types of therapy or other recommendations will you prescribe?

CASE B.   Mrs. S. is a 40-year-old black schoolteacher who is referred to you after attending a local health fair. Among the many blood tests performed, the most notable showed she had a serum cholesterol level of 370 mg per deciliter. Mrs. S. is deeply concerned about this and has been reading about hypercholesterolemia and its association with heart disease in the newspaper and other press. She comes in today demanding an electrocardiogram and exercise stress test and inquiring about drugs that will lower her cholesterol level.

After taking a complete history, you find that Mrs. S. has a history of cholelithiasis that is currently asymptomatic and spastic colon. She continues to menstruate regularly. Past medical history is otherwise unremarkable. Family history is significant for a mother and maternal grandmother with adult-onset diabetes mellitus. The remainder of the history is unremarkable, and the physical examination is within normal limits.

You decide to repeat the patient's serum cholesterol measurement and get back a value of 390. On further evaluation, you find that Mrs. S. has type IIa hyperlipidemia.

What will you tell Mrs. S. about her risk of developing coronary heart disease? Would you initiate treatment and, if so, with what? What would you tell Mrs. S. if she were age 65? Before attempting to answer these questions, let's take a step back and review the data on the relationship between serum cholesterol levels and coronary heart disease.

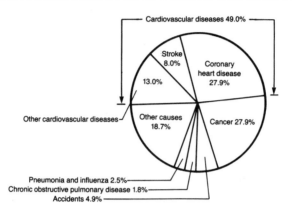

Fig. 6-1. Deaths by cause as percentage of total deaths in the United States, 1982. Causes of death for 1982 classified by the Ninth Revision of the International Classification of Diseases Adapted for Use in the United States. Data for 1982 are provisional. (From the National Center for Health Statistics, Division of Vital Statistics.)

Coronary Heart Disease

EPIDEMIOLOGY

Cardiovascular disease is the leading cause of death in the United States, still accounting for nearly 50 percent of all deaths. Coronary heart disease (CHD) is responsible for 26 percent of all deaths or 540,000 deaths in the United States each year. It continues to account for more deaths each year than all forms of cancer combined (Fig. 6-1) [1].

CHD costs the United States more than $60 billion each year in direct health care costs, lost wages, and productivity. It ranks first as a Social Security disability and second only to arthritis for limitation in all activities. CHD ranks second only to all forms of cancer for total hospital bed days [2].

Because CHD has such high morbidity and mortality, many health experts have focused attention on primary prevention of this disease—that is, on identifying populations at risk for developing CHD and intervening in some way *before* evidence of CHD is present.

NATIONAL INSTITUTES OF HEALTH RECOMMENDATIONS

A large body of evidence associates elevated blood cholesterol with subsequent development of CHD. Questions have been posed regarding the cause and effect relationship between cholesterol and heart disease, the steps that should be taken to treat elevated blood cholesterol, and the attempts that should be made to reduce the blood cholesterol levels of the general population. To address these issues, the National Heart, Lung, and Blood Institute and the National Institutes of Health (NIH) Office of Medical Applications of Research convened a Consensus Development Conference on lowering blood cholesterol to prevent heart disease. After hearing a series of presentations and reviewing the data, a panel of lipoprotein experts considered the evidence and came to the following conclusions [3]:

1. Elevated blood cholesterol is a major cause of CHD.
2. Lowering elevated blood cholesterol will reduce the risk of myocardial infarction owing to CHD.
3. Changing the American diet to a low-cholesterol diet will afford protection against CHD.

Inherent in these conclusions are the following assumptions:

1. Cholesterol affects men, women, and children in a similar manner.
2. There are no substantial adverse health effects of lowering serum cholesterol.
3. Lowering dietary cholesterol will reduce the risk of CHD.
4. Reductions in serum cholesterol below the current levels of most Americans will be beneficial.

This chapter will consider the data behind each of the questions, conclusions, and some of the underlying assumptions. In the end, you will be asked to evaluate this data and decide whether the NIH recommendations are well founded. Finally, you will be asked to apply your conclusions to Mr. L. and Mrs. S.

Cholesterol as a Contributory Cause of Coronary Heart Disease

The first step in proving a cause and effect relationship between cholesterol and CHD is to establish contributory cause. Contributory cause implies that (1) the cause is associated with the disease, (2) the cause precedes the disease (prior association), and (3) altering the cause alters the disease. Let us look at the evidence that cholesterol is associated with CHD.

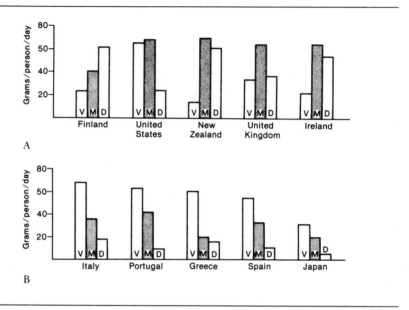

Fig. 6-2. Consumption of major types of food fats in certain countries with (*A*) high and (*B*) low coronary heart disease and deaths related to such disease. *V* = vegetable fats; *M* = meat fats; *D* = dairy fats. (From Keys [5].)

ECOLOGICAL OR GROUP STUDIES

Geographic studies have compared the dietary intake among representative countries and shown that countries with diets high in meat and dairy fats (the primary source of saturated fats and dietary cholesterol) have higher CHD mortality compared to countries whose dietary fat is derived chiefly from vegetables (Fig. 6-2). For instance, Finland and the United States are countries with high CHD mortality rates, and their populations consume relatively larger amounts of meats and dairy products. In contrast, Italian and Greek populations, which derive their major dietary fats from vegetables, have relatively low CHD mortality rates [4, 5]. When comparing average serum cholesterol levels of these same populations with CHD death, the association is again demonstrated: Those populations with higher average serum cholesterol levels also have higher CHD mortality and morbidity rates. Usually, the higher CHD and higher serum cholesterol populations are the same populations that consume larger amounts of meat and dairy fats.

What type of relationship between cholesterol and CHD is established by this data?

Now let us look at the evidence that an elevated cholesterol level is associated with CHD on an individual basis and that elevated cholesterol precedes the development of CHD.

PROSPECTIVE STUDIES
To establish whether the common types of hyperlipidemia are associated with subsequent CHD, a series of human population studies have prospectively investigated the relationship between elevated cholesterol and coronary artery disease [6–8]. These studies have addressed the question: Is individual elevation in cholesterol associated with subsequent CHD? The data from five of these studies have been combined in what has been called the Pooling Project, "Pool 5" [6]. Pool 5 includes data from the Albany Cardiovascular Health Center, Chicago Peoples Gas Co., Chicago Western Electric Co. [7], Framingham Heart Disease Epidemiology Study [8], and Tecumseh Community Study. Together these studies included more than 8000 white men, aged 40 to 64. The subjects had no history of angina pectoris or previous myocardial infarction and no electrocardiographic evidence of previous myocardial infarction on entry to the study. All the studies are prospective or cohort studies and, thus, are capable of establishing the existence of an association on an individual basis* and of establishing that the elevated cholesterol level precedes the CHD.

In addition, the data from the Pooling Project allow us to estimate the strength of the individual association between elevated cholesterol and CHD. The initial serum cholesterol levels and incidence of end points are shown in Table 6-1. End points were fatal and nonfatal myocardial infarctions and sudden CHD death over the 8.6-year follow-up period. Individuals with higher serum cholesterol had an increased incidence of CHD.

*The Pooling Project study design expresses incidence of end points by using age-standardized incidence ratios. These are expressions of relative incidence based on an average of 100 for all groups.

Table 6-1. Serum cholesterol level and incidence ratio of first cardiac event

Group	Serum cholesterol level (mg/dl)	Age-standardized incidence ratio for end points*
1	<194	72
2	194–218	61
3	218–240	78
4	240–268	129
5	>268	158

*Fatal and nonfatal myocardial infarctions and sudden death from coronary heart disease.
Source: Adapted from the Pooling Project Research Group [6].

Table 6-2. Reduction in cholesterol over years from the LRLC-LPPT Study

Time	Diet + placebo plasma total cholesterol (mg/dl)	Diet + cholestyramine plasma total cholesterol (mg/dl)
Initial	291.8	291.5
1 year later	275.4	238.6
7 years later	277.3	257.1
	4.9% change	13.4% change

Note: The percentage of change is compared for each individual and then averaged.
Source: Adapted from the Lipid Research Clinics Coronary Primary Prevention Trial [2].

CONTROLLED CLINICAL TRIALS

We have already provided some evidence that an elevated cholesterol level is associated with CHD and that the elevation precedes CHD. Contributory cause also requires that we establish that altering the cause (elevated cholesterol) alters the disease (CHD). Let us now look at the data that address this final criterion of contributory cause.

The Lipid Research Clinics Coronary Primary Prevention Trial (LRC-CPPT) was a multicenter, randomized, double-blind study designed to test the efficacy of lowering cholesterol in reducing the risk of CHD [2]. The study included more than 3800 asymptomatic men, aged 40 to 49, with primary hypercholesterolemia (type IIa). All study subjects had plasma cholesterol levels greater than or equal to 265 mg per deciliter after an outpatient trial of a low-cholesterol diet. Individuals were excluded if they had cardiac disease (history of myocardial infarction, an-

Table 6-3. Incidence of end points from the LRC-LPPT Study

End point	Diet + placebo (N = 1900)		Diet + cholestyramine (N = 1906)		% Reduction in risk[a]
	N	Incidence rate	N	Incidence rate	
Coronary heart disease death	38	0.02	30	0.016	$\dfrac{0.020 - 0.016}{0.020} = 24$
Definite nonfatal myocardial infarction[b]	158	0.083	130	0.068	$\dfrac{0.083 - 0.068}{0.083} = 19^{c}$
Total	187	0.098	155	0.081	$\dfrac{0.098 - 0.081}{0.098} = 19$

[a]Percentage of reductions in risk are adjusted for follow-up time and stratification.
[b]When definite and suspected myocardial infarctions are used, the numbers are larger and the results were similar.
[c]The 19-percent reduction in combined risk is significant at $p < .05$.
Source: Adapted from the Lipid Research Clinics Coronary Primary Prevention Trial [2].

gina, CHD), hypertension, obesity, or life-limiting diseases (i.e., diabetes mellitus, hepatic disease, or renal disease). Subjects within each of the eight strata or prognostic categories of increasing CHD risk were randomized to a diet and placebo or diet and cholestyramine group. Cholestyramine is a lipid-lowering drug that acts as a bile acid sequestrant. Follow-up at 7 to 10 years was achieved for 100 percent of participants.

The results of the study showed that the diet plus cholestyramine group experienced an average plasma total cholesterol reduction of 13.4 percent compared to 4.9 percent ($p < .001$) obtained in the diet plus placebo group (Table 6-2).

To determine whether the greater decrease in cholesterol in the cholestyramine group resulted in a decreased incidence of CHD, the primary end points of definite CHD death or definite nonfatal myocardial infarction were evaluated (Table 6-3).

STUDY QUESTION 6-2

Does the LRC-CPPT study satisfy the criteria to establish that cholesterol is a contributory cause of CHD among men with cholesterol levels greater than or equal to 265 mg per deciliter?

Cholesterol as a Risk Factor

Having established that cholesterol is a contributory cause of CHD, we must consider a number of other issues before we can recommend that individuals engage in an effort to lower cholesterol. First, we need to know how powerful a risk factor cholesterol is. In other words, what is the relative risk, attributable risk, and population attributable risk associated with elevated cholesterol levels?

RELATIVE RISK

Remember that relative risk assigns a numerical value to a risk factor and expresses the probability of disease (CHD) if the risk factor is present compared to its probability if the risk factor is absent.

$$\text{Relative risk } = \frac{\text{probability of developing disease if risk factor is present}}{\text{probability of developing disease if risk factor is absent}}$$

A relative risk of 1 would indicate no association between the risk factor and the disease.

In calculating the relative risk of an elevated cholesterol level, one needs to know the denominator, the probability of cardiac end points in those with a normal serum cholesterol level. We do not know, however, at what levels serum cholesterol is no longer a risk factor. We can compare the incidence rates of a CHD end point at each level of cholesterol compared to the CHD end point for those with cholesterol less than 194 mg per deciliter. For example, for group 2 (those with serum cholesterol between 194 and 218), the relative risk equals 61/72 or 0.85.

Group	Serum Cholesterol Level (mg/dl)	Age-Standardized Incidence Ratio	Relative Risk Compared to Group 1
1	<194	72	
2	194–218	61	61/72 = 0.85
3	218–240	78	
4	240–268	129	
5	>268	158	

--- STUDY QUESTION 6-3
Calculate the relative risks for each group, compare them to group 1, and insert those values into the table above.

Because the incidence of CHD began to increase at levels above 218, the Pooling Project investigators averaged the incidence ratios for groups 1 and 2 and used this as the denominator. Using this method, the relative risk for group 5, for example, equals $158/([61 + 72]/2)$.

--- STUDY QUESTION 6-4
Calculate the relative risk for groups 3 and 4 in this way and insert these values to the table below.

Group	Serum Cholesterol Level (mg/dl)	Age-Standardized Incidence Ratio	Relative Risk Compared to Groups 1 and 2
1	<194	72	
2	194–218	61	
3	218–240	78	
4	240–268	129	
5	>268	158	2.4

From the tabulated data, we can determine that the probability of developing CHD if the serum cholesterol level is greater than 268 mg per deciliter is approximately 2.4 times greater than the probability of developing CHD if the serum cholesterol level is less than 218. How impressive is a relative risk of elevated cholesterol of approximately 2.4? One way of answering this question is to examine the relative risks of other risk factors for CHD. The Pooling Project, in addition to studying serum cholesterol levels, also looked at blood pressure, cigarette smoking, and body weight, and their association with CHD over an 8.6-year follow-up period.* The relative risks for each of these factors in their study populations are tabulated below.

*Relative risks are computed for systolic blood pressure greater than 150 mm Hg compared to less than 130 mm Hg; for diastolic blood pressure greater than 94 mm Hg compared to less than 80 mm Hg; for cigarette smoking of more than 1 pack per day compared to nonsmokers; for body weight greater than 129 percent of desirable weight compared to less than 112 percent of desirable weight; and for serum cholesterol levels of greater than 268 mg/dl compared to less than 218 mg/dl. Adapted from the Pooling Project Research Grant [6].

Risk Factor	Relative Risk (adjusted)
Systolic blood pressure >150	1.9
Diastolic blood pressure >94	2.2
Cigarette smoking of >1 pack/day	3.2
Weight >129% desirable weight	1.3
Serum cholesterol level >268 mg/dl	2.4

These risk factors were assessed taking into account or adjusting for the other risk factors. Thus, the study attempted to assess the independent effect of each risk factor. When comparing serum cholesterol to other risk factors of CHD, the only risk factor with a greater relative risk is cigarette smoking of more than 1 pack per day.

ATTRIBUTABLE RISK
Let us calculate how much of the risk of CHD among those with high cholesterol can be attributed to cholesterol. This is the question of attributable risk. Another way to think of attributable risk is in terms of how much of the disease could potentially be eliminated, among those with elevated cholesterol, by lowering cholesterol, even without addressing other risk factors. The formula to calculate attributable risk is as follows:

$$\text{Attributable risk} = \frac{\text{incidence among those with the risk factor} - \text{incidence among those without the risk factor}}{\text{incidence among those with the risk factor}}$$

_____ STUDY QUESTION 6-5
Using the formula for calculating attributable risk and the data from Table 6-1, calculate the attributable risk for group 3 (i.e., those with a cholesterol level of 218 to 240 mg per deciliter).

The attributable risks for groups 4 and 5 are calculated in the same way and are 48.4 percent and 57.9 percent, respectively. These numbers imply that for individuals with blood cholesterol levels greater than 268, 57.9 percent is the maximum percentage that their incidence of CHD could be lowered if their blood cholesterol levels were reduced below 218. For those with cholesterol levels between 240 and 268, 48.4 percent is the maximum reduction in the risk of CHD that can be expected.

Table 6-4. Fiftieth and ninetieth percentiles for plasma total cholesterol concentrations for American adults by age and sex

Age (years)	Plasma total cholesterol (mg/dl) in men		Plasma total cholesterol (mg/dl) in women	
	50th percentile	90th percentile	50th percentile	90th percentile
20–29	172	215	164	207
30–39	194	234	176	219
40–49	206	254	195	241
50–59	211	261	222	275
60–69	210	258	228	280
70–79	205	249	228	280

Source: Adapted from the Lipid Research Clinics Coronary Primary Prevention Trial [2].

Remember, these estimates of attributable risk address the *potential* reduction in CHD for those with elevated cholesterol levels if their cholesterol were lowered.

POPULATION ATTRIBUTABLE RISK

In evaluating the potential impact of reduction of the cholesterol level on the incidence of CHD in an entire population, we need to know the population attributable risk (PAR). PAR, as opposed to attributable risk, answers the question: What proportion of the incidence of CHD in the population as a whole can *potentially* be eliminated by reducing elevated cholesterol levels? PAR differs from attributable risk because PAR looks at the population in general, which consists of individuals with and without the risk factor.

To calculate the PAR, we need to estimate the proportion of the population with elevated cholesterol. As Table 6-4 demonstrates, almost 10 percent of American men, aged 40 to 79, have plasma cholesterol levels exceeding 250 mg per deciliter.*

---

*Plasma total cholesterol values are 5 percent greater than their corresponding serum values. Thus, a plasma cholesterol level of 105 mg per deciliter is equal to a serum level of 100.

The formula for calculating PAR is:

$$PAR = \frac{b\,(RR - 1)}{b(RR - 1) + 1}$$

where b = the percentage of the population with the risk factor

RR = relative risk

_____ STUDY QUESTION 6-6
If 10 percent of the United States' male population, aged 40 to 79 years, have cholesterol levels exceeding 250 mg per deciliter and the relative risk for those with cholesterol in excess of 250 is approximately 2, what is the population attributable risk for men 40 to 79 years old?

If you have calculated correctly, the maximum potential reduction in the incidence of CHD among United States' men, aged 40 to 79, by eliminating elevated cholesterol alone is approximately 9 percent.

Note that the attributable risk is much greater than the PAR. This implies that despite the potential importance of elevated cholesterol for those who possess this risk factor, cholesterol alone accounts for only a small fraction of CHD in the male population older than 40.

_____ STUDY QUESTION 6-7
What are the implications of this modestly sized PAR for the association between cholesterol and CHD?

ABSOLUTE RISK
To appreciate the clinical importance of cholesterol elevation, let us take a look at the relationship between elevation in cholesterol and age. When looking at serum cholesterol level and risk of CHD by age group, the Pooling Project showed a decreasing relative risk with advancing age (Table 6-5).

To assess the clinical meaning of the reduced but still elevated relative risk for those older than 60, we must take into account relative risk, absolute risk, and the incidence of disease for those without the risk factor. We know that the incidence of CHD increases dramatically with age. This is a very important fact when thinking about the absolute risk.

Absolute risk is the probability that individuals with the risk factor will develop the disease.

Table 6-5. Relative risks for developing coronary heart
disease according to antecedent cholesterol levels and age

Age (years)	Relative risk
45–49	3.6
50–54	2.1
55–59	2.1
60–64	1.5

Relative risks computed for serum cholesterol levels greater than 268 mg per deciliter
compared to less than 218. Data for age group 40 to 44 years not given because of
lack of statistical significance.
Source: Adapted from the Pooling Project Research Group [6].

Absolute risk for those with the risk factor

= incidence of disease for those without the risk factor × relative risk

For example, let us assume that the 10-year incidence of CHD among
men in the 45- to 49-year-old group *without* elevated cholesterol is 0.1
percent or 1 per 1000. The absolute risk of CHD for an average man in
that age group with a serum cholesterol level greater than 268 is calculated as follows:

Absolute risk for those with the risk factor = 0.001 × 3.6 = 0.0036 = 0.36%

Thus, for a younger man with a cholesterol level exceeding 268, the risk
of CHD has increased from 0.1 to 0.36 percent, an absolute increase of
0.26 percent or 2.6 per 1000.

Now let us assume that the 10-year incidence of CHD in the 60- to 64-
year-olds without elevated cholesterol is 5 percent. The absolute risk of
CHD for a man in that age group with a similarly elevated serum cholesterol level is: 0.05 × 1.5 = 0.075 = 7.5 percent. For an older man,
the risk has increased from 5 to 7.5 percent, an absolute increase of 2.5
per 100. Thus, for the older man, the absolute increase in risk is nearly
10 times that for the younger man, despite the lower relative risk with
advancing age. The older man's absolute risk if he has a high cholesterol
level is much greater than the younger man's because of the dramatic
difference in the incidence of the disease at different ages. Although the
relative risk for a factor may appear small, its clinical importance de-

pends heavily on the incidence of the disease for those without the risk factor. Because moderately elevated cholesterol levels and CHD are both so prevalent in the United States, even fairly minor increases in relative risk above 1 may be associated with important increases in absolute risk.

Efficacy of Diet Versus Drugs for Reducing Cholesterol Levels

We have now established that cholesterol is a contributory cause of CHD at least among men aged 40 to 49 with an initial cholesterol level in excess of 265 mg per deciliter. We have also demonstrated that cholesterol is an important risk factor even at advanced age. Among those with elevated cholesterol levels, a substantial percentage of the incidence of CHD is attributable to the elevated cholesterol. The LRC-CPPT has shown that diet plus cholestyramine are effective in substantially reducing cholesterol and subsequent CHD [2].*

_____ STUDY QUESTION 6-8
Is there any risk associated with taking cholestyramine?

The Oslo diet heart study specifically addressed the question of whether a low-cholesterol diet will result in the reduction of plasma cholesterol and of CHD end points [10]. The study included 412 men aged 30 to 64 years up to 3 years after diagnosis of their first myocardial infarction. The men were randomized into two groups, a control group with no dietary change and a treatment group with a low-cholesterol diet. The cholesterol-lowering diet was 45.5 percent carbohydrates, 15 percent proteins, and 39 percent fats 8.5 percent saturated, 10.1 percent monounsaturated, and 20.7 percent polyunsaturated. Follow-up was obtained at 5 and 11 years (Tables 6-6, 6-7).

The men in the treatment group were reported to have a statistically significant and substantial decrease in their serum cholesterol. After 5 years, the incidence of CHD events, fatal, and nonfatal myocardial infarctions was substantially reduced (p <.05). After 11 years, there was a reduction in overall CHD and overall mortality, but only the difference in fatal myocardial infarctions was statistically significant (p = 0.004).

_____

*In addition, the Cholesterol Lowering Atherosclerosis Study (CLAS) has recently shown in a randomized placebo controlled trial that lowering cholesterol after coronary artery bypass grafts can partially reverse or at least retard the development of atheroma as visualized by angiography [9].

Table 6-6. Results of low-cholesterol dieting to reduce plasma cholesterol levels:
Follow-up at 5 years

	Initial serum cholesterol (mg/dl)	Mean reduction in serum cholesterol (mg/dl)	% Reduction in serum cholesterol
Control (N = 206)	296	11	3.7
Diet (N = 206)	296	52	17.6

Source: Adapted from the Oslo diet heart study [10].

Table 6-7. Results of low-cholesterol dieting to
reduce plasma cholesterol levels: Follow-up at 11 years

Mortality	Diet (N = 206)	Control (N = 206)	p Value
Fatal myocardial infarctions (MIs)	32	57	p = .004
Overall mortality	101	108	p = .35*
Overall coronary heart disease mortality (fatal MIs plus sudden death)	79	94	p = .097*

*For these categories, there is a reduction but it is not statistically significant. The
sample size in this study was calculated to enable the demonstration of statistically
significant results for common end points such as MI. Because of the large type II
error, one would not necessarily expect to demonstrate statistically significant
differences for less common events such as overall mortality.
Source: From the Oslo diet heart study [10].

STUDY QUESTION 6-9

Based on the data in Tables 6-3 and 6-7, do you think diet is as effective as drugs
in lowering blood cholesterol *and* CHD end points?

How Far Should Cholesterol be Lowered?

The Multiple Risk Factor Intervention Trials (MRFIT) beginning in November 1973 screened 356,222 men, aged 35 to 57 years, who were free
of a history of hospitalization for myocardial infarction [11]. Serum cho-

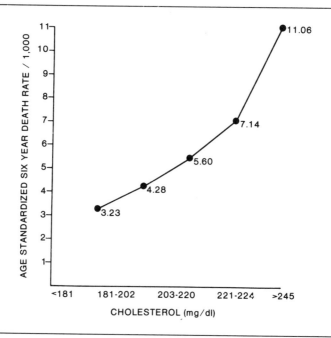

Fig. 6-3. Serum cholesterol levels related to 6-year mortality from coronary heart disease among men aged 35 to 57 years (N = 356,222). (From the Multiple Risk Factor Intervention Trials [11].)

lesterol levels were determined. Six-year CHD mortality data was collected for the entire cohort (Fig. 6-3). These data show that the lower the cholesterol, the lower the risk of CHD, a relationship that persists even at a blood cholesterol level of less than 200 mg per deciliter [10,12].

A second line of argument comes from the LRC-CPPT data [2]. The LRC-CPPT found that for an individual with an initial cholesterol level exceeding 265, a 1-percent decrease in plasma cholesterol produced approximately a 2-percent decrease in CHD risk. Despite the fact that this study did not examine the effect of lowering cholesterol for those with initial levels of less than 265, the LRC-CPPT did show a persistence of the 1 : 2 ratio with increasing reduction in cholesterol, as shown in Fig. 6-4. Thus, the LRC-CPPT demonstrated what has been called a constant percentage risk reduction [12]. In other words, the greater reduction in cholesterol produced a proportionately greater subsequent reduction in CHD.

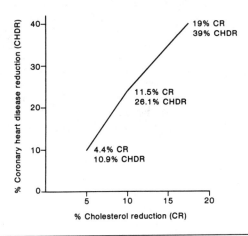

Fig. 6-4. Relation of reduction in total cholesterol to coronary heart disease. (From the Lipid Research Clinics Program [12].)

STUDY QUESTION 6-10

Are you convinced that the benefits of cholesterol reduction continue for those individuals with initial cholesterol levels lower than 265 mg per deciliter?

The NIH recommendations are, in essence, extrapolations from data such as the MRFIT data, which reveal that there is a need for cholesterol reduction even at levels lower than 265, and from the LRC-CPPT data, which demonstrate that the benefit continues the more the cholesterol level is lowered. The NIH consensus panel [3], having considered all the data, proposed the following recommendations:

1. Individuals with cholesterol levels above the ninetieth percentile should be treated by diet. If response is inadequate, appropriate drugs should be added.
2. Adults with cholesterol levels between the seventy-fifth and ninetieth percentiles (see Table 6-4) should be treated by diet. Only a small proportion should require drug treatment.
3. All Americans (except children under 2 years of age) should be advised to adopt a diet that reduces total dietary fat from 40 to 30 percent of total calories, decreases saturated fat to less than 10 percent

of total calories, increases polyunsaturated fat to no more than 10 percent of total calories, and reduces daily cholesterol intake to no more than 250 to 300 mg.

—————————————————————— STUDY QUESTION 6-11
Do you agree with the NIH conclusions?

Now let us return to our patients Mr. L. and Mrs. S. In light of what you have learned about elevated cholesterol, answer the following questions:

—————————————————————— STUDY QUESTION 6-12
What would you recommend in the case of Mr. L.?

—————————————————————— STUDY QUESTION 6-13
What would you recommend in the case of Mrs. S.?

—————————————————————— STUDY QUESTION 6-14
What would you recommend if Mrs. S. were 65 years old?

References

1. National Center for Health Statistics. Monthly vital statistics report. Annual summary of births, marriages, divorces, and death: United States, 1984. Vol. 33, No. 13.
2. Lipid Research Clinics Program. The Lipid Research Clinics Coronary Primary Prevention Trial results—reduction in incidence of coronary heart disease. JAMA 1984;251:351–364.
3. National Institutes of Health Consensus Development Conference Statement. Lowering blood cholesterol to prevent heart disease. Washington, DC: US Department of Health and Human Services, 1986. Vol. 5, No. 7.
4. Turpeinen O. Effect of cholesterol lowering diet on mortality from CHD and other causes. Circulation 1979;59:1–7.
5. Keys A. Coronary heart disease in seven countries. Circulation 1970;41:Suppl. 1.
6. Pooling Project Research Group. Relationship of blood pressure, serum cholesterol, smoking habit, relative weight and ECG abnormalities to incidence of major coronary events: final report of the Pooling Project. J. Chron Dis 1978;31:201.
7. Shekelle RB, et al. Diet, serum cholesterol, and coronary heart disease. The Western Electric Study. N Engl J Med 1981;304:65–70.
8. Kannel WB et al. Serum cholesterol, lipoproteins, and the risk of coronary heart disease. The Framingham Study. Ann Intern Med 1971;74:1-12.

9. Blankenhorn DH, Nessim SA, Johnson RL, et al. Beneficial effects of combined colestipol-niacin therapy on coronary atherosclerosis and coronary venous bypass grafts. JAMA 1987;257:3233-3240.
10. Leren P. The Oslo diet-heart study. Eleven year report. Circulation 1970;42:935-942.
11. Stamler J, et al. Is the relationship between serum cholesterol and risk of premature death from coronary heart disease continuous and graded? JAMA 1986;256:2823.
12. Lipid Research Clinic Program. The Lipid Research Clinics Coronary Primary Prevention Trial results. II. The relationship of reduction in incidence of coronary heart disease to cholesterol lowering. JAMA 1984;251:365–374.

The Primary Prevention of Osteoporosis: A Risk-Benefit Analysis of the Use of Calcium and Estrogen

CHAPTER SEVEN

ROBERT J. MELFI
TERESA M. SCHAER

CASE. Mrs. Nelson is a 78-year-old frail white woman who lived alone for several years after her husband died. She was active and independent, able to care for herself and her home without difficulty. While walking down her back steps one day, her foot caught on a loose board. She was able to break her fall but landed on her right hip. Unable to move, Mrs. Nelson tried to call for help. Finally, a neighbor found her, and she was brought to the nearest hospital.

In the emergency room, the physical examination revealed an externally rotated, foreshortened right leg, and hip x-rays confirmed the diagnosis of hip fracture despite the mild nature of the injury. Mrs. Nelson underwent surgical repair and had some difficulty postoperatively but finally was able to start physical therapy.

Although Mrs. Nelson learned to walk with a walker, she was unable to return to her home and ultimately required admission to a nursing home. Her ability to care for herself was limited owing to the difficulties she had with ambulation, and she became much more dependent on others for help.

A detailed history of Mrs. Nelson's past revealed that she was a housewife all her life and rarely exercised. Her diet included few dairy products; in fact, she drank little milk. She went through menopause at approximately age 49 and was never on estrogens. Since the age of 60, she noticed that she had gradually been "shrinking" in height and that she was not able to straighten her curved back.

It is clear that the hip fracture sustained by Mrs. Nelson was devastating not only in terms of dollars but also in terms of dramatic life changes. What was the cause of this fracture and how could it have been prevented? The purpose of this chapter is to discuss osteoporosis, a prevalent bone disease in the elderly, and analyze specific preventive measures.

Background Information on Osteoporosis

Osteoporosis is defined as a disorder in which decreased bone mass leads to an increased susceptibility to pathologic fractures. It is a very common disease and has an enormous impact on both society and the individual in terms of morbidity, mortality, and cost.

More than 1 million fractures per year in the United States are directly related to osteoporosis. The primary sites of these fractures include the vertebra, wrist, and hip. Vertebral and wrist fractures, although painful and limiting, are not as devastating as hip fractures, which lead to death in 12 to 20 percent of cases and long-term disability in 50 percent. More than $6 billion per year is spent in the care of patients who suffer the consequences of osteoporosis. Hip fractures are responsible for the largest percentage of this cost [1, 2].

CURRENT APPROACHES TO PREVENTING BONE LOSS
Over the past decade, there has been a marked increase in social awareness of the problems associated with osteoporosis. Emphasis has been placed on the prevention of bone loss before fracture occurs—that is, primary prevention. If fractures, particularly hip fractures, could be prevented, the cost savings to the individual and society would be dramatic.

Currently, research efforts are focused on multiple treatment regimens to prevent bone loss with age. Calcium supplementation and estrogen replacement therapy are currently receiving the most attention. Multiple studies have been completed to date, but the results are often vague, not statistically significant, or even contradictory. Because of this limitation in data, there are no clear answers. The practicing physician can merely analyze the information that exists and, together with the patient, make a decision.

To help with this difficult problem, the National Institutes of Health (NIH) held a consensus development conference on osteoporosis in April 1984. The conference resulted in a report that summarized study results, outlined conclusions, and presented recommendations regarding various modes of prevention, including both benefits and risks [1].

The plan of this chapter is to review these conclusions and recommendations, particularly with regard to calcium supplementation and estrogen replacement therapy, and to analyze the data on which they are based. The reader should thereby be able to devise a practical clinical approach to the primary prevention of osteoporosis and, in addition, be able to apply this approach to a variety of clinical situations.

PEAK BONE MASS AND LOSS OF BONE
Most of the literature on osteoporosis, including the NIH consensus report, agree on the following information and conclusions. The human body is composed of approximately 80 percent cortical bone, located primarily in the appendicular skeleton or long bones, and 20 percent trabecular bone, which predominates in the axial skeleton—that is, the

vertebrae and pelvis. Each of these undergoes continuous remodeling throughout life [1–3].

Peak bone mass is achieved at approximately 30. Nutrition (especially calcium intake), genetics, exercise, and health status influence this peak bone mass [1, 2]. In general, men have a peak bone mass that is approximately 30 percent higher than that of women, and darker races have a peak bone mass that is approximately 10 percent higher than in the fair-skinned races [4].

Once bone has achieved its peak mass, it begins to lose mineral and organic matrix, resulting in a decline in bone mass with age. This occurs at a rate of from 0.3 to 0.5 percent per year, with much individual variation [1, 5]. Superimposed on this slow phase of bone loss is an accelerated phase that occurs in women following menopause. During the postmenopausal period, bone mass is lost initially at a rate of 2 to 3 percent per year, a rate that slows over the next 10 years until the curve resumes its gradual age-related decline [2, 5]. Figure 7-1 illustrates these concepts of sex-related and race-related loss of bone mass over time. For women and the fair-skinned races, who in general have a genetically determined low peak bone density, the bone loss over time is particularly critical in that their bones will reach a critical fracture threshold at a much earlier age than men and the darker-skinned races, who start out with a higher peak bone mass.

Fig. 7-1. Loss of bone mass over time in relation to an individual's race and sex.

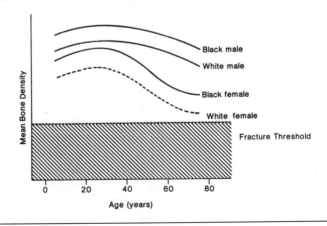

There are many additional factors that play a role in the achievement of peak bone mass and the loss of bone over time. Bone mass is somewhat lower in individuals with a reduced activity level, a thin body build, or a family history of osteoporosis, and in those who smoke, drink alcohol, or have a high caffeine intake and reduced amounts of protein in their diet [1, 5]. Certain diseases and medications can markedly affect bone mass and its rate of loss. Among the diseases are malabsorption syndromes, hyperparathyroidism, and multiple myeloma, and medications such as long-term systemic corticosteroids, heparin, and aluminum-containing antacids used extensively [1, 5].

A Basic Approach to Prevention of Osteoporosis

In light of this information, how do we approach the task of preventing osteoporosis? The first step is to identify the population most at risk. We then need to identify contributory causes that can be changed and to attempt to eliminate or reduce their effect so that for as long as possible the curve for bone loss does not reach or cross the fracture threshold.

It is generally agreed that in the absence of disease, the population most at risk for developing osteoporosis is the thin white woman [1, 5]. Although it is clear that fractures are not limited to this group, women have substantially higher rates of wrist, vertebral, and hip fractures. Furthermore, most of the research has been done on white women. Therefore, this is the population we will address.

Risk factors that can be changed include calcium deficiency, loss of estrogen at the time of menopause, lack of exercise, and smoking, alcohol, and caffeine intake [1, 5]. Of these, the most controversial factors are the first two and, because data is not clear-cut, any decision to treat patients with calcium or estrogen requires much thought and analysis.

CALCIUM AND ESTROGEN DEFICIENCIES: CONTRIBUTORY CAUSES OF BONE LOSS?

Establishing Association and "Cause" Precedes "Effect"

In the terminology of the NIH consensus report, "calcium deficiency has been implicated in the pathogenesis" of osteoporosis [1]. This statement is based on the following information: An inadequate intake of calcium coupled with obligatory fecal, urinary, and skin losses results in a daily negative calcium balance [3, 6]. In other words, calcium intake is less than calcium loss. Zero calcium balance occurs when intake equals loss. Positive balance occurs when calcium intake is greater than calcium loss.

Since the concentration of ionized calcium in the blood must be maintained at a relatively constant level, a net calcium loss requires the body to resorb calcium from bone, where 99 percent of the body's calcium is stored. It is presumed, therefore, that this leads to a gradual loss of bone mass with time [6].

How valid is this presumption? Why is the NIH wording about this so vague? Recall that a factor can be called a contributory cause if it fulfills three criteria: (1) The cause is associated with the disease; (2) the cause precedes the disease; and (3) altering the cause alters the disease. Any analysis of these three criteria with respect to calcium first requires an understanding of exactly what constitutes a low, adequate, and high calcium intake.

At present, the United States Recommended Daily Allowance (RDA) is equal to 800 mg of elemental calcium per day [1]. A major metabolic balance study done by Heaney and colleagues [7] indicated that the RDA for calcium underestimates the amount needed to maintain a positive calcium balance. Based on Heaney's data, most of the literature now advocates that premenopausal women require at least 1000 mg of elemental calcium per day and postmenopausal women require 1500 mg [1, 2].* In addition, Heaney's study and other epidemiologic studies demonstrate that the average daily intake of calcium in both women and men in the United States is below the RDA of 800 mg per day [6].

The pertinent information we have thus far can be summarized as follows:

1. Women lose bone mass with age and are most at risk for developing osteoporosis.
2. Women need 1000 to 1500 mg of elemental calcium per day to maintain a zero calcium balance.
3. Most women have a chronically low calcium intake.

If we can accept each of these statements as independently valid, together they demonstrate that calcium deficiency is *associated* with osteoporosis and that it *precedes the disease.* Thus, calcium deficiency fulfills the first two criteria for establishing a contributory cause.

---

*At the time of this writing, the blanket acceptance of Heaney's data is being questioned, and further research as to the amount of calcium needed to maintain a zero calcium balance is being encouraged.

Similarly, it is widely held that estrogen deficiency fulfills these first two criteria. In fact, few clues to mechanisms and potentials for prevention of osteoporosis stand out as clearly as the association of the menopause with the time of accelerated bone loss in women.

In 1984, Richelson and co-workers [8] attempted to quantitate the role of estrogen deprivation in bone loss by comparing bone density in three groups of women: (1) fourteen women between the ages of 50 and 55 who had undergone bilateral oophorectory 15 to 25 years before the time of natural menopause; (2) fourteen perimenopausal women, matched for age alone, who had not undergone oophorectomy; and (3) fourteen older women matched for years after menopause, (i.e., 15 to 25 years after natural menopause).

Bone mineral density, as determined by photon absorptiometry, at the midradius, lumbar spine, and proximal femur was lower in the oophorectomized and post–natural menopausal women compared with the perimenopausal group. In addition, both groups with the lower bone density had essentially the same absolute bone mass, despite an average age difference of 19 years. Since the two groups had been matched for years after menopause, be it natural or surgical, the study concluded that most of the bone loss that occurs in the first 20 years after estrogen deprivation is owing to estrogen deficiency rather than the effects of age.

STUDY QUESTION 7-1

Do the data establish lack of estrogen as a contributory cause of osteoporosis?

Establishing a Cause and Effect Relationship

If we accept that both calcium and estrogen deficiencies fulfill the first two criteria for a contributory cause, the third must now be addressed. Several randomized controlled clinical trials that have been completed or are now in progress attempt to do just this. One such study was published by Recker and associates in 1977 [9]. They assessed the effects of replacement therapy (ERT) and calcium supplementation on bone density over a 3-year period—that is, they attempted to alter the cause to alter the effect. The subjects in this study were 60 white Roman Catholic nuns 55 to 65 years old. They were randomly divided into three groups: control, hormone-treated, and calcium-treated. The average dietary intake for each group was 500 mg of elemental calcium per day. At the beginning of the study and at 6-month intervals, single photon absorp-

Table 7-1. Mineral content loss at distal
radius as measured by single photon absorptiometry

Group	N	Treatment	Mean rate of mineral content loss/24 months (gm/sq cm)	% Reduction of bone mass over 2 years
1	20	Control	0.046	5.76
2	20	Estrogen	0.012	1.5
3	20	Calcium	0.034	4.25

Source: Adapted from Recker and colleagues [9].

tiometry was used to determine the mineral content of the distal radius. The results are summarized in Table 7-1.

Analysis of the data reveals that there is a statistically significant loss of bone mass over time in the control (p <.01) and the calcium-treated (p <.025) groups. The differences, however, between the control and treatment groups and between the two treatment groups, do not achieve statistical significance. From this study, the authors concluded that ERT measurably decreases bone loss and that calcium supplementation produces the same effect but to a lesser degree.

_____ STUDY QUESTION 7-2

(a) Although the differences between the study groups were not statistically significant, does this mean that the data should be disregarded? (b) What may explain the lack of statistical significance in this study?

Another study that evaluated the effectiveness of ERT and calcium supplementation in preventing osteoporosis was conducted by Riggs and colleagues at the Mayo Clinic [10]. Riggs's group took a different approach from that of Recker and associates. Rather than measure bone mass itself, they looked at the effects on fracture rate, specifically vertebral fracture rate. The subjects included 165 postmenopausal women who were sequentially assigned to one of five treatment groups* and followed prospectively over a 12-year period.

---

*The authors state that they used "prospective assignment to consecutive treatment groups, using identical selection criteria . . . as a practical and appropriate alternative to a concurrent randomized study" [11].

Table 7-2. Effect of estrogen replacement therapy
and calcium supplementation on fracture rate

Group	N	Treatment	No. of fractures/1000 patient-years*
1	45	Control	834
2	27	Calcium	419
3	32	Estrogen and calcium	181

*p <.001
Source: Adapted from Riggs and colleagues [10].

A control group was compared with each of four other groups treated
with various combinations of calcium, estrogen, vitamin D, and fluoride
[10]. By comparing serial vertebral spine roentgenograms, the number
of new vertebral fractures occurring over the 12-year treatment period
was determined for each patient. New fractures were defined by specific
criteria. The fracture rate associated with each treatment was expressed
as the number of new fractures detected per 1000 patient-years of observation for each treatment group. The results with regard to treatment
with and without estrogen and calcium, summarized in Table 7-2, demonstrates a dramatic and statistically significant protective effect associated with both forms of treatment [10].

The benefits of ERT and calcium therapy are apparent in the preceding two studies, and in general, the conclusions have been confirmed in
several other studies [1, 2].* Most authorities would therefore agree that
estrogen and calcium deficiencies satisfy the three criteria required to
be considered contributory causes of osteoporosis.

PRIMARY GOAL: THE PREVENTION OF HIP FRACTURES
The main fracture syndromes associated with osteoporosis are Colles'
fractures of the distal radius, vertebral crush fractures, and fractures of
the proximal femur. The Recker study [9] previously described measured bone density specifically at the distal radius, which is made up
predominantly of cortical bone and only 25 percent trabecular bone. It

*At the time of this writing, the efficacy of calcium supplementation alone when begun
in the perimenopausal period is being critically challenged by a few studies with preliminary results revealing that it does little to slow the rate of bone loss. Long-term studies
on several different populations, both male and female, are needed before definitive
conclusions can be drawn [12, 13].

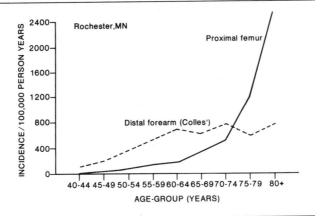

Fig. 7-2. Comparison of the rates of wrist (Colles') fractures (*broken line*) and hip fractures (*solid line*). Note that both increase at the menopause (45 to 54 years), but the slope of Colles' fractures is substantially steeper. (Adapted from Riggs and Melton [15].)

has been demonstrated that cortical bone thickness measurements are not a good indicator of bone loss and that single photon absorptiometry of the distal radius does not effectively predict bone loss at sites with a higher percentage of trabecular bone (i.e., the vertebrae and proximal femur) [14].

Whether information regarding wrist (Colles') fractures can be extrapolated to hip fractures is also controversial. Furthermore, it is unclear whether estrogen deficiency plays a major role in causing bone loss in the proximal femur [15]. Rochester Minnesota data depicted in Figure 7-2 reveal that there is an acceleration in the rate of both types of fractures at the menopause, but the slope for Colles' fractures is substantially steeper than that for hip fractures [15]. In addition, the male-to-female ratio for patients sustaining wrist fractures is 6 : 1, whereas the ratio for those with hip fractures is 2 : 1.

These data suggest that the acceleration in bone loss associated with the menopause may play a more substantial role in the attainment of fracture threshold at the distal radius than at the hip. An alternative reason has been proposed for the later age at which the incidence of hip fracture rises. The loss of trabecular bone in weight-bearing bones (e.g., femur and vertebra) may occur differently from in non-weight-bearing bones such as the wrist. In the femur, loss of the secondary horizontal struts (also called trabeculae) seems to occur first, with simultaneous reinforcement of the primary vertical struts (or trabeculae), which are lost later [Jensen PS, personal communication, 1987]. This may be the mechanism responsible for delaying hip fractures until a substantial proportion of trabecular bone is lost and implies that loss of bone in the femur may indeed be related to estrogen deficiency.

An Ideal Controlled Clinical Trial
To determine whether ERT and calcium supplementation in fact decrease the rate of hip fractures, one would ideally perform a controlled clinical trial in which perimenopausal women were randomly and blindly assigned to one of three groups: one treated with estrogen, one with calcium, and one with placebo. These patients would then be followed for a prolonged period of time, and hip fracture rates in the three groups would then be compared in such a way to produce a relative risk (RR) for hip fractures associated with either ERT or estrogen deprivation (ED), and calcium supplementation (CS) or calcium deficiency (CD). The relative risks would be calculated as follows:

$$RR_{ERT} = \frac{\text{hip fracture rate on ERT}}{\text{hip fracture rate on placebo}}$$

$$RR_{ED} = \text{the inverse of } RR_{ERT} = 1 \div RR_{ERT}$$

$$RR_{CS} = \frac{\text{hip fracture rate on CS}}{\text{hip fracture rate on placebo}}$$

$$RR_{CD} = \text{the inverse of } RR_{CS} = 1 \div RR_{CS}$$

Recall that as a probability ratio, the relative risk does not indicate the magnitude of risk. It can be used, however, to calculate the attributable risk (AR) and population attributable risk (PAR) associated with a given risk factor.

$$AR = \frac{RR - 1}{RR}$$

$$PAR = \frac{(RR - 1)}{b(RR - 1) + 1}$$

where RR = RR_{ED} or RR_{CD}

   b = the proportion of the population that has the risk factor

The attributable risk represents the proportion of the disease among those with a given risk factor (e.g., estrogen deprivation or calcium deficiency) that is attributable to the risk factor. If a contributory cause exists, then the attributable risk represents the maximum percentage of the disease that can be eliminated by removal of the risk factor. By taking into account the percentage of the population who possess the risk factor, the population attributable risk represents the maximum percentage of disease that can be eliminated in a particular population made up of individuals with and without the risk factor. (Note that as the prevalence approaches 100 percent [i.e., b = 1], the PAR approaches the AR.)

Using these formulas and given the baseline hip fracture rate and the baseline prevalence of calcium and estrogen deficiency in the population of our hypothetical study, the potential reduction in hip fracture rate through either calcium or estrogen replacement in that population could be estimated.

_____ STUDY QUESTION 7-3
What study design problems make this ideal study difficult?

An Ideal Case-Control Study
A feasible alternative to a controlled clinical trial is a case-control study designed to estimate the impact of estrogen and calcium therapy on hip fracture rates. In such studies, the relative risk* for hip fracture associated with estrogen is estimated by comparing prior estrogen use in two similar groups of patients: one (the cases) consisting of postmenopausal women with a history of hip fracture, the other (the controls) consisting of postmenopausal women without fracture.

In 1981, Paganini-Hill and colleagues [16] compared 91 cases of hip fractures that occurred in a retirement community, whose population's average age was 72, to 166 controls from the same community. Data on calcium intake, history of diabetes mellitus, tobacco use, age at menopause, history of oophorectomy, and history of exogenous estrogen use was collected by both interviews and medical record reviews. The relative risks of hip fracture were determined for each variable and are listed in Table 7-3.

_____
*Although commonly referred to as relative risks, the outcome measures determined in such studies are actually odds ratios which, in most well-designed case-control studies, are an estimation of the relative risk.

Table 7-3. Relative risk of hip fracture associated with specific variables in an elderly population

Variable	Relative risk of hip fracture
Age at menopause (years)	
<44	1.00
45–49	0.78 (0.56)*
>49	0.61 (0.47)*
History of tobacco use after menopause	
1–10 cigarettes/day	0.85 (1.05)*
>10 cigarettes/day	1.65 (1.96)*
History of diabetes mellitus	2.70 (3.28)*
History of calcium supplements for 61 months	0.62
History of estrogen replacement therapy for 61 months	0.42

*Adjusted for estrogen use and oophorectomy.
Source: Adapted from Paganini-Hill and co-workers [16].

The relative risk associated with calcium supplementation and the net relative risk associated with ERT are similar to those determined in other retrospective studies [17, 18]. In this particular study, because neither estrogen nor calcium were found to be associated with any of the other variables, the RR relative risk determined for each of them reflects their independent relation to hip fractures.

── STUDY QUESTION 7-4
What are the relative risks and attributable risk of estrogen deficiency based on the data in Table 7-3?

Based on the relative risks determined in this study, one can calculate an attributable risk of 58 percent for calcium deficiency and 38 percent for estrogen deprivation, which may be interpreted as follows. If a cause and effect relationship holds, a maximum of 58 percent of hip fractures among women with ED may be prevented by ERT and a maximum of 38 percent of hip fractures among women with CD may be prevented by calcium replacement. Since the data on which these percentages are based come from a study of white postmenopausal women, these values are applicable only to that specific subset of the population at risk for developing osteoporosis. However, since all postmenopausal women are estrogen-deficient and the majority are also calcium-deficient, the population attributable risk for white women is nearly as large as the attributable risk.

Limitations of the Findings
Although the results of the preceding analysis are very encouraging, they are limited by certain aspects of the data on which they are based. First, the study population in Paganini-Hill's study [16] and all similar studies includes oophorectomized women. The relative risk of hip fracture for ERT, listed in Table 7-3, combines the relative risk associated with ERT in both oophorectomized and nonoophorectomized women. Separating the two reveals that the relative risk is 0.14 in the former and 0.86 in the latter group, suggesting that the protective effect of estrogens is much greater in women who have undergone oophorectomy.

The relative risk for each group, however, was determined relative to nonoophorectomized women who had never taken exogenous estrogens. The oophorectomized women treated with ERT should ideally be compared with untreated oophorectomized women, a group that does not exist since standard practice is treatment with estrogens. If the protection offered the oophorectomized women by ERT was owing solely to the restoration of normal hormonal status at the time of oophorectomy, the risk ratio as calculated should have been 1. It appears that the continued use of ERT beyond the age of natural menopause afforded these women protection against more than the effects of oophorectomy. Perhaps these patients are an example of the maximum protection affordable by the avoidance of estrogen deficiency. Because their surgical menopause began at a specific point in time, they received estrogen replacement before experiencing *any* estrogen deficiency. On the other hand, those who underwent natural menopause may have spent a few years in relative estrogen deficiency with accelerated bone loss before the institution of ERT.

This is one possible interpretation of the results, but it has not yet been fully substantiated. It suggests that the potential benefits of ERT are even greater than that suggested by the relative risk of 0.46. On the other hand, if one uses only the raw data, a much smaller maximum benefit is suggested by relative risk of 0.86 in nonoophorectomized women.

A further consideration is that today a growing percentage of postmenopausal women have already increased their estrogen and calcium use, and the future benefits of additional increased use may not be as dramatic as these numbers suggest. Finally, it is important to recognize that the benefits of estrogen and calcium administration may or may not be addictive. Ettinger [13] showed that low dosage estrogen and calcium supplements may be at least synergistic.

Benefits of Estrogen Replacement Therapy and Calcium Supplementation: NIH Conclusions and Recommendations

In the 1984 NIH consensus report on osteoporosis [1] that was alluded to earlier, the panel concluded the following with regard to the efficacy of ERT and calcium supplementation in preventing osteoporosis: (1) "Estrogen replacement therapy is highly effective for preventing osteoporosis in women." (2) "It seems likely that an increase in calcium intake to 1000 to 1500 mg per day beginning well before the menopause will reduce the incidence of osteoporosis in postmenopausal women."

Their *recommendations* were as follows [1]:

1. Cyclic estrogen therapy should be given to women whose ovaries are removed before age 50 in whom there are no specific contraindications. Women who have had natural menopause also should be considered for cyclic estrogen replacement if they have no contraindications and if they understand the risks and agree to regular medical evaluation. The decision to treat women of [racial backgrounds other than white] should be determined on a case-by-case basis.
2. For those unable to take 1000 to 1500 mg calcium by diet, supplementation with calcium tablets is recommended, with special attention to their elemental calcium content.

As we begin to read between the lines of the official recommendations, we find that the panel's final conclusions and recommendations with regard to calcium supplementation and estrogen replacement differ considerably. The conclusions about calcium are a bit vague, but the recommendations are specific and definitive. In contrast are the firmer conclusions about the benefits associated with the use of ERT followed by more vague recommendations for its use, leaving the decision to the individual physician and patient.

The differences in conviction between the conclusions with regard to each therapy may reflect the less impressive effect of calcium as compared to estrogen in the various studies we have reviewed. The basis of the differences in the panel's final recommendations, on the other hand, must lie beyond the issue of relative efficacy. Indeed, to understand these recommendations one must compare the risks associated with the use of these two very different forms of therapy.

RISKS OF ESTROGEN REPLACEMENT THERAPY
In addition to their prominent role in the growth, development, and function of breast and endometrial tissue, endogenous estrogens affect numerous metabolic processes throughout the body in ways that are not fully understood (Table 7-4) [19]. As a result, the use of exogenous estrogen is associated with several metabolic changes that may ultimately affect the organism either beneficially or deleteriously.

Many studies, mostly retrospective, have investigated the relationship between ERT and various disease processes. To date, only endometrial cancer has been consistently shown to be positively associated with ERT to an extent that might offset its benefits with regard to osteoporosis. Numerous clinico-pathologic phenomena suggest the biologic plausibility of a causal relationship between estrogen excess and endometrial cancer [20]:

Estrogen-secreting ganulosa-theca cell tumors are associated with endometrial cancer.

Women with ovarian agenesis rarely have endometrial cancer.

Table 7-4. Effect of endogenous estrogens throughout the body

Site	Effect	Possible result
Endometrium	Stimulate growth	Cancer
Breast	Stimulate growth	Cancer progression
Lipoproteins	Increase ratios of high-density to low-density lipoproteins	Decreased rate of atherosclerotic cardiovascular disease
Coagulation	Increase thrombogenicity	Increased rate of thromboembolic disease
Blood pressure	Increase blood pressure	Increased rate of atherosclerotic cardiovascular disease
Bile	Increase gallstone formation	Increased rate of cholecystitis

Source: Adapted from Judd and colleagues [19].

There is an association of infertility, nulliparity, and anovulatory cycles with endometrial cancer.

There is an association of endometrial cancer with forms of endometrial hyperplasia believed to be secondary to hyperestrogenism (e.g., adenomatous and atypical hyperplasia).

In the middle to late 1970s, a number of case-control retrospective studies reported an association between the use of estrogens during menopause and the subsequent development of endometrial cancer [21–23]. Despite differences in study design, findings were generally consistent, yielding relative risk estimates of 4 to 8 associated with ERT.

In 1979, Antunes and colleagues [24], in one of the better-designed studies of the type just described, looked at rates of exposure to estrogen in cases of endometrial cancer and compared them to rates of exposure in two control groups, one derived from a gynecologic service and the other derived from other nongynecologic services, both made up of in-hospital patients. The relative risk varied according to the control group used, being 2.1 and 6.0, respectively. The study was important because it helped answer several questions pertaining to the effects of study design on the association being reported. The use of two control groups, for example, illustrated the influence of control group selection on the relative risk determined by a given study. Indeed, with the publication of this study, the association of ERT with endometrial cancer was well accepted.

The range of relative risks from 4 to 8 reported in the various studies of ERT and endometrial cancer correspond to attributable risks of 75 to 87 percent. Thus, it would appear that in the patient on ERT, most of the risk of developing endometrial cancer is associated with that therapy. Although these are striking figures, it is important to realize that they do not tell us about the absolute magnitude of the risk of endometrial carcinoma. This is particularly important with regard to a risk-benefit analysis, in which the ultimate issue is whether the benefit of decreasing the incidence of one disease (hip fracture) is offset by a concomitant increase in the incidence of another disease (endometrial cancer) associated with that therapy. Remember that the absolute risk equals the relative risk times the incidence of the disease in the absence of the risk factor. For the individual, the absolute risk is dependent on the individual's other risk factors. Thus, an individual's risk of fracture would be increased if that subject had a history of frequent falls, smoking, excessive alcohol intake, or a family history of osteoporosis. Similarly, the individual's risk of endometrial cancer would be increased if there were a history of other risk factors for endometrial cancer such as obesity, younger age at menarche, older age at menopause, low gravidity and parity, or a history of dysfunctional uterine bleeding and possibly hypertension and diabetes.

It would appear that a quantitative approach to weighing the risks and benefits of ERT would be tedious, complex, and impractical for the primary care physician to perform for each of his or her patients. Eventually, computer programs allowing bedside decision analysis may help us to make such calculations. For the present, a less quantitative approach is possible with the help of two important considerations.

The Lesser of Two Evils

In a risk-benefit analysis, changes in the absolute risk and incidence of diseases must be looked at in light of the morbidity, mortality, and cost of each disease in question. Increased risk of a disease of lesser severity can generally be accepted if it accompanies a substantial decrease in the risk of a disease of much greater severity.

In their study of endometrial cancer and ERT, Antunes and co-workers [24] determined the relative risk for the various pathologic stages of endometrial cancer (Table 7-5). The higher relative risks for earlier stages of cancer suggest that the forms of cancer associated with ERT are either relatively nonaggressive or become symptomatic earlier in their history, leading to detection at an early stage. Whichever is the case, the implication is that much of the disease caused by ERT may be cured. Therefore, with regular medical evaluation, there may be substantially less morbidity, mortality, and cost from endometrial carcinoma than from hip fractures potentially prevented by such therapy.

In other studies of this type, a similar association has been reported [23]. In order for this relationship to hold true in clinical practice, how-

Table 7-5. Relative risk for the various pathologic stages of endometrial cancer

Stage	Relative risk	95% Confidence interval*
0	10.0	2.3–90
1	7.2	3.6–14.5
2–4	4.0	1.0–22

*Exact confidence limits.
Source: Adapted from Antunes and co-workers [24].

ever, close follow-up and aggressive management would be necessary. The extent to which this could be achieved would vary from patient to patient and physician to physician. Compliance thus becomes a consideration in individual decision making. In a given case, then, if such follow-up seemed assured, it would appear likely that any endometrial disease that might occur as a result of ERT would probably (although not definitely) be curable and substantially less severe than the hip fracture potentially being prevented. Remember, however, that for a perimenopausal woman, the risk of endometrial carcinoma begins many years before the risk of hip fracture.

Progestogens: A Medical Curettage
It is generally accepted that estrogen administration leads to endometrial cancer through the induction of precancerous forms of endometrial hyperplasia. In the normal menstruating woman, this potential effect of estrogen is prevented by the regular sloughing of the endometrium during menses. The orderly, essentially complete nature of this biologic curettage is the net effect of complementary influences of both estrogen and progesterone on the endometrium during the luteal phase of the menstrual cycle. Hence, it would seem biologically plausible that the administration of progesterone along with estrogen in postmenopausal women can prevent the development of endometrial cancer.

Since the 1970s, many authors have reported on the observation that endometrial hyperplasia induced by unopposed exogenous estrogens can be reversed by various progesterone regimens [25]. Other authors have compared the incidence of precancerous endometrial hyperplasia in routine endometrial biopsies in women given estrogen alone to the incidence in women given estrogen with progesterone, and they found a substantially higher incidence of precancerous endometrial hyperplasia among the estrogen group [26].

In cause and effect terms, these studies have merely demonstrated the biologic plausibility of the concept that progesterone can prevent estrogen-induced endometrial cancer. To demonstrate clinical efficacy, controlled clinical trials of combined estrogen-progesterone regimens, or at least case-control studies similar to that of Antunes and colleagues [24], are required. Unfortunately, good studies of this type are not available because there is much less clinical experience with such regimens than there is with estrogen alone.

In 1979, Gambrell and co-workers [27] published a cohort study in which a population of postmenopausal women at a United States Air

Table 7-6. Incidence of cancer in a group of
postmenopausal women on various hormonal regimens

Treatment	Patient-years	No. of cancer cases	Cancer incidence/1000 patient-years
Estrogen	2088	8	3.8
Estrogen-Progesterone	3792	2	0.5
Vaginal Cream	574	1	1.7
Other	201	0	0
None	1515	3	2.0

Source: Adapted from Gambrell and colleagues [27].

Force base on various hormonal regimens were followed for 3 years. Regimens included unopposed cyclic estrogen, estrogen-progesterone, estrogen vaginal cream, and no therapy. For each regimen, the total number of patient-years (number of patients times number of years followed) observed for the 3-year period was reported along with the number of incident cases of endometrial cancer for each regimen and corresponding computed incidence per 1000 patient-years. The results are presented in Table 7-6. In this study, details about individual patient regimens throughout the 3 years were reported for the cases of cancer only. The authors did report that there was a steady decline in the number of women with intact uteri who used only estrogens during the 3-year period: 1060 in 1975, 635 in 1976, and 394 in 1977. Thus, one may assume that the patient groups referred to in the results did not include the same individuals throughout the 3 years of the study.

This "migration" of patients between treatment groups detracted from the value of Gambrell's study. Because of it, the authors could not control for various confounding variables, such as gravidity or parity that could bias the results. In addition, disease rates in groups of patients on various regimens could not be analyzed, and values such as relative risk or attributable risk could not be calculated. Instead, the results were expressed in terms of patient-years of experience with regimens applied to different patients over varying periods of time. Such data are difficult to interpret and apply to clinical practice because they are not generated from circumstances representative of a true clinical situation, one in which a given patient is treated with one regimen over a prolonged period of time.

It is also important to note that the follow-up period in this study was

fairly short. Photoabsorption studies on bone suggest that the postmenopausal acceleration of bone loss resumes when estrogen replacement is
stopped. ERT must therefore be a lifelong prescription if it is to be max-
imally effective. Its effects, both beneficial and deleterious, thus need to
be assessed for longer than the 3 years of this study, since the average
lifespan of a perimenopausal woman is 23 years.

Gambrell's study [27] is, at the time of this writing, the most commonly
sited clinical study supporting the safety of estrogen-progesterone regimens in postmenopausal women. Clearly, the clinical data available for
long-term estrogen-progesterone replacement are limited. Indeed, the
NIH consensus panel stated that although the addition of progesterone
to ERT regimens *may* protect against the development of endometrial
cancer, there is little information available about the safety of long-term
use of progestogens in postmenopausal women. In addition, they
pointed out that some data suggest that progestogens may blunt the beneficial effect of estrogens on the ratio of high-density to low-density lipoproteins and that younger patients receiving progestogens in oral
contraceptives experience an increased risk of hypertension and cardiovascular disease [1].

It would appear that the reluctance of the NIH panel to make firm
recommendations regarding ERT results from the limited and confusing clinical data available. On the one hand, there is a large body of
evidence supporting the notion that ERT prevents a substantial proportion of hip fractures in postmenopausal women. On the other hand, a
similarly persuasive set of data implicates estrogen as a cause of endometrial cancer. Biologic models rather compellingly suggest that progesterone therapy can effectively combat this problem, but clinical experience with its use in the postmenopausal age group is limited. Therefore,
we are left to speculate on what the actual clinical impact of progesterone
will be as well as what complications may be seen with long-term therapy.
Nonetheless, we are compelled by the severity of the potential complications of osteoporosis to consider the use of estrogen and estrogen-
progesterone regimens in each of our perimenopausal patients at risk.

RISKS OF CALCIUM SUPPLEMENTATION
The NIH consensus panel's stronger recommendations regarding the
use of calcium supplementation suggest that less risk is associated with
this therapy than with ERT [1]. In addition, since the available data suggest that calcium supplementation is somewhat less effective in prevent-

ing the problems associated with osteoporosis than ERT, one would tend to accept less associated risk before choosing to institute it.

There are two potential sources for complications associated with oral calcium therapy: hypercalcemia and hypercalciuria. Only a few studies have looked at the risk of hypercalcemia in persons taking supplemental calcium, and these were conducted several years ago when the milk-alkali syndrome was first described [6, 28, 29]. These studies, in general, showed that in any person with normal renal function, a high calcium intake does not result in hypercalcemia, especially if the calcium intake is only as high as 1000 to 1400 mg per day [6]. In the face of renal insufficiency, however, the risk of developing hypercalcemia can be considerable.

There are other underlying disease states in which hypercalcemia is a manifestation of the disease process. These include hyperparathyroidism, breast cancer, multiple myeloma, hyperthyroidism, and sarcoidosis. If one of these were present, it is reasonable to assume that hypercalcemia could be precipitated or exacerbated by the intake of dietary calcium supplements.

Another potential risk of taking calcium supplements is hypercalciuria which, over time, may lead to nephrocalcinosis or nephrolithiasis. Although no study has looked specifically at this issue, a few studies include data on urinary calcium levels at the time of increased calcium intake [30–32]. Before analyzing this data, it is important to recall that hypercalciuria is defined as 4 mg of calcium per kilogram of body weight per 24-hour urine. This, on average, is equal to approximately 300 mg of calcium per 24-hour urine in men and 250 mg of calcium per 24-hour urine in women.

One of the studies, published by Hunt and Johnson [32], was designed to look at calcium absorption as a function of gastric acid secretion, using urinary calcium as proof that the calcium was absorbed. The subjects were 12 young healthy volunteers. Each was instructed to take calcium carbonate with 500 mg of elemental calcium orally 3 times daily for 2 days. Urinary output of calcium was determined on day 0 (predose) and day 2 of the treatment regimen. The results were as follows: Four individuals were found to have low gastric acid and were poor absorbers of calcium. Eight subjects were found to have normal absorption of calcium. In this group, the mean 24-hour urinary calcium output before treatment was 177 mg, with a range of 112 to 236 mg. During treatment with calcium, this rose to a mean of 275 mg, with a range of 158 to 390 mg per 24-hour urine. In terms of potential side effects of calcium supplements, this study demonstrates that some individuals may indeed develop hypercalciuria while taking oral calcium.

Several unanswered questions remain. Which individuals are most at risk for developing hypercalciuria and, more importantly, nephrocalcinosis or nephrolithiasis? It seems reasonable to assume that those persons with a baseline hypercalciuria, such as persons with familial hypercalciuria or with a history of renal calculi, may be more at risk of developing these complications than the average person if placed on calcium supplements. Other situations known to predispose to hypercalciuria include weightlessness and bed rest [6, 33]. It has been documented that astronauts living in an atmosphere without gravity develop high urinary calcium levels owing to increased bone resorption. This is much like the hypercalciuria that has been shown to develop in any individual, young or old, who is placed at bed rest with minimal activity. [33] One might therefore assume that the bedridden person should not be placed on calcium supplements so as to avoid worsening the hypercalciuria. However, this has not been demonstrated, and alternatively, one might speculate that calcium supplements may prevent the marked bone resorption that occurs at bed rest and is responsible for the hypercalciuria.

Other data that are not yet available but that would be useful include the percentage of persons who will develop hypercalciuria while taking 1 to 1.5 gm of calcium per day, and the percentage of those persons who develop hypercalciuria on calcium supplements who will also develop nephrolithiasis or nephrocalcinosis.

_____ STUDY QUESTION 7-5
Why would it be difficult to perform a study designed to provide the missing data on the percentage of those persons who develop hypercalciuria who will also develop nephrolithiasis or nephrocalcinosis?

The Decision-Making Process
It has been shown that with respect to calcium supplementation, there is little data available to help quantitate the potential risks involved. Yet the NIH panel recommends wide use of calcium. This probably reflects the assumption on the part of the panel that the potential complications of calcium supplementation are unlikely to occur at a frequency sufficient to offset the benefit of preventing the complications of osteopo-

rosis. This assumption points up the great difference in severity between the potential complications of calcium therapy (i.e., renal calculi) and osteoporosis (i.e., hip fractures).

We have also seen that in the case of ERT, where the potential complications of therapy may be more severe (endometrial cancer), the panel did not make strong recommendations favoring therapy. Thus, it is left to the physician to make the difficult decisions regarding treatment of the individual by weighing the risks and benefits on a case-by-case basis.

Having reviewed some of the pertinent available data and considered how the NIH panel may have reached their conclusions, we have in essence outlined a practical approach to such a decision-making process. Initially, the benefit to be obtained was identified, substantiated, and quantified to the extent allowed by available data. Based on the known effects of available therapy, potential complications were identified and then substantiated and quantified in a similar fashion. Owing to gaps in the data available, it remains necessary to make clinical judgments taking into account both the severity of the disease being prevented and the severity of the complications of therapy. Basically, this means recommending therapy in patients most at risk for hip fractures and least at risk for the more severe complications of therapy.

Weighing the benefits and risks for individual patients is not an easy task, but it is a necessary one. Let us see how well you can cope with the uncertainty as you make recommendations for therapy for the following patients. Using the preceding approach and the data presented, consider various options for treating these patients.

_____ STUDY QUESTION 7-6
What would you recommend for a 30-year-old white woman who has just undergone bilateral oophorectomy?

_____ STUDY QUESTION 7-7
What would you recommend for a 55-year-old obese, nulliparous white woman with a history of heavy tobacco use, a strong family history of myocardial infarction, and no family history of osteoporosis?

_____ STUDY QUESTION 7-8
What are your recommendations for a 53-year-old thin, inactive white woman who bore three children from as many pregnancies and has a 30-pack-per-year history of smoking and a negative family history for myocardial infarction?

_____ STUDY QUESTION 7-9

What would you recommend to a 55-year-old thin, inactive white woman who had a hysterectomy in the past, bore one child, and has diabetes mellitus, a 30-pack-per-year history of smoking, and a positive family history of myocardial infarction?

_____ STUDY QUESTION 7-10

What recommendations would you make for a 55-year-old thin black woman in good health with no history of tobacco use and no family history of myocardial infarction?

_____ STUDY QUESTION 7-11

What would you recommend in the case of a 70-year-old white woman with vertebral crush fractures and a recent right wrist fracture?

_____ STUDY QUESTION 7-12

What recommendations would you make for a 76-year-old white man with vertebral crush fractures?

_____ STUDY QUESTION 7-13

Would a history of renal calculi change your decision with regard to calcium supplementation in any of the patients described in the preceding study questions?

References

1. National Institutes of Health. Osteoporosis—consensus development conference statement. Washington, D.C.: U.S. Government Printing Office 1984:421–432.
2. Riggs BL, Melton LJ. Involutional osteoporosis. N Engl J Med 1986;314:1676–1684.
3. Altken M. Osteoporosis in clinical practice. Bristol, England: John Wright and Sons, 1984.
4. DeLuca HF (Coordinator). Tenth Steenbock Symposium, 1980, University of Wisconsin. Baltimore: University Park Press, 1981.
5. Heaney RP. Prevention of age-related osteoporosis in women. In: Avioli LV, ed. The osteoporotic syndrome: detection and prevention. New York: Grune & Stratton. 1983:123–144.
6. Heaney RP, Gallagher JC, Johnston CC, et al. Calcium nutrition and bone health in the elderly. Am J Clin Nutr 1977;30:986–1013.
7. Heaney RP, Recker RR, Saville PD. Calcium balance and calcium requirements in middle-aged women. Am J Clin Nutr 1977;30:1603–1611.
8. Richelson LS, Wahner HW, Melton LJ, Riggs BL. Relative contributions of aging and estrogen deficiency to postmenopausal bone loss. N Engl J Med 1984;311:1273–1275.

9. Recker, RR, Saville PD, Heaney RP. Effect of estrogens and calcium carbonate on bone loss in postmenopausal women. Ann Intern Med 1977;87:649–655.

10. Riggs BL, Seeman EE, Hodgson SF, et al. Effect of the fluoride/calcium regimen on vertebral fracture occurrence in postmenopausal osteoporosis. N Engl J Med 1982;306:446–450.

11. Riggs BL, Hodgson SF, O'Fallon WM. Letter to the editor. N Engl J Med 1982;307:442.

12. Ettinger B. Preventing postmenopausal osteoporosis with estrogen replacement therapy. Int J Fertil 1986;Suppl:15–20.

13. Ettinger B, Genant HK, Cann CE. Postmenopausal bone loss is prevented by treatment with low-dosage estrogen with calcium. Ann Intern Med 1987;106:40–45.

14. Mazess RB, Cameron JR. Densitometry of appendicular bone in osteoporosis (letter). JAMA 1985;307:442.

15. Riggs BL, Melton LJ. Evidence for two distinct syndromes of involutional osteoporosis. Am J Med 1983;899–901.

16. Paganini-Hill A, Ross RK, Gerkins VR, et al. Menopausal estrogen therapy and hip fractures. Ann Intern Med 1981;95:28–31.

17. Hutchinson TA, Polansky SM, Feinstein AR. Postmenopausal oestrogens protect against fractures of hip and distal radius. Lancet 1979;(2):705–708.

18. Weiss NS, Ure CL, Ballard JH, et al. Decreased risk of fractures of the hip and lower forearm with postmenopausal use of estrogen. N Engl J Med 1980;303:1195–1198.

19. Judd HL, Meldrum DR, Deftos LJ, Henderson BE. Estrogen replacement therapy: indications and complications. Ann Intern Med 1983;98:195–205.

20. Robbins SL, Cotran RS. Female genital tract. In: Robbins SL, Cotran RS, eds. Pathological basis of disease. Philadelphia: Saunders, 1979:1241–1304.

21. Smith DC, Prentice R, Thompson DJ, Herrman WL. Association of exogenous estrogen and endometrial carcinoma. N Engl J Med 1975;293:1164–1167.

22. Mack TM, Pike MC, Henderson BE, et al. Estrogens and endometrial cancer in a retirement community. N Engl J Med 1976;294:1262–1267.

23. Weiss NS, Szekely DP, English DR, Schweid AI. Endometrial cancer in relation to patterns of menopausal estrogen use. JAMA 1979;242:261–264.

24. Antunes CM, Stolley PD, Rosenshein NB, et al. Endometrial cancer and estrogen use. N Engl J Med 1979;300:9–13.

25. Thom MH, White PJ, Williams RM, et al. Prevention and treatment of endometrial disease in climacteric women receiving estrogen therapy. Lancet 1979;(2)455–457.

26. Paterson M, Wade-Evans T, Sturdee DW, et al. Endometrial disease after treatment with oestrogens and progestogens in the climacteric. Br Med J 1980;280:822–824.

27. Gambrell RD, Massey FM, Castaneda TA, et al. Reduced incidence of endometrial cancer among postmenopausal women treated with progestogens. J Am Geriatr Soc 1979;27:389–394.
28. Burnett CH, Commons RR, Albright F, Howard JE. Hypercalcemia without hypercalciuria or hypophosphatemia, calcinosis and renal insufficiency: a syndrome following prolonged intake of milk and alkali. N Engl J Med 1949;240:787–794.
29. McMillan DE, Freeman RB. The milk alkali syndrome: a study of the acute disorder with comments on the development of the chronic condition. Medicine (Baltimore) 1965;44:485.
30. Vincent PC, Radcliff FJ. The effect of large doses of calcium carbonate on serum and urinary calcium. Am J Dig Dis 1966;11:286–295.
31. DeQueker J, Heylen H, VanSteenkiste J, Vroninkx R. Urinary total hydroxyproline, calcium and phosphorus excretion after administration of calcium and oestrogen to postmenopausal women. Pharmacology 1972;7:321–326.
32. Hunt JN, Johnson C. Relation between gastric secretion of acid and urinary excretion of calcium after oral supplements of calcium. Dig Dis Sci 1983;28:417–421.
33. Mazess RB, Whedon GD. Immobilization and bone. Calcif Tissue Int 1983;35:265–267.

Varicella: Control, Prevention, and Remaining Dilemmas

CHAPTER EIGHT

JAMES F. CAWLEY
HOWARD J. BENNETT

Varicella (chickenpox) is an acute communicable disease caused by *herpesvirus varicellae* (the varicella-zoster virus). The disease occurs primarily among preschool and school-aged children, with 95 percent of cases occurring before 15 years of age. Varicella is usually a mild illness, but it can produce serious and even fatal complications.

Clinical Characteristics

The clinical features of varicella appear after an average incubation period of 14 days (range, 10 to 21 days). The illness begins with fever, malaise, and a rash that is generally pruritic. The rash is concentrated on the trunk but also involves the face, scalp, and extremities. Individual lesions progress rapidly from macule to papule to vesicle to crust. A characteristic feature of varicella is that several stages of lesions are present at the same time. New lesions erupt over a 4- to 5-day period, typically reaching 100 to 300 in number, and scabs fall off after a 1- to 2-week period. Constitutional symptoms such as headache, fever, malaise, and anorexia usually parallel the severity of the rash. Temperatures generally range from 100 to 102.5°F but may reach 104°F [1]. The typical course of varicella is illustrated in Figure 8-1.

The principal route of spread appears to be by aerosolized small droplet rather than by direct contact with vesicular fluid or with the dried crusts of skin lesions. Paradoxically, virus is difficult to detect in oropharyngeal secretions but is present in high titer in vesicular fluid from the lesions [2].

In normal children outside of the neonatal period, varicella is almost always a benign illness. Encephalitis occurs occasionally, but the most serious apparent complication is Reye's syndrome. Although the nature of the relationship between varicella and Reye's syndrome is uncertain, it is clear that varicella either plays a direct role in the pathogenesis of the syndrome or acts as a surrogate or marker for some concurrent condition that predisposes children to the disorder (Fig. 8-2).

Adults are much more likely to experience significant morbidity or even mortality owing to varicella. Varicella pneumonia, which may or may not be complicated by secondary bacterial pneumonia, is the prin-

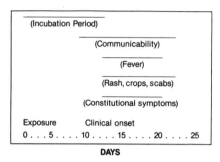

Fig. 8-1. Typical course of varicella illness.

cipal complication in adults, although encephalitis also occurs. Varicella-zoster virus shares with other members of the herpesvirus group the property of persistence or latency. In the case of varicella-zoster, the sensory ganglia have been suggested as the principal site of latency. Reactivation of the virus secondary to advancing age, stress, immunosuppression, and perhaps other factors results in herpes zoster (shingles), a painful and prolonged eruption of lesions involving dermatome(s) supplied by the affected ganglion. Generalized dissemination, involvement of motor neurons, and meningoencephalitis also may complicate typical herpes zoster [2–4].

Epidemiology
Chickenpox is second only to gonorrhea among the reportable infectious diseases in the United States. In 1982, the incidence rate of chickenpox (reported) was 94.3 per 100,000 persons. It is safe to assume that many cases go unreported, and overall estimates range from 3.0 to 3.7 million cases annually. In the United States, 32 percent of cases occur between 1 and 4 years of age, and 50 percent occur between 5 and 9 years [5]. Estimates suggest that between 100 and 200 varicella-associated deaths occur yearly in the United States [6, 7].

In temperate zones, varicella is seen most frequently in the winter and spring months. The customary explanation for this seasonal pattern relates to the aggregation of susceptible children in schools in the fall, the introduction of the agent, and its subsequent dissemination to contacts in the classroom and to susceptible siblings in the home (Fig. 8-3).

As mentioned, varicella is highly contagious. Secondary clinical attack

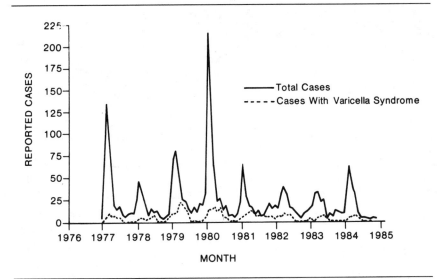

Fig. 8-2. Cases of Reye's syndrome, by month of hospitalization, in the United States from December 1976 through November 1984. (From Centers for Disease Control. Annual summary, 1984: reported morbidity in the United States. MMWR 1986;32:54.)

Fig. 8-3. Incidence rates of varicella, by month, in the United States from 1980 through 1984. (From Centers for Disease Control. Annual summary, 1984: reported morbidity in the United States. MMWR 1986;32:54.)

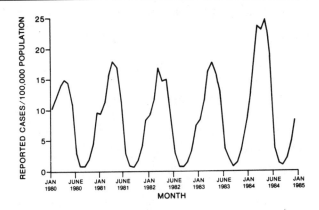

Table 8-1. Distribution of cases of varicella in the United States

Age	Percentage of all cases	No. of cases
<1	2	75,767
1–4	20	757,667
5–14	73	2,767,486
15–24	4	151,534
25–59	0.9	34,095
≥60	0.1	3,788
All ages	100	3,790,337

Source: From the Institute of Medicine [5].

rates of approximately 90 percent follow exposure of household contacts. The incubation period is most commonly 12 to 14 days. The period of communicability is estimated to be 1 to 2 days before the onset of the rash until 5 to 6 days after the rash onset. Persons with severe varicella may be contagious for longer periods, presumably because their immune response is depressed to some degree, allowing viral replication to persist.

It is not known why chickenpox is more severe in adults, but it is an aspect of infection not restricted to chickenpox. The same type of phenomemon is seen in measles, polio, infectious hepatitis, and many other communicable diseases (Table 8-1).

Complications
Although usually benign, varicella can produce serious complications, including the following:

Progressive varicella

Disseminated varicella

Bullous varicella (secondary *Staphylococcus aureus* infection)

Varicella pneumonia

Bacterial superinfection

Hepatitis

Encephalitis

Optic neuritis

Reye's syndrome

The risk of complications from varicella infection usually is related to host immunity. In the immunocompromised patient, varicella infection may take a hemorrhagic progressive or disseminated course. These patients have widespread disease with visceral involvement, hemorrhagic lesions, and prolonged illness.

The most commonly reported complications are encephalitis, Reye's syndrome, secondary bacterial infections, and pneumonia. The Centers for Disease Control (CDC) estimate that there are approximately 6500 hospitalizations annually for complications associated with varicella. Of these, 80 percent are for children aged 1 to 14, and only 4 percent are for children with an underlying malignancy [6].

The risks of complications from varicella are much higher in immunocompromised children and normal adults. Children with congenital or acquired immunodeficiency syndromes, leukemia, lymphoma, or other types of malignancy, and those on immunosuppressive drugs have much more severe cases of varicella and higher mortality. Among leukemic children with varicella, 30 percent have visceral involvement, and 7 percent die of the disease.

The risk of encephalitis following varicella is estimated to be 1.7 per 100,000 cases in children from 1 to 14 years and 15 per 100,000 cases in persons older than 20 years [6]. The CDC estimates that approximately 900 cases of Reye's syndrome occur annually in the United States and that 25 percent (225) are associated with varicella. Almost half of the survivors of Reye's syndrome are estimated to suffer mild to severe chronic neuropsychologic problems (e.g., mental retardation, cranial nerve palsies, motor dysfunction). Reye's syndrome is also strongly associated with administration of aspirin. Reductions in the use of aspirin among children with chickenpox is currently resulting in a reduced incidence of Reye's syndrome.

Overall, the risk of death from complications associated with varicella is estimated to be 2.0 per 100,000 cases in children aged 1 to 14 and 50 per 100,000 in persons aged 20 years or older. Infants younger than 1 year are estimated to account for 7 percent of all deaths [5].

Varicella Immunization

In the last 30 years, many vaccines have been developed that have successfully reduced the morbidity and mortality associated with previously common childhood diseases. Recommendations for immunization are made only after considerable study regarding the efficacy, risks, and benefits of the vaccine in question. Although varicella is usually a benign disease, the potential complications seen in certain individuals makes a strong argument for the development of an effective vaccine. In this chapter, we will examine the issues surrounding the development and implementation of a vaccine to control the spread of varicella.

DEVELOPMENT OF THE LIVE-VIRUS VARICELLA VACCINE
In the vast majority of cases, chickenpox is a mild illness of little clinical importance. Thus, vaccine research in the past has focused on those infectious diseases with more serious outcomes (i.e., polio, hepatitis, and measles). Another factor is that the varicella virus is a member of the herpesvirus group, and concern existed regarding the not-well-understood biologic properties of these viruses. Herpesviruses are well known for their capacity to persist in the host and recur after a period of dormancy. The use of an attenuated live-virus varicella vaccine might initially prevent chickenpox but later lead to increased development of shingles. Moreover, if protection against varicella were short-lived or if immunization rates were suboptimal, the vaccine could convert a childhood illness to one of adulthood, with an age-associated increase in both morbidity and risk of congenital infection.

_____ STUDY QUESTION 8-1
What information is necessary to assess the value of a varicella vaccine?

VACCINE TRIALS
Progress in the development of an attenuated live-virus varicella vaccine began in 1974 when Takahashi and colleagues [8] perfected a vaccine that could be tested in human subjects, the only host for the disease. Research in Japan was conducted in a stepwise manner by administering the vaccine first to immunologically normal children, then to children with some degree of immunosuppression [8], and later to children with an underlying malignancy who were highly immunocompromised [9]. The early studies from Japan revealed the vaccine to be immunogenic and to produce few serious immediate side effects. The vaccine induced protective levels of antibody among immunocompetent children, but little information was available on its overall protective efficacy.

There was considerable controversy among American academic pediatricians regarding the clinical testing and overall value of a varicella vaccine [10]. Experts raised several troublesome questions regarding implementation of varicella immunizations. Was the vaccine needed in the first place? After all, varicella-zoster immune globulin could be used to prevent varicella in high-risk groups, and chickenpox in normal children is fairly benign. Would the vaccine virus itself produce herpes zoster? The implication of this question was that follow-up periods of 60 years or more would be needed to answer questions about postimmunization decline in immunity and the effect of an attentuated member of the herpesvirus family on the occurrence and natural history of zoster.

_____ STUDY QUESTION 8-2
Short of a 60-year follow-up, would there be any way of determining the risk of herpes zoster among immunized subjects?

Despite the controversy, vaccine testing began in this country amid an attitude of cautious optimism. It was first administered to normal children [11] and adults [12] and then to leukemic children who were no longer receiving chemotherapy [13, 14]. Subsequently, the vaccine was administered to children with leukemia, in remission for at least 1 year, who were still receiving maintenance chemotherapy.

Vaccine Trials in Healthy Children
The results of a large-scale clinical trial of the varicella vaccine in healthy children were reported in 1984. Weibel and associates [15], using Oka/ Merck varicella vaccine, set up a randomized doubleblind, placebo-controlled trial among 956 healthy children between the ages of 1 and 14 with a negative clinical history of varicella. Of the 914 who were found to be serologically susceptible to varicella, 468 received the vaccine and 446 received placebo. The vaccine produced few clinical reactions and was well tolerated.

Eight weeks after vaccination, 94 percent of the initially seronegative children who received the vaccine had detectible antibody to varicella. The groups were followed over a 9-month surveillance period. During this time, 39 cases of varicella were observed, 38 of which were confirmed by laboratory tests. All 39 occurred among placebo recipients. No child who received the vaccine contracted varicella.

The results of the trial were as follows:

	No. of Children	*Varicella Cases*
Placebo	446	38
Vaccine	468	0

——————————————————————— STUDY QUESTION 8-3
What is the relative risk or protective efficacy ratio of varicella for those receiving placebo versus those receiving vaccine?

Another way of looking at the efficacy of the varicella vaccine is to consider attributable risk. In vaccine trials, attributable risk is often called the protective efficacy rate. Using the data from Weibel's trial, recall the formula for attributable risk.

$$\text{Attributable risk} = \frac{\text{incidence in the placebo group} - \text{incidence in the vaccine group}}{\text{incidence in the placebo group}}$$

$$= \frac{38/446 - 0/468}{38/446} = 100\%$$

Attributable risk is the maximum percentage of cases of a disease that can be potentially eliminated by administration of the vaccine. This type of result is not expected in most vaccine trials. A protective efficacy rate of more than 90 percent is a characteristic of some of the more useful vaccines (i.e., hepatitis B) and suggests that the vaccine will be protective, at least initially, in the majority of individuals who are immunized.

The most direct means of assessing the efficacy of the vaccine is to assess how well it protects those children with known household contacts with chickenpox. The data from the household contacts of participants in the Weibel trial are presented in Table 8-2.

——————————————————————— STUDY QUESTION 8-4
What do you conclude from these data?

Although the results of this early vaccine trial are very impressive, the follow-up period of the study was only 9 months. Further studies are warranted to determine the long-term safety of the vaccine, the incidence of herpes zoster in recipients, and the duration of immunity provided by the vaccine in comparison to immunity from natural disease.

Vaccine Trials in Immunocompromised Patients
While varicella vaccine trials in healthy children were undertaken, the efficacy of the vaccine was also being tested in groups of high-risk immunocompromised children. Gershon and colleagues [14] examined a group of 240 leukemic children in remission for at least 1 year. With one

Table 8-2. Disease rate in immunized and nonimmunized children exposed to varicella in the household

	Placebo group	Varicella vaccine group
No. of subjects	9	33
No. of study subjects who developed varicella	4	0
Secondary attack rate	4/9 (44%)	0/33 (0%)

Source: Adapted from Weibel and colleagues [15].

dose of vaccine, 80 percent produced detectable levels of antibody, and 90 percent had antibody after a second dose. In this uncontrolled study, Gershon was able to follow 191 of these children who had completed their chemotherapeutic regimen or whose chemotherapy had been suspended. The major side effect of vaccination was a rash, the incidence and severity of which was dependent on the state of immunocompetence. Maculopapular rashes occurred after the first dose in 54 (36 percent) of 149 children in whom chemotherapy had been suspended. Rashes occurred approximately 1 month after immunization, when vaccinees were at risk (10 percent) of transmitting the virus to others. Twenty-two vaccinees subsequently had household exposure to varicella. The attack rate of varicella was 18 percent, far lower than the expected rate of 90 percent in susceptible individuals with household exposure [14].

To assess the risk of herpes zoster development after varicella immunization, Brunell and co-workers [16] compared zoster rates in leukemic children receiving the varicella vaccine with a similar group of leukemic children with naturally occurring varicella. It was observed that 15 of 73 children who had previously contracted varicella subsequently developed herpes zoster, whereas none of the 34 children who had received the vaccine developed zoster. Both groups were followed for a period of approximately 4 years.

The risk of contagion in leukemic children receiving varicella vaccine is an important clinical point. Approximately 10 percent are at risk of spreading the disease to others, and examination of viral deoxyribonucleic acid in nonleukemic contacts of vaccine recipients indicates that the virus is of vaccine origin. The disease experienced by the contacts, however, is milder than chickenpox and is not believed to be associated with varicella complications.

It is estimated that, overall, the varicella vaccine has a protective efficacy rate of approximately 80 percent in preventing clinical varicella in immunocompromised children.

PASSIVE IMMUNIZATION

Aside from the promising live-virus varicella vaccine, which is not yet licensed for use, another clinical option for varicella control is varicella-zoster immune globulin (VZIG).

Available since 1981, VZIG is prepared from plasma found in routine screening of normal blood donors. Human VZIG is a form of passive immunization that aims to prevent or modify clinical illness, particularly in immunocompromised patients exposed to varicella. VZIG is of maximum benefit when given as soon as possible after exposure. It is not useful once clinical varicella or zoster is present. Protection lasts for at least 3 weeks. VZIG is very safe, the most common adverse reaction being pain and redness at the injection site in fewer than 1 percent of patients. It must be noted that VZIG supplies currently are limited and that the cost of an adult dose is approximately $400.00. The indiscriminate use of VZIG would quickly exhaust supplies. Thus, the CDC has developed a series of recommendations for the use of VZIG.

_____ STUDY QUESTION 8-5
What general criteria should be satisfied before administering VZIG to a particular patient?

To aid clinicians in the appropriate use of VZIG, the immunization Practices Advisory Committee (ACIP) of the CDC has issued a series of guidelines [17]. The initial clinical determination is that of susceptibility to varicella: Is the child or adult immune or susceptible? The clinical history is most important in making this assessment. In the presence of a positive recollection of infection, it is highly probable that one is immune. Approximately 85 to 95 percent of adults with negative or unknown histories of varicella are immune.

When there is doubt regarding the accuracy of the history, laboratory assays for varicella antibody may be necessary, but such tests have an unacceptable rate of false negative reactions and are not commonly available. In addition, it is difficult to interpret the results of antibody assays in immunocompromised persons. Low levels of such antibodies have been detected in the sera of immunocompromised persons lacking a history of chickenpox who subsequently developed clinical varicella.

Table 8-3. Exposure criteria for which
varicella-zoster immune globulin (VZIG) is indicated

One of the following types of exposure to persons with chickenpox or herpes
   zoster:
Continuous household contact
Playmate contact (generally >1 hour of play indoors)
Hospital contact (in the same 2- to 4-bed room, or adjacent beds in a large
   ward, or prolonged face-to-face contact with an infectious staff member or
   patient)
Newborn contact (newborn or other who had onset of chickenpox 5 days or
   less before delivery or within 48 hours after delivery)

and

Time elapsed from exposure to administration of VZIG 96 hours or less

---

Source: From the Centers for Disease Control [17].

Although present, their antibodies did not prevent illness. It is believed
that these patients received some amount of passive antibody as a result
of transfusions of blood or blood products during the course of their
underlying illness.

Several types of exposures are likely to place a susceptible person at
risk for varicella. Persons continuously exposed in the household to patients with varicella are at greatest risk. More than 90 percent of such
exposed susceptible patients contract varicella after a single exposure.
The risk after playmate exposure or hospital room exposure is approximately one-fifth the risk of household exposure (Table 8-3).

Once questions of susceptibility and exposure have been answered,
the clinician must then decide whether an individual falls into a high-
risk group. High-risk groups are composed mostly of children with primary immunodeficiencies or neoplasia, children receiving immunosuppressive therapy, newborns of mothers who develop chickenpox shortly
before delivery, and premature infants (Table 8-4).

The CDC recommends administration of VZIG to all who fulfill the
eligibility, exposure, *and* high-risk criteria. For immunocompromised
patients 15 years of age or older, the decision is made on an individual
basis. Let us look at some individual cases.

CASE A.   A healthy 30-year-old executive with no history of chickenpox and a
negative antibody test has a 13-year-old son with varicella, diagnosed 48 hours
previously. The executive is worried about getting varicella and is willing to pay
for VZIG out of his pocket.

Table 8-4. Candidates for whom varicella-zoster
immune globulin (VZIG) is indicated

Susceptible to varicella-zoster

Significant exposure

Age of <15 years, with administration to immunocompromised adolescents
    and adults and to other older patients on an individual basis (see text)

and

One of the following underlying illnesses or conditions that connote high risk:
    Leukemia or lymphoma
    Congenital or acquired immunodeficiency
    Immunosuppressive therapy
    Newborn of mother who had onset of chickenpox within 5 days before
        delivery or within 48 hours after delivery
    Premature infants (<28 weeks' gestation or <1000 gm), regardless of
        maternal history

Source: From the Centers for Disease Control [17].

STUDY QUESTION 8-6

How would you manage the patient in case A? Should he receive VZIG?

CASE B.   A 35-year-old woman is on immunosuppressive therapy for lymphoma. She has no recollection of having chickenpox. She was briefly exposed
almost 4 days ago to a hospital employee who has chickenpox.

STUDY QUESTION 8-7

(a) Would this patient benefit from VZIG? (b) From vaccine? (c) Would you consider her susceptible since she cannot recall having chickenpox?

Let us assume that an inexpensive vaccine has been approved that has
an 80-percent efficacy rate among immunosuppressed patients and has
been shown to be safe regarding short-term side effects. Let us consider
the advantages and disadvantages of using this vaccine as opposed to
using VZIG in high-risk individuals.

CASE C.   Joe Smith is an 8-year-old boy who developed minimal change ne-
phrotic syndrome when he was 6 years old. Initial treatment with salt restriction
and high-dose prednisone (2 mg per kilogram 4 times daily) resulted in a prompt
regression of his proteinuria. After 4 weeks, Joe's prednisone was reduced to 1.5
mg per kilogram every other day. Joe remained well over the next 4 weeks, and
his prednisone was discontinued over an additional 2-week period. Since his
initial presentation, Joe has relapsed twice, each episode responding to treat-

ment with prednisone. His last relapse was 4 weeks ago, and he is currently taking 1.5 mg of prednisone per kilogram of body weight every other day.

_____ STUDY QUESTION 8-8

(a) In Joe's case, what are the advantages and disadvantages of use of the vaccine? (b) Of the use of VZIG?

PROJECTING THE EPIDEMIOLOGIC IMPACT

In assessing the effect of widespread use of a chickenpox vaccine in healthy children, additional factors need to be taken into account. Even if it is feasible to reduce dramatically the incidence of chickenpox, we need to assess the potential long-term effects of widespread vaccinations of healthy children. First, one needs to consider whether it is feasible to reach an adequate percentage of a population to interrupt the spread of the disease.

With certain infectious diseases, immunization of a certain proportion of the susceptible population confers protection against the disease even among nonimmunized individuals. This epidemiologic concept is known as herd immunity. Herd immunity is believed to be an important factor underlying the dynamics of propagated epidemics and the periodicity of common viral infections. If, in a population, a sufficient number of individuals contract the disease (thus becoming immune), the likelihood of effective contact between patients with the disease and remaining susceptible individuals declines. This may limit the spread of the disease: For example, if 70 percent of the population is immune, either through contracting the disease or by immunization, the remaining 30 percent are unlikely to contract the disease. In vaccine epidemiology, this means that it is not necessary to achieve 100 percent immunity in the population to control the spread of disease. In general, the more contagious the disease, the higher the level of immunity that is required. Just how far short of 100 percent is enough to control the disease is, of course, the crucial question. It has been customary to cite a figure of 70 percent for diphtheria, but for other diseases such as measles or rubella, the figure may be 85 or 90 percent, and even in populations achieving that level of immunization, outbreaks have occurred.

In terms of varicella, there is little evidence that herd immunity is a major factor in its epidemiology [5]. The universally contagious nature of the disease is such that very high levels of immunity would be necessary to control the disease.

It is possible that the widespread application of a varicella vaccine

Table 8-5. Age distribution and reported
cases of measles in the United States, 1983–1985

Age (years)	1983 Cases		1984 Cases		1985 Cases	
	No.	%	No.	%	No.	%
0–4	451	31.5	622	24.5	466	25.9
5–9	160	11.2	283	11.1	152	8.4
10–14	195	13.6	679	26.7	319	17.7
15–19	382	26.7	650	25.6	603	33.5
20–24	163	11.4	173	6.8	175	9.7
≥25	80	5.6	136	5.3	86	4.8
Total	1431	100.0	2543	100.0	1801	100.0

Source: From the Centers for Disease Control [18, 19].

could change the existing epidemiology of varicella. With a vaccine, extensive control of varicella would be likely in the pediatric age groups. If the vaccine merely delays the occurrence of disease, this could result in an increase in varicella among adults, with a resultant increase in varicella mortality and morbidity. This concern has gained attention in view of recent experiences with the measles vaccine.

Measles is a common childhood infection that is usually benign but does have serious consequences in certain patient groups. The licensure of live-virus measles vaccine in 1963 has reduced the annual number of cases from approximately 500,000 to 2534 cases in 1984 [18]. Analysis of reported cases shows that the age distribution of measles appears to be rising (Table 8-5). Prior to 1983, the highest incidence rates were seen in preschoolers. Beginning around 1984, the percentage of cases in the 10- to 14-year age group began to rise, as did the percentage of cases in the 15- to 19-year age group. In fact, the latter group had the highest percentage of reported cases of measles [19]. These figures corroborate reports of outbreaks of measles on college campuses [20]. Thus, it would appear that the epidemiology of measles is changing somewhat and that the institution of the measles vaccine program has shifted the distribution of measles to older persons (albeit at much lower case rates).

In assessing the consequences of the institution of a nationwide varicella vaccine program, it is important to consider that the measles experience could prove to be analogous.

STUDY QUESTION 8-9
What factors would determine whether a varicella immunization program would result in an increased incidence of chickenpox among adults?

Toward Control of Varicella

Although trials with the varicella vaccine have thus far yielded favorable results in both healthy and immunocompromised persons, important questions regarding its implementation still remain. Moreover, new questions have been raised, as a result of recent vaccine studies, that challenge some fundamental concepts of viral immunology and immunity.

As we have discussed, the issue of the length of protective immunity to varicella is a major consideration. We know that 5- and 10-year follow-up studies from Japan indicated the presence of antibody (humoral immunity) among vaccinees and a very low rate of either varicella or herpes zoster among these patients [21, 22]. However, it is not certain that the presence of antibodies to varicella-zoster virus necessarily protects against infection, or more accurately, reinfection.

It has long been assumed that in most viral diseases the presence of humoral antibody, obtained either by immunization or by contracting the disease, confers lifelong protection. This was believed to be the case with varicella until reports of exogenous clinical reinfection in patients known to have been immunized began to surface [23–25]. Gershon and colleagues [23] describe 8 patients in whom varicella-zoster antibody was present up to 10 months before the clinical reappearance of varicella. One of these patients had received the varicella vaccine and had demonstrated specific antibody and cellular immunity to the vaccine virus, but subsequently developed clinical varicella. By studying the viral DNA by restriction-endonuclease techniques, this vaccine was shown to be infected with wild-type varicella-zoster virus, not vaccine virus. Thus, even in the presence of specific antibody to varicella, exogenous clinical reinfection can occur.

In herpesvirus infections, immunity is obviously complex and does not appear to follow patterns observed in other viral infections. It is not known whether immunization or the acquisition of natural infection can confer lifelong protection.

Another issue involves acceptance if the vaccine were to become licensed. Although it has been shown that the varicella vaccine could be given routinely with the measles-mumps-rubella immunizations at age

15 months without side effects [26], some pediatricians and parents may still hesitate to use a live herpesvirus vaccine, particularly when varicella usually is such a mild disease in normal children. Acceptance and use would appear to be more clear-cut in immunocompromised children and perhaps in high-risk adult patients.

_____ STUDY QUESTION 8-10
Summarize the major conclusion that can be drawn from the data on varicella vaccine. Faced with unanswered questions about the long-term safety and effectiveness of varicella vaccine, would this affect your recommendations on use of the vaccine?

_____ STUDY QUESTION 8-11
Assume a chickenpox vaccine is licensed with the following characteristics: (1) 99 percent protective efficacy rate in normal children; (2) 80-percent protective efficacy rate in immunocompromised children; (3) very small incidence of herpes zoster in healthy and immunocompromised children older than 10 years; and (4) demonstrated protection against chickenpox for at least 10 years in healthy and immunocompromised children. Who should receive this vaccine?

References

1. Krugman S, Katz K, Gershon AA, et al. Infectious disease of children (8th ed.). St. Louis: Mosby, 1985.
2. Weller TH. Varicella and herpes zoster: changing concepts of the natural history, control and importance of a not-so-benign virus. N Engl J Med 1983;309:1362–68, 1434–1440.
3. Weller TH. Varicella–herpes zoster virus. In: Evans AS, ed. Viral infections of humans. 2nd ed. New York: Plenum, 1984.
4. Straus SE, Reinhold W, Smith H, et al. Endonuclease analysis of viral DNA from varicella and subsequent zoster infections in the same patient. N Engl J Med 1984;311:1362–1364.
5. Institute of Medicine. _New vaccine development: establishing priorities. Vol. 1, diseases of importance in the United States._ Washington, D.C.: National Academy Press, 1985.
6. Preblud SR. Age-specific risks of varicella complications. Pediatrics 1981;68:14–17.
7. Preblud SR, D'Angelo LJ. Chickenpox in the United States, 1972–1977. J Infect Dis 1979;140:256–260.
8. Takahashi M, Otsuka T, Okna Y, et al. Live vaccine used to prevent the spread of varicella in children in the hospital. Lancet 1974;2:1288–1290.
9. Izawa T, Ihara T, Hattori A, et al. Application of a live varicella vaccine in

children with acute leukemia or other malignant diseases. Pediatrics 1977;60:805–809.

10. McIntosh K. Varicella vaccine: decisions a little nearer. N Engl J Med 1984;310:1456.

11. Arbeter AA, Star SE, Weibel RE, Plotkin SA. Live attenuated varicella vaccine: immunization of healthy children with the OKA strain. J Pediatr 1982;100:886–893.

12. LaRussa P, Hammerschlag M, Steinberg S, et al. Varicella vaccine: use to prevent varicella in susceptible adults. Pediatr Res 1982;16:15A.

13. Brunell PA, Shehab Z, Geiser C, Waugh JE. Administration of live varicella vaccine to children with leukemia. Lancet 1982;2:1069–1072.

14. Gershon AA, Steinberg SP, Gelb L, et al. Live attenuated varicella vaccine: efficacy for children with leukemia in remission. JAMA 1984;252:355–362.

15. Weibel RE, Neff BJ, Juter BJ, et al. Live attenuated varicella vaccine: efficacy trial in healthy children. N Engl J Med 1984;310:1409–1415.

16. Brunell P, Taylor-Wiedeman J, Gleiser C, et al. Risk of herpes zoster in children with leukemia: varicella vaccine compared with history of chickenpox. Pediatrics 1986;77:53–56.

17. Centers for Disease Control. Advisory Committee on Immunization Practices. Varicella-zoster immune globulin for the prevention of chickenpox. ACIP, MMWR 1984;33:81–96.

18. Centers for Disease Control. Measles, United States, 1984. MMWR 1985;34:308–312.

19. Centers for Disease Control. Measles, United States, first 26 weeks, 1986. MMWR 1986;35:525–533.

20. Centers for Disease Control. Measles on college campuses, United States, 1985. MMWR 1985;34:445–449.

21. Asano Y, Nagai T, Miyata T, et al. Long-term protective immunity of the recipients of the OKA strain live attenuated varicella vaccine. Pediatrics 1985;75:667–671.

22. Takahashi M. Clinical overview of varicella vaccine: development and early studies. Pediatrics 1986;78(suppl):736–741.

23. Gershon AA, Steinberg SP, Gelb L, et al. Clinical reinfection with varicella-zoster virus. J Infect Dis 1984;149:137–142.

24. Martin JLT, Dohner DE, Wellinghoff WJ, Gelb L. Restriction endonuclease analysis of varicella-zoster vaccine virus and wild type DNAs. J Med Virol 1982;9:69–76.

25. Palmer SR, Donald DE, Caul EO, et al. An outbreak of shingles. Lancet 1985;4:1108–1110.

26. Taylor-Wiedman J, Novelli V, Brunell PA, et al. Combined measles-mumps-rubella-varicella vaccine in children. Pediatr Res 1985;19:306A.

Pneumococcal Vaccine

CHAPTER NINE

RICHARD K. RIEGELMAN

As a practicing physician, you are constantly receiving stacks of mail promoting new therapies. On the bottom of your daily pile of mail you come across a promotion for a new vaccine directed against pneumococcal disease. Why, you ask, would anyone want to use a vaccine when a disease can be cured? Why subject large numbers of patients to the potential side effects of a therapy when it is possible to cure the disease in the few patients who actually contract the illness. Prevention, you say, has surely gone too far!

Before you insert this information in your circular file, let us take a look at the reasons one might want to develop a vaccine directed against pneumococcal disease. Then, let us look at the risks and benefits of pneumococcal vaccine and, finally, at the cost effectiveness of this form of preventive therapy.

This chapter will illustrate the ways we assess data on vaccines. It will also demonstrate the need to be on the lookout for new data that challenge underlying assumptions contained in official recommendations.

Basic Information on Streptococcus Pneumoniae

The bacteria *Streptococcus pneumoniae*, often referred to as pneumococci, is a common cause of human disease. Pneumococci are gram-positive streptococci that possess an antigenic capsule. There are more than 80 antigenic subtypes; however, only a minority of these are known to be capable of causing human infection. Pneumococcal disease is most frequently expressed as a lobar pneumonia. Pneumococcal pneumonia may progress to bacteremia, which is associated with a high incidence of complications and death, especially among the elderly and those with underlying cardiopulmonary disease. The overall case-fatality rate for untreated pneumococcal pneumonia is approximately 28 percent. The case-fatality rate dramatically increases for bacteremic elderly patients. *Streptococcus pneumoniae* is capable of colonizing the nasopharynx without causing disease. Pneumonia is believed to occur when nasopharyngeal organisms are aspirated into the lungs and defense mechanisms are incapable of clearing the organisms. Another important risk factor for pneumococcal pneumonia is the absence of splenic function, including sickle-cell patients and those with surgical removal of the spleen. Pneumococcal pneumonia may occur in apparently normal healthy young people, especially as a complication of influenza infections. *Streptococcus pneumoniae* is associated with a series of other complications, including

145

empyema, meningitis, endocarditis, pericarditis, peritonitis, and septic arthritis.

Treatment of pneumococcal pneumonia in the preantibiotic era included the use of type-specific antisera directed against the pneumococcal capsular antigens. Research in the 1930s and 1940s suggested some effectiveness of type-specific sera. However, the mass production of penicillin and the recognition of its effects against pneumococcal pneumonia resulted in a discontinuation of research and production of type-specific sera.

The obvious overall success of penicillin in curing the vast majority of pneumococcal pneumonia cases caused a delay in fully recognizing the fact that individuals older than 50 and those with severe cardiopulmonary disease, cirrhosis, diabetes, and renal diseases continued to experience increased mortality despite antibiotic therapy. Approximately 15 to 20 percent of hospitalized patients with bacteremic pneumococcal pneumonia continue to die despite appropriate antibiotic therapy.

An additional limitation of antibiotic therapy developed in the 1970s. Resistance to high levels of penicillin began to appear and increase in frequency. Strains resistant to many other antibiotics have now been detected and also are increasing in frequency.

As a result of the recognition of the failures of and increasing resistance to antibiotics, efforts were resumed to develop vaccines effective against streptococcal pneumonia. This chapter is designed to help you think through the problems inherent in designing, evaluating, developing, and implementing recommendations for the use of pneumococcal vaccine.

Inherent Limitations of a Pneumococcal Vaccine

Technical limitations require that a vaccine use only a small fraction of the more than 80 known pneumococcal subtypes. Thus, one must identify the subtypes that are the most common causes of pneumococcal disease. Among the possible methods for determining which type-specific organisms to include in the vaccine are: (1) use of the most common organisms isolated from the nasopharynx, (2) use of the most common organisms isolated from sputum of individuals with pneumonia, and (3) use of the most common organisms isolated from the blood.

_____ STUDY QUESTION 9-1

Which of these sources of *Streptococcus pneumoniae* would you choose as the basis for developing the vaccine?

Two versions of the vaccine have been produced, an initial 14-valent vaccine and a newer 23-valent vaccine. The 14-valent vaccine was directed against subtypes associated with approximately 75 percent of the cases of bacteremic disease, whereas the 23-valent vaccine is directed against subtypes associated with approximately 90 percent of the cases of bacteremic disease. Thus, if the vaccine has a 100 percent efficacy against the types included in the vaccine, it will still have only a 90 percent efficacy in preventing cases of bacteremic infection.

Another problem inherent in the development of the pneumococcal vaccine is that the vaccine actually represents a series of vaccines, one for each of the capsular subtypes contained in it.

_____ STUDY QUESTION 9-2
Assume that each antigen in a 14-valent vaccine has a 98 percent efficacy against pneumococcal disease caused by that particular subtype. What proportion of disease caused by these 14 subtypes would potentially be prevented by the vaccine?

The vaccine is also limited in that it provides an inadequate response in individuals younger than 2 years. On the other hand, individuals should receive pneumococcal vaccine only once, since severe reaction can occur with repeated vaccination. Therefore, those who previously received the 14-valent vaccine should not receive the newer 23-valent vaccine.

Efficacy

Studies of the experimental efficacy of pneumococcal vaccine have utilized populations of individuals at high risk for disease. Young healthy South African gold miners have an extraordinarily high incidence of pneumococcal pneumonia, reported to be as high as 9 percent annually. This group has been used repeatedly as an initial population for studying the efficacy of pneumococcal vaccine.

_____ STUDY QUESTION 9-3
Why is it desirable to study the efficacy of a treatment on a high-risk population?

In one of the initial efficacy studies of pneumococcal vaccine performed on South African gold miners by Austrian and colleagues [1], 1493 subjects were immunized, and 3007 subjects received placebos. The diagnosis of pneumococcal pneumonia was defined as radiologic evidence of pneumonia with a positive streptococcal pneumonia culture from the blood, deep sputum, or nasopharynx. The data are as follows:

	Pneumococcal pneumonia	No pneumococcal pneumonia	
Vaccinated subjects	17	1476	1493
Placebo subjects	160	2847	3007

The results for vaccinated subjects were statistically significant (p <.0001).

_____ STUDY QUESTION 9-4
(a) What is the relative risk of pneumococcal pneumonia for those receiving the placebo versus those receiving the vaccine? (b) How do you interpret this relative risk from a vaccine trial?

_____ STUDY QUESTION 9-5
Can you think of any reason why this calculation might inaccurately estimate the true protection afforded by the vaccine?

_____ STUDY QUESTION 9-6
To calculate the absolute risk for a population, what other information besides relative risk is required?

_____ STUDY QUESTION 9-7
In this vaccine trial, what percentages of the disease was eliminated by use of the vaccine?

Because of the difficulties in definitively diagnosing pneumococcal pneumonia, precise estimates of incidence are difficult to obtain. Estimates based on community studies by Mufson and colleagues [2] and Felice and co-workers [3] found bacteremic rates of approximately 8 per 100,000 persons per year or 0.08 per 1000 persons per year. Estimates of pneumococcal pneumonia based on sputum analysis suggest a rate between 1.5 and 2.3 cases per 1000 persons per year. These differences can be reconciled if one assumes that only 5 percent or less of individuals with pneumococcal pneumonia develop bacteremia. There is still a great degree of uncertainty about the true incidence rate of pneumococcal pneumonia.

Effectiveness

In vaccine trials attributable risk is often called the protective efficacy rate. Attributable risk serves as an estimate of the maximum overall efficacy of the vaccine. To determine whether the vaccine lives up to this maximum efficacy estimate in clinical practice, let us take a look at the data on use of the vaccine in a United States population.

The efficacy of pneumococcal vaccine in a controlled clinical trial should be distinguished from the effectiveness of the vaccine when used in clinical practice in the United States.

CASE-CONTROL STUDIES IN CLINICAL PRACTICE

Shapiro and Clemens [4] have employed a retrospective or case-control study to examine the effectiveness in practice. In this study, they used a special form of matching, called pairing, for selecting their cases and their controls.* They began by identifying 90 individuals who experienced bacteremic pneumococcal disease. The investigators determined the age and indication, if any, for recommending the vaccine for each of these individuals. They then identified an individual to pair with each of the 90 subjects. The individual in the control group was approximately the same age as the diseased subject and possessed the same indication for recommending pneumococcal vaccine. Thus, the investigators identified 90 cases and controls paired for age and indication for the pneumococcal vaccine. For each pair, Shapiro and Clemens determined whether the case and the control had actually received the pneumococcal vaccine before the time of the study. On the basis of these determinations, each pair was classified into one of four categories, labeled a through d: (a) case and control both vaccinated; (b) case vaccinated and control unvaccinated; (c) case unvaccinated and control vaccinated; and (d) case and control both unvaccinated. The data from the study may be summarized as follows:

	Vaccinated controls	Unvaccinated controls
Vaccinated cases	a = 1	b = 5
Unvaccinated cases	c = 15	d = 69
	a + c = 16	b + d = 74

*Matching may be done by merely assuring that the average age or other characteristic of the case group approximates that of the control group: This is group matching. The form of matching used here, in contrast, is called pairing.

As in all retrospective or case-control studies, the odds ratio is used as an estimate of relative risk. In paired studies, the odds ratio is measured using only pairs in which cases and controls differed according to their vaccination status. These discordant pairs are made up of a case who did not receive vaccine and its pair who did receive vaccine, or vice versa. Pairing means that individuals from the cases and the controls are compared pair by pair. Statistical tests for matched data are applicable only to this special type of matching called pairing. The formula for an odds ratio in this situation is: c/b = 15/5 = 3 (p <.05). This indicates that the study found a 3-fold increase in vaccination among those without pneumococcal bacteremia compared to paired individuals with pneumococcal bacteremia. The odds ratio can be used as an estimate of the relative risk or protective efficacy ratio. This odds ratio is consistent with the protective effect of vaccination found among the South African miners.

A study of the effectiveness of the 14-valent pneumococcal vaccine against pneumococcal pneumonia and pneumococcal bronchitis in a United States population was conducted as a Veterans Administration cooperative study [5]. The investigators randomized 2295 individuals who were older than 55 years and had one or more of the following potential indications for pneumococcal vaccine: chronic renal, hepatic, cardiac, or pulmonary disease, alcoholism, or diabetes mellitus. The study was designed to include enough individuals to assess whether the pneumococcal vaccine was capable of providing protection against pneumococcal pneumonia and bronchitis in these high-risk individuals.

The Veterans Administration study did not require bacteremia to establish a probable pneumococcal infection [5]. A probable pneumococcal pneumonia was defined as the presence of clinical and roentgenographic features of pneumonia in association with the recovery of *Streptococcus pneumoniae* from sputum. The sputum was required to contain more than 25 white cells and fewer than 10 epithelial cells per 100-power field, with gram-positive diplococci predominating. In addition, the clinical and roentgenographic evaluation must have shown a response to antibiotic therapy.

The investigators followed patients for an average of nearly 3 years. Among the vaccine recipients, they found a total of 28 pneumococcal infections in the placebo group and 43 pneumococcal infections in the vaccine group. This difference in the direction opposite the hypothesized effectiveness of the vaccine was not statistically significant. They also found that a majority of the vaccine recipients who subsequently developed pneumococcal infection did not obtain or sustain a substantial rise in serum antibody to the infectious pneumococcal subtype associated with the infection.

_____ STUDY QUESTION 9-8
How can you reconcile the findings of this controlled clinical trial with the previously cited case-control study?

CENTERS FOR DISEASE CONTROL RECOMMENDATIONS
Prior to the publication of the VA study, the Centers for Disease Control (CDC) [6] made recommendations for the use of pneumococcal vaccine. Their indications included adults with chronic illnesses that predispose to pneumococcal infections, such as cardiovascular disease, chronic pulmonary disease, cirrhosis, and renal failure.

_____ STUDY QUESTION 9-9
What do you think about this recommendation in light of the Veterans Administration study [5]?

The CDC also recommended pneumococcal vaccination for adults with immunosuppressive disease, such as Hodgkin's disease and multiple myeloma, as well as sickle-cell patients and others with splenic dysfunction.

_____ STUDY QUESTION 9-10
What else would you like to know about the efficacy of the pneumococcal vaccine for those with immunosuppressive disease or immune dysfunction?

BALANCING BENEFITS AND RISKS
It is important to balance the benefits of therapy against the risk. In a controlled clinical trial, it is difficult to evaluate the risks of therapy since only a limited number of individuals receive the vaccine. Thus, one cannot expect to identify rare but serious side effects of the vaccine. The rule of three provides a guide to how much information on safety can be obtained from a controlled clinical trial. If 1500 individuals receive the vaccine and no one develops a serious side effect, then one can be 95 percent confident that a serious side effect will occur no more frequently than once in 500 cases.

The safety of a therapy requires additional evaluation after it has been employed in practice. Data are available based on the first 4 million uses of the vaccine. Approximately 5 of every 100 vaccinees develop fever, and approximately 1 per 100,000 vaccinees develop severe generalized symptoms that are self-limited. Three cases of anaphylaxis have been reported. The Food and Drug Administration, which is responsible for monitoring side effects, reports that Guillain-Barré syndrome has rarely been reported in temporal association with pneumococcal vaccine but that no cause and effect relationship has been established [7].

_____ STUDY QUESTION 9-11
Assume that pneumococcal vaccine is very effective against the development of pneumococcal bacteremia but that it is not effective in preventing the primary bronchitis or pneumonia. How would that affect your use of the vaccine?

Cost Effectiveness
The CDC has also recommended use of pneumococcal vaccine for healthy individuals aged 65 years or older who do not have any special risk factors for pneumococcal disease or its complications. Those older than 65 are believed to have a 2-fold increase in the incidence of pneumococcal disease and have several times the risk of death if they do develop pneumococcal pneumonia. They are also believed to be generally capable of providing an adequate antibody response to the vaccine. This population includes more than 25 million Americans and thus represents by far the largest high-risk group. In 1979, Congress approved coverage for pneumococcal vaccine under Medicare. This is the only vaccine for which Medicare will reimburse. While approval for pneumococcal vaccine reimbursement was pending, Congress requested that the Congressional Office of Technology Assessment (OTA) perform a cost-effectiveness analysis of pneumococcal vaccine [8]. In 1984, OTA updated this analysis [9]. Let us look at how OTA went about performing a cost-effectiveness analysis, the assumptions they made, and the conclusions they reached.

OTA's cost-effectiveness analysis was done from the viewpoint of the Medicare program. It took into account the immediate costs and benefits of administration of the vaccine. However, since it was concerned with the long-term implications for the Medicare program, it also took into account the costs of treating future illness among those whose lives are prolonged as a result of vaccination (Ci). When considering effectiveness, it took into account the fact that elderly persons are likely to develop other diseases even if they escape the consequences of pneumococcal disease. Thus, they subtracted from the effectiveness the morbidity from future illnesses among vaccinees whose lives are prolonged as a result of vaccination (Ei).

In developing its cost-effectiveness analysis, OTA used the following formula:

$$\frac{\text{Net medical costs (dollars)}}{\text{Net health effects (years of healthy life)}} = \frac{(Cp + Cse) - Ct + Ci}{(Ely + Em) - Ese - Ei}$$

where Cp = cost of preventive vaccination

Cse = cost of treating vaccinees' side effects

Ct = cost of treating pneumococcal pneumonia prevented by vaccination

Ci = cost of treating other future illness not prevented by vaccination among patients whose lives are prolonged as a result of vaccinations

Ely = years gained from vaccination

Em = quality-adjusted life years (QALY) of morbidity prevented by vaccination

ESE = QALY of morbidity and mortality associated with vaccinee's side effects

Ei = QALY of morbidity from future illness not prevented by vaccination among vaccinees whose lives are prolonged as a result of vaccination

OTA also used available clinical and economic literature to make educated guesses for each of these variables. These were included in their "base case" estimates. Because of the uncertainty inherent in most of these estimates, the OTA group also made low and high case estimates, reflecting reasonable guesses about the possible inaccuracy of their base case estimates. This allowed the group to perform sensitivity analyses to see how dependent OTA's conclusions were on changes or inaccuracies in any of the estimates. Among the base case assumptions made in the OTA update report are the following:

1. The incidence of pneumococcal pneumonia is approximately 2.2 cases per 1000 per year.

2. Seventy-five percent of pneumococcal pneumonia is caused by sub-types included in the vaccine.
3. The vaccine has an 80-percent efficacy against disease caused by sub-types included in the vaccine.
4. Vaccine side effects include 1 case of severe systemic reaction per 100,000 vaccinates and 5 cases of fever per 100 vaccinates.
5. A year of healthy life is valued at 1, compared to 0.4 for bed disability and 0.6 for non–bed disability, whereas death is valued at 0.
6. The average duration of immunity for the elderly is 8 years.

Given these and a series of economic assumptions, OTA's initial cost-effective analysis, based on the base case estimate, found that administration of the pneumococcal vaccine to the healthy elderly would actually be cost saving. That is, the saving in medical care costs to the Medicare program would more than offset the costs of administering the vaccine and treating the side effects of the vaccine, even taking into account the later need to treat those kept alive.

The sensitivity analysis performed by OTA sheds additional light on the issue of cost effectiveness. The OTA study assumed that a vaccine effective against pneumococcal bacteremia would be effective against pneumococcal pneumonia. OTA then performed a sensitivity analysis to see how the results might differ if the true incidence of pneumococcal pneumonia was lower. It also studied the effect on the results if the duration of immunity was not as long as originally estimated.

The OTA update report calculated the cost of a quality-adjusted life year (life at full health) if one assumes that (1) the incidence of pneumococcal pneumonia among the elderly is only 1.4 cases per 1000 per year (rather than 2.2 cases per 1000 per year), and (2) the average duration of immunity is only 3 years (rather than 8 years). Taking into account both these new assumptions, OTA found that the net cost per quality-adjusted life year gained was approximately $6000.

_____ STUDY QUESTION 9-12
What is the meaning of a quality-adjusted life year gained?

_____ STUDY QUESTION 9-13
The OTA data assumed that the pneumococcal vaccine was effective against pneumococcal pneumonia and not just against pneumococcal bacteremia. If one concludes from the Veterans Administration cooperative study [5] that the vaccine is only effective in preventing bacteremia, how would this effect alter the cost-effectiveness analysis?

———————————————————————————— STUDY QUESTION 9-14
(a) If the net cost per healthy year gained is $6000, should pneumococcal vaccine
be recommended for all healthy elderly persons? (b) What if the net cost per
healthy year gained is $50,000, or $500,000?

References

1. Austrian R, Douglas RM, Schiffman C, et al. Prevention of pneumococcal
   pneumonia by vaccination. Trans Assoc Am Physicians. 1976;89:184–194.
2. Mufson MA, Oley G, Hogney D. Pneumococcal disease in a medium-sized
   community in the United States. JAMA 1982;248:1416–1419.
3. Felice GA, Darby CP, Fraser DW. Pneumococcal bacteremia in Charleston
   County, S.C. Am J Epidemiol 1980;112:828–35.
4. Shapiro ED, Clemens ED. A controlled evaluation of the protective efficacy
   of pneumococcal vaccine for patients at high risk for serious pneumococcal
   infections. Ann Intern Med 1984;101:325–330.
5. Simberkoff MS, Cross AP, Al-Ibrahim M. Efficacy of pneumococcal vaccine
   in high risk patients: results of a Veterans Administration cooperative study.
   N Engl J Med 1986;315:1318–1327.
6. Centers for Disease Control. Update: pneumococcal polysaccharide vaccine
   usage—United States: recommendations of the Immunization Practices Advisory Committee. MMWR 1984;33:273–281.
7. Schwartz JS. Pneumococcal vaccine: clinical efficacy and effectiveness. Ann
   Intern Med 1982;96:208–220.
8. U.S. Congress, Office of Technology Assessment. A review of selected federal
   vaccine and immunization policies. Washington, D.C.: Government Printing
   Office, 1979.
9. U.S. Congress, Office of Technology Assessment. Update of federal activities
   regarding the use of pneumococcal vaccine. Washington, D.C.: Government
   Printing Office, 1984.

Asbestos

CHAPTER TEN

EVE BARGMANN

At first, Mrs. A.* thought she had pulled a muscle. The brief dull pain gripped her right side as she carried a load of laundry up from the basement. When she stopped to rest for a moment and her breathing slowed down, the pain subsided.

She thought no more of it, or at least she tried not to think about it. It was hard not to notice, as it seemed to be a stubborn injury, hurting even more after 2 weeks had passed. As she reached over to unlock the car door when she picked her son up from school, she turned her face away involuntarily so he would not see her wince.

It wasn't clear what came next. Before she was even conscious of her short-windedness, she may have been aware of the ache of fear in her stomach. She paused halfway up the stairs from the basement and remembered her father.

Her father had paused in this same way, first after a flight of stairs, then after walking from the car to the house. For many years his doctor had told him to stop smoking; and he nodded, mainly to humor the doctor, and continued to buy his cigarettes as before. Smoking was the manly thing to do, and he wasn't going to give it up easily, least of all when giving it up meant admitting that he was sick. A year later, he was dead. He had spent his last month in the hospital, a frail skeleton of a man, wearing a blank face to hide his pain.

It was her father that Mrs. A. remembered as she paused on the stairs. Not until later, when the pain gnawing at her side had grown more intense and more insistent, did she think about her mother.

Mrs. A.'s mother did not smoke. In fact, she quietly disapproved of her husband's smoking and made rather too much of a show of cleaning the ashtrays. Mrs. A.'s mother was a neat woman, and she kept a neat house, which was no mean feat. Her husband was a pipe insulator at a shipyard. When he walked home after work, his clothing gave off little sprays of white dust with every step he took. On warm days, his wife greeted him outside the front door with a brush. On cold days, she took him downstairs into the laundry room, where he nearly disappeared into great white clouds of dust as she brushed down his work clothes.

No one was entirely surprised when Mrs. A.'s father died of lung cancer, but when Mrs. A.'s mother began to suffer from chest pain and shortness of breath years later, cancer was the last thing on anyone's mind. Her doctor treated her for pneumonia and drew large volumes of fluid from outside her lung, first with a needle and then with a chest tube. But the fluid kept coming back, and the shadows grew outside her lung.

Mrs. A.'s mother had mesothelioma—cancer of the pleura—a cancer so rare as to be almost unheard of except after asbestos exposure. She had never worked

---

*This is a fictionalization of an actual case. It is an unusual case, as most mesothelioma patients do not have a family member with mesothelioma.

outside the home; her only asbestos exposure had been outside the front door and downstairs in the laundry room, surrounded by clouds of white asbestos dust. The doctors could do nothing. She was dead in 6 months.

At first, Mrs. A.'s doctor could not believe the roentgenogram. He repeated it to make sure. Then he went to the hospital to look at her chest roentgenogram from 5 years before, to confirm that it had really been normal. He went over her history in detail. Had she worked at the shipyard, insulated her house, done any work on the plumbing? No, she was a housewife. She had helped her mother in the laundry room, shaking out her father's clothes that were still laden with dust.

Less than 1 year later, Mrs. A. was dead. The autopsy confirmed her doctor's diagnosis: Asbestos fibers filled her lungs, and her right lung was squeezed in the grasp of a massive mesothelioma.

You are a doctor in Mrs. A.'s community. Mrs. A. was your patient. Her tragedy, an extreme among those of asbestos victims, is one you won't easily forget. Among your patients now are many who have worked or who continue to work with asbestos. Which patients are at risk? How great is their risk? What can you do to protect them? To find out more, you go to the literature. You will try to determine (1) which workers are, or have been, exposed to asbestos, and for what diseases they are at risk as a result; (2) how great their risk is; (3) how you can help those who have already been exposed; and (4) what you can do to help those who are still working with asbestos.

Asbestos-Associated Disease: Who Is at Risk? What Can Happen?

Between 8 and 11 million people in the United States have been exposed to asbestos since 1940, 4 to 5 million of them in shipyards during World War II [1]. More than 375,000 workers currently are exposed to substantial levels of asbestos [2].

Asbestos insulation workers are by no means the only persons exposed. Asbestos miners and workers in manufacturing plants—plants that make asbestos products, including tiles, insulation, gaskets, and cement—handle the fibers daily. Automobile repairmen doing frequent brake repairs inhale asbestos dust from brake shoes. Construction and maintenance workers, especially those who install and repair asbestos-containing pipes and insulation and those involved in demolition of buildings, face considerable asbestos exposure. Shipbuilders and ship repairmen are likewise exposed [2].

Asbestos-associated disease has appeared not only in heavily exposed workers but also in those who had short-term exposure to the fibers many years ago. Shipbuilders during World War II, who often worked with asbestos for only one or a few months, are a classic example.

Asbestos exposure has been associated with a variety of diseases. Nonmalignant asbestos-associated diseases include the following:

Pleural plaques, which appear 20 or more years after exposure begins and do not cause symptoms.

Pleural fibrosis (far less common than plaques), which can cause pain, pleural effusions, dyspnea, and cor pulmonale.

Exudative pleural effusion, with pleuritic chest pain, which can appear within 10 years after exposure begins.

Asbestosis (progressive pulmonary fibrosis), which develops 20 or more years after asbestos exposure begins. Although it can be severe and disabling, it is not the primary cause of death.

Malignant asbestos-associated diseases include mesothelioma, bronchogenic carcinoma, and gastrointestinal cancers. Gastrointestinal cancers have been found to occur more commonly in asbestos-exposed workers than in the U.S. population as a whole. Although the increase in gastrointestinal cancers in these studies is less than 2-fold, they are fairly common cancers, so this increased risk could account for a substantial number of asbestos-associated deaths. Because more studies have looked at mesothelioma and bronchogenic cancer, the discussion in this chapter will focus on these.

The latency period of mesothelioma is long. It appears 25 or more years after asbestos exposure (Fig. 10-1) [3]. No effective treatment exists for this cancer, and patients die within a few months to a few years of diagnosis. From this disease, we know that asbestos exposure has not always stopped at the work place as mesothelioma has been found not only in workers but also in their wives and children [4]. Mesothelioma bears no relationship to cigarette smoking. Smokers and nonsmokers are equally at risk.

Bronchogenic Cancer: How Great Is the Risk?

Much of the controversy surrounding asbestos exposure has centered on its relationship to bronchogenic cancer. Bronchogenic cancer is the

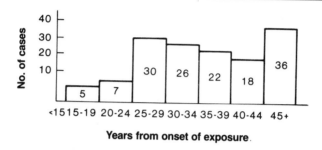

Fig. 10-1. Years from asbestos exposure to death from pleural or peritoneal mesothelioma. (Adapted from Selikoff [3].)

number one killer among asbestos-associated diseases. Its latency period, like mesothelioma's, is long; lung cancer rarely appears less than 15 years after onset of exposure and it may follow exposure by more than 40 years. In general, the lower the exposure, the longer the latency period [5].

As you know, the only way to establish causation definitively is with a well-designed randomized controlled trial. However, for suspected hazards, such a study is ethically out of the question. The next alternative is a cohort or prospective study, which will help you to determine that an association exists and that cause precedes effect, the first two criteria for establishing contributory cause.

Dr. Irving Selikoff [6] has followed 17,000 asbestos insulation workers, of whom 12,051 were first exposed to asbestos 20 or more years before the study began. During an average of 6.4 years of follow-up, 450 men in this group died of lung cancer. Deaths from lung cancer were expected to total 81.7.

_____ STUDY QUESTION 10-1
The mortality ratio in a study like the one just summarized can be used as an estimate of relative risk. What is the mortality ratio from lung cancer among these asbestos workers compared to unexposed persons?

Table 10-1 provides the death rates and mortality ratios from lung cancer with respect to cigarette smoking (the other major risk factor for

Table 10-1. Age-standardized death rates for lung
cancer associated with smoking and asbestos exposure

Group	Death rate	Mortality difference	Mortality ratio
Nonsmokers, unexposed	11.3	0.0	1.00
Nonsmokers, asbestos workers	58.4	+47.1	5.17
Smokers, unexposed	122.6	+111.3	10.85
Smokers, asbestos workers	601.6	+590.3	53.24

Source: Data from Hammond and colleagues [7].

lung cancer) and asbestos exposure, standardizing for age because lung
cancer is age-related.

STUDY QUESTION 10-2

What does Table 10-1 tell you about the numerical interaction of cigarette smoking and asbestos exposure?

The mortality ratio from Selikoff's data [6] approximates the relative
risk: 1.00 is the risk in nonsmokers not exposed to asbestos. By reading
the study report more closely, you discover that 97.5 percent of these
workers were current or past cigarette smokers (all included in the smokers category). Using this information, you can calculate the attributable
risk for asbestos exposure, which determines how much of the lung cancer in this group of asbestos workers can be attributed to their asbestos
exposure. Remember that

$$\text{Attributable risk} = \frac{\begin{array}{c}\text{incidence of an event} \\ \text{or disease among those} \\ \text{with the risk factor}\end{array} - \begin{array}{c}\text{incidence of the event} \\ \text{or disease among those} \\ \text{without the risk factor}\end{array}}{\begin{array}{c}\text{incidence of the disease among those} \\ \text{with the risk factor}\end{array}}$$

The event here is death from lung cancer. Table 10-1 gives age-standardized death rates per 100,000 person-years of follow-up. Knowing
that 97.5 percent of your population smokes or has smoked, you can
come to a reasonable approximation by looking at the figures for smokers only.

Attributable risk

$$= \frac{\begin{matrix}\text{death rate of smoking} \\ \text{asbestos workers}\end{matrix} - \begin{matrix}\text{death rate of smoking} \\ \text{unexposed men}\end{matrix}}{\text{death rate of smoking asbestos workers}} = \frac{601.6 - 122.6}{601.6} = 79.6\%$$

Aha! you say. Eighty percent of their lung cancers were caused entirely by asbestos! But this conclusion is wrong. The attributable risk tells you only the maximum proportion of their lung cancer deaths that might have been prevented by removing this single risk factor. This will make more sense if you ask: In this same group of asbestos workers, what is the attributable risk from cigarette smoking? That is, what percentage of lung cancer deaths could you potentially prevent if you eliminated cigarette smoking entirely without altering asbestos exposure? The attributable risk for the group of smokers who work with asbestos is as follows:

$$\text{Attributable risk} = \frac{\begin{matrix}\text{death rate of} \\ \text{smoking asbestos} \\ \text{workers}\end{matrix} - \begin{matrix}\text{death rate of} \\ \text{nonsmoking asbestos} \\ \text{workers}\end{matrix}}{\text{death rate of smoking asbestos workers}}$$

$$= \frac{601.6 - 58.4}{601.6} = 90.3\%$$

Keep in mind, though, that smokers make up 97.5 percent of your exposed population, and this attributable risk applies only to them. The 2.5 percent of people who do not smoke will not have any lung cancers attributable to smoking. Thus, the attributable risk from cigarette smoking among those asbestos workers who smoke is approximately 90 percent.

_____ STUDY QUESTION 10-3
What percentage of lung cancer deaths could you potentially prevent in this asbestos-exposed population if you could eliminate both smoking and asbestos exposure?

How Can You Help People Who Have Been Exposed in the Past?
CLINICAL INVESTIGATION AND CASE FINDING
Case finding means obtaining careful occupational histories from patients, keeping in mind that work place carcinogens such as asbestos do

their damage 15, 25, 35, or more years after exposure begins. Discovering work place carcinogens often depends on exceptionally alert clinicians, such as the ones who first reported cases of asbestosis and lung cancer in 1935, or on very unusual diseases, such as mesothelioma. Both patients and doctors need to know about past exposures, so that they can watch for early illness and avoid doing more damage. For people exposed to asbestos only in the past, avoiding damage means avoiding other lung carcinogens: Above all, smoking is absolutely taboo.

COMMUNITY EDUCATION

Physicians can play an active role in community education by publicizing the risk of asbestos exposure and pinpointing the sites where workers have been exposed. This allows many people at risk to discover this fact for themselves.

COMPENSATION

Patients with cancer have vast medical bills and generally are unable to support themselves or their families. Will you encourage them to seek legal help? You may want to think about the following questions:

1. *Who is responsible* for the injuries? Table 10-2 suggests that industries and government agencies knew of the risk well before they acted to reduce it. On the other hand, do workers share responsibility if they continued to smoke cigarettes well after the United States Surgeon General's report was published?

2. *Who benefits* from the production and use of asbestos? Certainly the asbestos industry stands to benefit, as do industries that use asbestos, including builders who use it for insulation and automobile makers who use it for brake linings. Workers benefit by having jobs. Society at large also benefits, if there are no better alternatives, as it has gaskets for its machinery and brake linings to stop its cars.

3. *Who should pay?* Should it be all those who benefit from asbestos, or only those who knew or should have known of the risk, could have prevented further harm, and did not? Should the workers who become sick have to bear all or part of the cost, or should only workers who smoke have to pay? To answer these questions, you need to consider more than attributable risk; these are not merely practical decisions but also moral choices.

4. *How effective are compensation systems?* Consider that one study looked at the effectiveness of state workmen's compensation systems in

Table 10-2. Chronology of scientific, industrial, and government action on asbestos

Scientific	Industry	Government
1906: First documented death from asbestosis [8] 1928–29: Twelve articles on asbestosis in British literature 1933: First report of lung cancer and asbestosis [9]		
	1935: Industry-sponsored Lanza study finds asbestosis in 53% of workers [10]	
		1938: U.S. Public Health Service recommends 5 mppcf (approximately 30 f/cc) as voluntary standard
1943: First report links asbestos to mesothelioma [11] 1946: JAMA article lists asbestos as a cause of lung cancer [12]		
	1949–50: Schepers compiles cases of cancer and mesothelioma in Canadian asbestos workers. Johns Manville (a major U.S. and Canada asbestos manufacturer) asks him to suppress the report	
1955: Doll report finds 10-fold increase in lung cancer in asbestos workers [13] 1964: Selikoff finds lung cancer, mesothelioma, and gastrointestinal cancer in asbestos workers [14]		

1971: OSHA is created and issues 5-f/c emergency standard
1972: OSHA rules that by 1976 standard will be 2 f/cc
1976: New standard—2 f/cc—in effect
1983: OSHA issues 0.5-f/cc emergency temporary standard

1972: Industry groups oppose OSHA standard, saying 2 f/cc "unreasonable," "would force us out of business"
1982: Johns Manville files for bankruptcy over workers' asbestos suits
1983: Johns Manville sues United States government over payment to workers with asbestos suits. Asbestos Information Association sues OSHA over emergency standard

mppcf = millions of particles per cubic foot of air; f/cc = fibers per cubic centimeter.

helping asbestos victims. Only 33 percent of injured workers filed work-men's compensation claims, and only 15 percent received any benefits prior to death [2]. An alternative route is litigation, but this too has its drawbacks. A recent study showed that companies spent so much on fighting these lawsuits and plaintiffs' lawyers fees were so great that, in total $3.40 went to legal fees for every $1.00 that went to asbestos victims.

How Can We Protect Workers Now?
To what extent can or should we protect workers now from further risk of illness? To answer this question, we need to decide (1) whether a dose-response relationship exists that will help us estimate workers' risks at various levels of exposure; (2) how much of a risk we can, morally or legally, ask workers to accept; and (3) what options are available—tech-nically, socially, and individually—to help potentially exposed workers.

IS THERE A DOSE-RESPONSE RELATIONSHIP?
We ask about dose-response relationships because, in part, such a rela-tionship fulfills an ancillary criterion for establishing contributory cause. When we are trying to make small- and large-scale decisions about pro-tecting workers, we want to try to define and quantify, even if roughly, the risk that various levels of exposure poses to workers.

In an attempt to arrive at a dose-response curve for various cancers related to asbestos, the U.S. Occupational Safety and Health Administra-tion (OSHA) has analyzed the findings of 11 different studies of lung cancer in asbestos workers and 4 studies of mesothelioma [2]. Each study was entirely independent, conducted by different investigators in differ-ent work places. Let's look at a few of the studies.

Table 10-3 shows the ratio of observed to expected deaths from lung cancer (expressed as the percentage of men who would have been ex-pected to die of lung cancer) in 820 men followed for up to 35 years from the onset of exposure to asbestos in a factory [5]. The longer they worked in the factory, the greater the relative risk. Exposure was esti-mated by the number of asbestos fibers per milliliter of air (also called fibers per cubic centimeter, or f/cc) multiplied by the number of years worked.

Table 10-4 shows the ratio of observed to expected deaths from respi-ratory cancer for a group of production and maintenance employees of

Table 10-3. Observed and expected lung cancer death
5 to 35 years after onset of exposure in an Amosite factory

No. of months of exposure	Average no. of years of exposure	Estimated average dose (f/cc-yr)	Expected % deaths	Observed % deaths	Mortality ratio
<1	0.04	1.4	2.95	6.07	2.06
1–2	0.09	3.2	2.70	7.34	2.72
2–3	0.17	5.9	2.79	7.42	2.66
4–6	0.29	10.2	2.47	5.90	2.38
6–12	0.59	20.5	2.15	10.21	4.74
12–24	1.28	44.8	2.02	12.41	6.14
25+	4.77	166.9	2.34	18.51	7.91

f/cc = fibers per cubic centimeter.
Source: Data from Seidman et al. [5].

Table 10-4. Deaths from respiratory cancer in 1075 men
retired from an asbestos company 1941–67, followed through 1973

Total exposure (mppcf-yr)	Average exposure (mppcf-yr)	Observed no. of deaths	Expected no. of deaths	Mortality ratio
<125	62	19	9.6	1.98
125–249	182	9	5.0	1.80
250–499	352	19	5.8	3.28
500–749	606	9	2.0	4.50
750+	976	7	0.9	7.78

mppcf = millions of particles per cubic foot of air.
Source: Data from Henderson and Enterline [15].

an asbestos company [15]. Exposure here is estimated in millions of particles per cubic foot of air (mppcf) multiplied by years. This measurement can only be loosely translated into fibers per cubic centimeter; for asbestos textiles, for instance, 1 mppcf equals somewhere between 1 and 6 f/cc.

Both studies do find a dose-response relationship between asbestos exposure and lung cancer death. Combining these studies, along with nine others of lung cancer and four of mesothelioma, into a single risk estimate will introduce some predictable imprecision. The individual studies could be critiqued on the basis of:

Data reliability: How accurate are the exposure figures?

Confounding variables: Mortality rates in each study were compared to expected figures. Were these corrected for employment status? For smoking history?

Follow-up: For how long after exposure were subjects followed? Because of the lung latency of occupational cancer, follow-up should continue for decades. How many workers were lost to follow-up? Why?

When you combine the studies, even more critiques are possible. Should you give more weight to better-designed studies? Should you combine exposure to different forms of asbestos, when asbestos could be more dangerous in some forms than in others?

Despite the limitations inherent in a single dose-response estimate, such a figure is undeniably helpful for policy decisions. Therefore, OSHA combined the studies and determined a best estimate of the dose-response relationship. In its estimate, OSHA assumed that the relationship was linear. Estimates often assume a relationship is linear for the sake of simplicity and because data may fit such a line fairly well. At lower exposure levels, the actual risk may be greater or less. If the curve is linear, the number of excess deaths is the same for 1000 workers exposed for 45 years as for 10,000 workers exposed for 4.5 years (Table 10-5).

OSHA estimated in 1983 that workers were being exposed to average levels of up to 2 fibers per cubic centimeter, with occasional exposures of up to 20 fibers per cubic centimeter [2]. If all exposures could be reduced from these varying levels to 0.1 fibers per cubic centimeter for the entire exposed work force of 375,000 persons, OSHA estimated that 9162 cancer deaths would be prevented. Assuming these estimates are reasonable, a new standard at this level would thus prevent approximately 25 cancer deaths for every 1000 workers exposed for a 45-year working lifetime.

HOW MUCH RISK TO WORKERS IS ACCEPTABLE?
When the U.S. Congress created OSHA, it gave this agency an explicit legal duty: to set standards "to assure, so far as possible, safe and health-

Table 10-5. Excess cancer deaths per 100,000 workers exposed to asbestos

Type of cancer	Level of exposure (f/cc) over 45 years				
	0.1	0.2	0.5	2.0	5.0
Lung cancer	231	460	1143	4416	10,318
Mesothelioma	82	162	447	1554	3547
Gastrointestinal cancer	23	46	114	442	1032
Total cancer	336	668	1704	6412	14,897

f/cc = fibers per cubic centimeter.
Source: Data from OSHA [2].

ful working conditions for every American worker over the period of his or her working lifetime."

A recent Supreme Court decision about another occupational hazard, benzene, provided one example of the type of work place risks that the Court considers great enough to warrant regulatory action. The Court wrote: "If the odds are one in a thousand that regular inhalation of gasoline vapors that are 2% benzene will be fatal, a reasonable person might well consider the risk significant and take the appropriate steps to decrease or eliminate it" [16]. This sets at least an upper limit of a legally acceptable work place risk: A 1 in 1000 risk of predictable death is too high. The morally acceptable risk is a different matter; the Supreme Court rules on laws, not morality.

OSHA's risk assessment roughly estimates that 25 cancer deaths per 1000 workers exposed for a working lifetime could be prevented by lowering (not eliminating) asbestos exposure from current levels.

_____ STUDY QUESTION 10-4
Do you think this meets the Supreme Court's definition of a risk that calls for action?

What constitutes a morally acceptable risk is different here than for other cases in this book. We allow people to take a substantial risk for themselves only, whether they are smoking or skydiving, because we value free choice, but we restrict people's freedom to subject others to risks by, for instance, forbidding automobile companies to sell manifestly unsafe cars and air traffic controllers to work if they are drunk. A

worker may be free to choose to take risks, but a company is not necessarily free to force its workers to take risks.

Can we allow workers to choose risky occupations? Not always. To pick
an extreme case, we will not allow people to commit suicide, no matter
how well they are paid. However, even in ordinary situations, most workers have a limited selection of jobs. If their community's major employer
is an asbestos industry, they can either take the risk or have no job. Moreover, the vast majority of workers do not have enough knowledge about
work place hazards to make an informed choice. Under these conditions, allowing work places to be unsafe will limit, rather than increase,
workers' choices.

HOW WELL, AND IN WHAT WAY, CAN WORKERS BE PROTECTED?
Prevention of asbestos-related illness and death depends on reducing or
eliminating worker exposure to asbestos. You can approach this problem
from several different angles: by asking about technical options (what is
possible?), policy options (what should society as a whole do?), and individual physicians' options (what should I do?).

Technical Options
To reduce or eliminate workers' exposure to asbestos, you could make a
number of changes. These include (1) banning the use of asbestos in any
form; (2) using engineering controls to reduce substantially the concentration of asbestos in work place air; and (3) requiring workers to wear
protective equipment, including rubber air-filtering masks called
respirators.

_____ STUDY QUESTION 10-5
What are the pros and cons of each method? Consider practical and ethical issues as well as cost.

Policy Options
Given that it is technically feasible to reduce work place asbestos exposure substantially, we still need to determine the best way to bring about
a reduction in exposure. Here are some alternatives:

1. *Individual action only*: Such a method leaves work place controls up to
   the preference of the companies and individual protection up to the

worker. Neither government agencies nor the courts intervene to protect workers.

2. *Compensation and individual litigation*: Through these, workers injured by work place hazards can appeal to state workmen's compensation systems or bring lawsuits after they become ill. Only the courts intervene; no laws or regulations act to prevent injury or illness.

3. *Group action and litigation*: Unions, other workers' groups, or public interest groups may negotiate, bring lawsuits, or both to make work places safer and to compensate workers who have already been endangered or injured.

4. *Regulation*: Laws or regulations can compel industries to reduce or eliminate workers' exposure to asbestos.

_____ STUDY QUESTION 10-6
What are the pros and cons of each strategy? Consider practical and ethical issues as well as cost.

Individual Physicians' Options
As an individual physician, you can choose not to act at all. If you do choose to act, you can potentially play a role in each of the previously mentioned strategies.

_____ STUDY QUESTION 10-7
What can you as an individual physician do to prevent asbestos-related illness and death?

References

1. Fontana RS. Lung cancer and asbestos-related pulmonary disease. Chicago: American College of Chest Physicians, 1981:23–24,34.
2. OSHA. Occupational exposure to asbestos. The Federal Register 1984 Apr 10;49(70):14133, 14134, 14137.
3. Selikoff IJ, Cancer risk of asbestos exposure. In: Hiatt HH, et al, eds. Origins of human cancer. Cold Spring Harbor: Cold Spring Harbor Laboratory, 1977:1764–1784.
4. Vianna NJ, Polan AK. Non-occupational exposure to asbestos and malignant mesothelioma in females. Lancet 1978;1:1061–1063.
5. Seidman H, Selikoff IJ, Hammond EC. Short-term asbestos exposure and long-term observation. Ann NY Acad Sci 1979;330:61–89.
6. Selikoff IJ, Hammond EC, Seidman H. Mortality experience of insulation

workers in the United States and Canada, 1943–1976. Ann NY Acad Sci 1979;330:91–116.

7. Hammond EC, Selikoff IJ, Seidman H. Asbestos exposure, cigarette smoking and death rates. Ann NY Acad Sci 1979;330:473–490.

8. Murray HM. Departmental Committee on Compensation for Industrial Disease minutes of evidence. Appendices and index. London: Wyman and Sons, 1907:127–128.

9. Gloyne SR. The morbid anatomy and histology of asbestosis. Tubercle 1933;14:550–558.

10. Lanza A. Effects of asbestos dust on the lung. Pub Health Rep 1935;50:1.

11. Wedler HW. Asbestose and Lungenkrebs. Bull Hyg 1944;19:362.

12. Hueper WC. Industrial management and occupational cancer. JAMA 1946;131:738–741.

13. Doll RL. Mortality from lung cancer in asbestos workers. Br J Ind Med 1955;12:81–86.

14. Selikoff IJ, Hammond EC, Churg, J. Asbestos exposure and neoplasia. JAMA 1964;188:22–26.

15. Henderson VL, Enterline PE. Asbestos exposure: factors associated with excess cancer and respiratory disease mortality. Ann NY Acad Sci 1979;330:117–126.

16. Industrial Union Department. AFL-CIO. American Petroleum Institute. 488 U.S. 601, 65 L. Ed. 2d 1010, 100 Sup. Ct. 2844 (1980) at 655.

Child Restraints

CHAPTER ELEVEN

TEEKIE WAGNER
MARK I. WEISSMAN

Jamie, a 3-year-old white boy, was admitted to a hospital's intensive care unit with head trauma suffered in an automobile crash. Jamie was riding in the front seat, unsecured by a lap belt or child restraint, when the car his mother was driving was struck head on. Both cars were traveling at 30 to 35 miles per hour (mph) at the time of the frontal collision. Jamie never regained consciousness and died 60 days later. His mother and two siblings, who were unbuckled in the back seat, received minor injuries.

What were the chances that Jamie would die in an automobile crash? The greatest risk of death or brain damage to a healthy 3-year-old child is the automobile. As a matter of fact, the number one cause of death in every pediatric age group beyond the neonatal period is motor vehicle crashes (MVCs). Approximately 4500 children younger than 14 years old are killed each year in the United States in automobile crashes, compared with the number two killer, cancer, which claims approximately 2500 victims per year [1]. (Table 11-1, Fig. 11-1).

_____ STUDY QUESTION 11-1

(a) Who is at greater risk of death from automobile accidents, the young or the old? (b) Which group (young or old) had the greater number of years of life lost from accidents?

To Buckle Up or Not to Buckle Up

Was Jamie's death preventable? Under what conditions do 3-year-olds die in automobile crashes? Dr. Robert Scherz [3], by reviewing in detail fatalities in the years 1977, 1978, and 1979, developed an epidemiologic profile of the under-4-year-old MVC victim. He found that children less than 4 years of age are killed during the day (8 AM to 3 PM), in good weather conditions, and at low speeds (less than 40 mph), and that such accidents are unrelated to alcohol, whereas teenagers and adults die at night, at high speed, and alcohol often is associated. Scherz's profile [3] of fatal motor vehicle accidents involving children in Washington state from 1977 through 1979 may be summarized as follows:

Vehicles involved

Family car and another motor vehicle

Neither with significant mechanical defects

Table 11-1. Death rates from accidents per 100,000 population

Age (yr)	Death rate per 100,000		Proportionate mortality for accidents (%)
	All causes	Automobile accidents	
1–14	70	28.2	40.0
65–74	3190	65.5	2.1

Source: From the National Center for Health Statistics [2].

Driver
    Mother or father
    Had not been drinking
    Was not using a seat belt
Child riding unrestrained in front seat
Accident conditions
    Low speed (<65 kilometers per hour or 40 mph)
    State route
    Near home
    Daylight (between 8 AM and 3 PM)
    Dry weather

This epidemiologic profile is consistent with the testing of child restraint systems at 35 mph required by the National Highway Traffic Safety Administration (NHTSA). NHTSA has required dynamic testing of child restraints since 1978. The dynamic testing involves a simulated crash test at 35 mph using a doll or dummy. Each child restraint must pass this test to be approved and, thus, allowed to be sold in the United States market. Consequently, since 1978, all child restraints, *if used properly,* give protection at 35 mph in laboratory tests by preventing the child from hitting the windshield or dash board or being thrown out of the car. But do child restraints work in real-life situations? How could you study this, knowing that it is impossible and unethical to slam children, buckled up or not buckled up, into a wall at 35 mph?

Scherz [3] tried to show the difference in mortality between children who were buckled up and those who were not in real-life situations. His study design involved reviewing all reported motor vehicle accidents in Washington state that occurred between 1970 and 1979. "Investigation

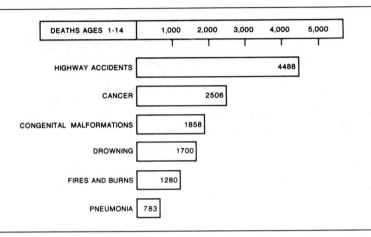

Fig. 11-1. The highway accident epidemic in the 1- to 14-year-old population in the United States. (From the National Safety Council [1].)

of motor vehicle accidents in Washington state is required for all injury-producing accidents and for all accidents that entail property damage of $300.00 or more. The report form includes information relative to the use of seat belts by the driver and all other passengers. However, the reports did not differentiate between seat belt, seat belts and shoulder belt, and child restraint (or between proper and improper use)" [3]. The results of Scherz's study were as follows: There were approximately 39,500 child passengers, aged 0 to 4 years, involved in motor vehicle accidents in Washington state from 1970 through 1979. Of these, 148 (0.4 percent) were killed outright or subsequently died. Approximately 6300 of the children (16 percent) were wearing some type of safety restraint, and only 2 of these (1 : 3150) were killed. In contrast, 33,200 were not wearing restraints, and 146 (1 : 227) were killed.

	No. of Children	Deaths
Buckled up	6,300	2
Not buckled up	33,200	146

STUDY QUESTION 11-2

What is the relative risk of a child less than 4 years of age being killed in an automobile accident if he or she is not buckled up?

──────────────────────────────── STUDY QUESTION 11-3
What percentage of the automobile accident deaths among children younger than 4 might have been prevented if the children had been buckled up? (In other words, what is the attributable risk associated with failure to wear seat belts?)

──────────────────────────────── STUDY QUESTION 11-4
Scherz chose a retrospective, epidemiologic study to show effectiveness of child restraints in preventing deaths in automobile crashes. Why did he choose a retrospective study rather than a prospective study?

──────────────────────────────── STUDY QUESTION 11-5
Speed is a factor known to contribute to the severity of injuries in automobile crashes. Was this study controlled for the speed at which accidents occurred?

Intervention Methods to Encourage Use of Child Restraints
Both in the laboratory (in simulated tests with dummies) and on the road, child restraints seem to give good protection, especially at low speeds (less than 35 mph). Why wasn't Jamie buckled up? Was his mother unaware of the protective effect of child restraints? Did she know about restraints and still not use them? If child restraints could decrease mortality among children under 4 who do not use child restraints by up to 93 percent, as Scherz claims, how can pediatricians motivate parents to buckle up their kids? What method of intervention should be used; an informational strategy, a motivational strategy, or an obligatory strategy?

INFORMATION AND MOTIVATION
Education and counseling have always been desirable and acceptable methods of changing behavior. Physicians have used education as an informational strategy that allows voluntary choice. At times, physicians try to counsel or persuade patients by strong personal recommendations designed as a motivational strategy. For some patients, gaining the physician's approval may be an effective motivation. Let us see how well education works in the case of child restraints. Would Jamie have been buckled up if his physician had informed his mother of the protective effects of a child restraint?

In the mid-1970s, two articles were published in the pediatric literature describing (1) the need for pediatricians to educate their patients to use child restraints and (2) the increase in usage of child restraints with counseling. Kanthor [4] tried to determine whether prenatal counseling by a pediatrician could increase usage of child restraints. His study design was as follows: Over 1½ years, 40 expectant third-trimester mothers scheduled prenatal counseling with the investigator, Kanthor. Car safety education was provided to every other woman at the conclusion of the visit and consisted of: (1) a *brief description* of the importance of using infant restraint systems and their effectiveness in protecting the new baby; (2) the distribution of a *pamphlet* ("Stop Risking Your Child's Life"), reiterating the necessity of using a child restraint; and (3) the strong *recommendation to purchase* either of two approved infant carriers.

The alternate group (the control group) received no counseling, and no woman in the noncounseled group asked for this information. No further mention was made of car safety until the 6-week well-child visit. At that time, Kanthor asked the mother how she had restrained the infant in the car on her trip to the pediatrician's office that day. The women in the study and control groups were similar in age, race, and socioeconomic status.

The results of Kanthor's study of these 40 mothers, 35 of whom returned for a 6-week visit (1 child died and 4 mothers changed pediatricians), are summarized below.

	Counseled (No. = 16)		Noncounseled Women (No. = 19)	
Restraint	No.	%	No.	%
Safe	11	69	8	42
Unsafe	5	31	11	58

STUDY QUESTION 11-6

What problems can you identify in Kanthor's study?

In 1978, Reisinger and Williams [5] conducted a study to evaluate programs designed to increase usage of child restraints based on education and counseling. Their study was set up in the following way: During a 6-month period, all women who delivered babies in consecutive-day periods were asked to participate in a study. The women were divided into four groups:

Group 1   No education (including no literature) was given to this control group. An approved child restraint seat was available in the gift shop, but mothers were not specifically advised of this.

Group 2   A pamphlet describing the importance of child restraint usage was given to each mother. Mothers were told child restraints were available in the gift shop.

Group 3   A pamphlet describing the importance of child restraint usage was given to each mother. Mothers were told child restraints were available in the gift shop. A health educator visited each mother to discuss car safety.

Group 4   A pamphlet describing the importance of child restraint usage was given to each mother. A free approved infant carrier was given to each mother with a demonstration of correct usage.

Participants were to return "to have their ears checked" at 2- and 4-month intervals. They were guaranteed free parking, and an observer was stationed at the parking lot attendant's booth to record child restraint usage.

Of the 1103 babies in the study, 955 were observed at discharge. In all groups, approximately 90 percent of infants were held in someone's arms. Six percent in control group 1 buckled up, compared to 11 percent in group 4 (Table 11-2). Child restraint usage rates at 2-month and 4-month visits are outlined in Table 11-3.

_____ STUDY QUESTION 11-7

What makes this study by Reisinger and Williams better than that by Kanthor?

_____ STUDY QUESTION 11-8

What can you conclude about the effectiveness of the informational and motivational approaches in changing behavior in the Reisinger and Williams study [5]?

OBLIGATION

Many safety experts, disenchanted with education and counseling as a means of increasing child restraint usage, turned to legislation. In January 1978, the first state law requiring children to buckle up was passed in Tennessee. The Tennessee Child Restraint Law required "parent or legal guardians of children less than 4 years old residing in Tennessee to use child restraint systems when transporting their children in motor vehicles owned by the parents, and to ensure that the restraints were used *properly*" [6].

To study the effectiveness of the Tennessee Child Restraint Law in increasing child restraint usage, Williams [6, 7] made observations of child restraint usage in four different cities, two in Tennessee (Knoxville and Nashville), 4 months before the law was enacted and again 4 months

Table 11-2. Observed child restraint use at hospital discharge

Group	Total no. observed	Method of restraint	
		No. (%) properly using infant carrier	No. (%) being held in someone's arms
1 (no literature)	239	15 (6)	217 (91)
2 (literature)	236	18 (8)	213 (90)
3 (literature and personal discussion)	262	21 (8)	233 (89)
4 (literature and free infant carrier)	218	24 (11)	189 (87)

Source: Data from Reisinger and Williams [5].

Table 11-3. Observed child restraint use
at 2 to 4 months after hospital discharge

Group	Total no. observed	No. (%) using infant carrier
1 (no literature)	174	36 (21)
2 (literature)	175	39 (22)
3 (literature and personal discussion)	205	41 (20)
4 (literature and free infant carrier)	180	51 (28)

Source: Data from Reisinger and Williams [5].

and 2½ years after the law was enacted. The two other cities were in Kentucky (Louisville and Lexington), where no seat belt laws existed; these were controls.

Observations were made at stop signs and traffic lights at exits from the same shopping centers in the same cities in the prelaw and two post-law surveys. If cars stopping at these exits contained one or more children who appeared to be younger than 4 years old, information was obtained from the drivers about the ages of the children and their relationship to the driver, and observations on how the children were traveling were made and recorded. If child restraints were in use, it was noted whether they were anchored by vehicle seat belts, because this anchorage is an essential component of the safety of restraints.

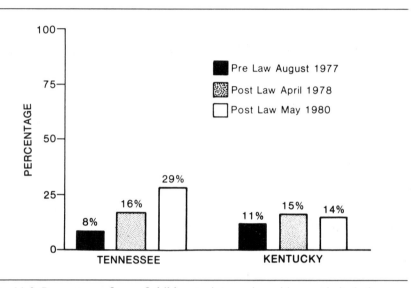

Fig. 11-2. Percentage of use of child restraints anchored by seat belts before and after enactment of Tennessee Child Restraint Law. (From T Wagner. Accident Prevention Newsletter, Vol. 1, pp. 1–5. Washington, DC Chapter of the Academy of Pediatrics.)

———————————————————————— STUDY QUESTION 11-9
What does the Kentucky control group, observed at the same time, add to this study?

Williams observed approximately 4917 automobile passengers less than 4 years old in Tennessee and Kentucky, in August 1977 (prelaw) and in April 1978 (4 months postlaw). He showed that child restraint use increased from 8 percent in 1977 (prior to the law) to 16 percent in April 1978 (4 months after the law) and finally to 29 percent by May 1980 (15 months postlaw) (Fig. 11-2).

———————————————————————— STUDY QUESTION 11-10
What do you conclude from Williams's study?

The Insurance Institute of Highway Safety noted a concomitant decrease in mortality in the state of Tennessee, from an average of 22 to 25 deaths in the less-than-4-years age group per year before 1977 to 14 deaths in the same group in the year 1980. The conclusion, however, that the law caused the decline in deaths was controversial.

To see why one must be very careful in drawing conclusions from data using small numbers, let us take a look at the data from Michigan [8] on fatalities among 0- to 3-year-old automobile occupants in crashes that occurred 3 years before to 1 year after the child restraint law took effect in that state:

Time	No. of Fatalities
3 years before law	10
2 years before law	20
1 year before law	9
1 year after law	12

The number of child occupants killed *increases or decreases* 30 to 50 percent from year to year *without any major change in policy or program*. The expected effect of a child restraint law is only in the 20 to 30-percent range. Without an appreciation of this variability, one might even be tempted to conclude that the Michigan Child Restraint Law was detrimental because child fatalities increased 33 percent during the first year that the law was in effect. Few researchers, however, would base a conclusion concerning the effectiveness of the law on three additional fatalities during a 1-year period.

A published study took another approach to assessing the effectiveness of the 1982 Michigan Child Restraint Law [8]. The investigators assessed usage rates and morbidity by using the number of children injured, not the number of children killed. This allowed for a much larger and, therefore, much more reliable number of outcome events. The Michigan study reported that child restraint use among children younger than 4 years of age injured in crashes increased from 12 percent before the Michigan Child Restraint Law to 51 percent after the law was implemented. More importantly, a 25-percent *decrease* (from 180 to 130 injured per month) in the number of children younger than 4 years of age injured in crashes was associated with the law (Figs. 11-3, 11-4).

This Michigan study is one of the most sophisticated studies to date in evaluating the effectiveness of child restraint laws. Not only did investigators obtain a large sample by using injuries rather than deaths, but

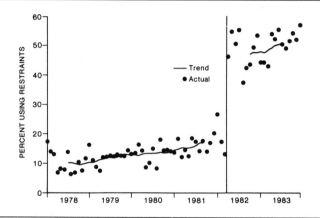

Fig. 11-3. Child restraint use among injured motor vehicle occupants, aged 0 to 3 years, before and after implementation of the 1982 Michigan Child Restraint Law. (From Wagenaar and Webster [9].)

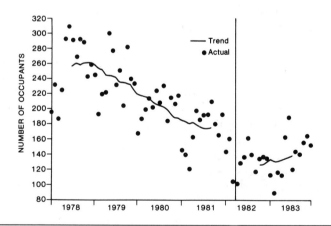

Fig. 11-4. Number of injured motor vehicle occupants, aged 0 to 3 years, before and after implementation of the 1982 Michigan Child Restraint Law. (From Wagenaar and Webster [9].)

they also tried to determine the effectiveness of child restraints in preventing severe injuries as well as minor ones. Therefore, the injured children were separated into two groups for analysis: moderate nonincapacitating injury and severe incapacitating injury (requiring hospitalization) or resulting in death. "A decline of 32 percent in the number of children experiencing moderate injuries was associated with the law, whereas the decrease in the number of severely injured was 22 percent" [8].

Another way to compare the effectiveness of the child restraint law in moderate and severe automobile crashes is to use the level of car damage. "The Child Restraint Law was associated with a 37-percent decrease in the number of children injured in vehicles with low levels of damage, a 27-percent decrease in the number of injured in medium-damaged vehicles, and no significant decrease in the number of children injured in high-damage vehicles" [8].

_____ STUDY QUESTION 11-11
What are possible explanations for the decreased effectiveness of child restraints in more severe crashes?

_____ STUDY QUESTION 11-12
(a) What are your conclusions about the effectiveness of child restraint laws? (b) Do these studies guarantee that the observed effectiveness will continue at the same level?

Preventing Adolescent Automobile-Related Deaths

Now let us take a look at the problem of automobile accidents in another age group, adolescents. An adolescent has an even higher risk or probability of dying in an automobile crash than does a child younger than 4. The epidemiology of automobile crashes involving teenagers is very different. Such accidents occur at night, at high speeds, and are often related to alcohol. Adolescents have the highest automobile-related death rates—36.5 deaths per 100,000 population (Fig. 11-5) [9]. Approximately 7000 teenagers are killed each year in motor vehicle crashes.

_____ STUDY QUESTION 11-13
Do you think a seat belt law will increase seat belt usage and decrease mortality and morbidity in the adolescent age group as the child restraint law did in the under 4 years of age group?

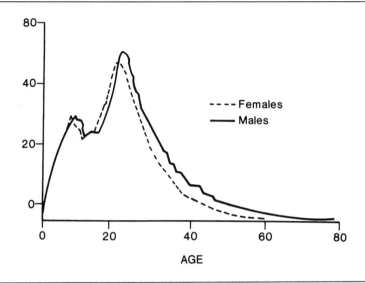

Fig. 11-5. Motor vehicle deaths as a percent of all deaths, by age, in the United States in 1977. Because of the low number of deaths from other causes, motor vehicle deaths increase as a percentage of all deaths well into the 20s. (From Hood [10].)

STUDY QUESTION 11-14

If seat belt laws are not likely to be effective in the adolescent population, what methods would you suggest to prevent automobile fatalities in this group

References

1. National Safety Council. Accident facts. Washington, D.C.: National Safety Council, 1978.
2. National Center for Health Statistics. Vital statistics of the United States, 1975, vol 11A. Washington, D.C.: U.S. Government Printing Office, 1979.
3. Scherz RG. Fatal motor vehicle accidents of child passengers from birth through 4 years of age in Washington state. Pediatrics 1981;68(4):572–575.
4. Kanthor HA. Car safety for infants: effectiveness of prenatal counseling. Pediatrics 1976;58(3):320–322.
5. Reisinger KS, Williams AF. Evaluation of programs designed to increase the protection of infants in cars. Pediatrics 1978;62:280–287.

6. Williams AF, Wells JK: The Tennessee child restraint law in its third year. Am J Public Health 1981;71(2):163–165.
7. Williams AF. Evaluation of the Tennessee child restraint law. Am J Public Health 1979;69:455–458.
8. Wagenaar AC, Webster DW. Preventing injuries to children through compulsory automobile safety seat use. Pediatrics 1986;78(4):662–672.
9. Hood P (ed). Status Report: Teenagers and autos: a deadly combination. Vol. 16, No. 14, Sept. 23, 1981.

Secondary Prevention

PART FIVE

Screening for Breast Cancer CHAPTER TWELVE

KATHLEEN K. DAVIS

Your next patient is a woman who has just turned 50. Having achieved this milestone in good health, she felt she should have a thorough check-up. This patient is ready to do whatever you recommend in order to remain healthy. Your history and physical examination confirm that she has no major illnesses that you can detect. Recently, you have been thinking about the value of screening tests for breast cancer. Breast examination and mammography are screening procedures you have considered.

How often do you advise this patient to return to your office for breast examination? Would you order a mammogram for her now? Remember from our earlier discussion of screening that there are four criteria that should be fulfilled before considering screening for a disease.

Criterion 1. The disease must have a substantial morbidity or mortality.

Criterion 2. There are risk factors that, if identified, will facilitate early detection.

Criterion 3. Early detection must improve outcome.

Criterion 4. Screening must be feasible and practical.

Criterion 1. Significant Disease
To advise your patient about the value of screening tests, you must know some facts about the epidemiology of breast cancer. The fact that breast cancer has a substantial morbidity and mortality cannot be disputed. Breast cancer and lung cancer have the highest mortality of all cancers among women in the United States. More than 100,000 new cases are diagnosed each year. Approximately 8 percent, or 1 in 12 American women, will die of breast cancer.

Criterion 2. Risk Factors
If we are to try to improve this statistic by screening, we need to decide which women will benefit most from screening. Thus, we need to ask: What are the risk factors for developing breast cancer? The most important risk factor is age. As can be seen from Table 12-1, the disease is rare under age 30 and becomes increasingly common after age 35. In fact, 75 percent of women with breast cancer have no risk factor except

Table 12-1. Average annual breast cancer incidence among
white females in the United States, 1969–1971

Age	Cases per 100,000
20–24	1.1
25–29	8.7
30–34	22.4
35–39	52.5
40–44	103.7
45–49	159.0
50–54	171.6
55–59	191.8
60–64	226.6
65–69	234.0
70–74	260.1
75–79	294.7
80–84	301.3
85+	306.8

Source: From Levin and Thomas [1].

age. There are, however, a few subgroups of women who are at higher risk than the general population, as noted in Table 12-2.

A positive family history, either in the maternal or paternal line, not only carries a higher risk but, if the family member has premenopausal disease, the woman is more likely to develop breast cancer at a younger age and have a more aggressive tumor.

Whether benign breast disease (so-called fibrocystic disease, or lumpy breasts) puts a woman at increased risk of breast cancer is a controversial issue. In a review of the literature in 1982, Love [2] makes the following points: As defined clinically, fibrocystic disease is "a condition in which there are palpable lumps in the breasts, usually associated with pain and tenderness, that fluctuate with the menstrual cycle and become progressively worse until menopause" [2]. This occurs in more than 50 percent of women of reproductive age. As a pathologic diagnosis, it has "been understood to include macrocysts, adenosis, apocrine change, fibrosis, fibroadenomas, or ductal hyperplasia" [2]. Looking at several autopsy studies of women without known breast disease, Love found that 58 to 89 percent had breast tissue that met this definition. Since fibrocystic disease is a condition that seems to apply to a majority of women, the

Table 12-2. Breast cancer risk factors

Factor	Relative risk*
Family history: Primary relative with breast cancer	1.2–3.0
Premenopausal	3.1
Premenopausal and bilateral	8.5–9.0
Postmenopausal	1.5
Postmenopausal and bilateral	4.0–5.4
Menstrual history	
Age at menarche <12	1.3
Age at menopause >55 with >40 menstrual years	1.48–2.0
Pregnancy	
First child after age 35	2.0–3.0
Nulliparous	3.0
Other neoplasms	
Contralateral breast cancer	5.0
Cancer of the major salivary gland	4.0
Cancer of the uterus	2.0
Benign breast disease	
Atypical lobular hyperplasia	4.0
Lobular carcinoma in situ	7.2

*General population risk is 1.0.
Source: From SM Love et al. Fibrocystic disease of the breast—a nondisease? *N Engl J Med* 1982;307:1010. Reprinted with permission.

question arises whether this should be considered a pathologic entity at all. Love reviewed previous studies that show an increased incidence of breast cancer in women who have had breast biopsies for benign breast disease. This increased incidence may be an artifact of more intense screening, since those with breast lumps usually are followed more closely with physical examination, breast self-examination, and mammography than those without breast complaints. Is there a subgroup of women with benign breast biopsies whom we can identify as being at particularly high risk? In the same review [2], Love concluded that there is. Those with atypical lobular hyperplasia and those with lobular carcinoma in situ were at substantially higher risk of developing breast cancer in the future than were those never biopsied.

To examine this question further, Dupont and Page [3], in a retrospective cohort study, looked at breast biopsies from 10,000 women. They then compared the pathology to the clinical outcome in 3000 of these women followed for 17 years (median follow-up). The average age

Table 12-3. Pathologic and clinical findings in
3000 women biopsied for benign breast masses

Type of lesion on biopsy	Relative risk of breast cancer[a]	% of Biopsies	p Value	% with Breast cancer within 15 yr of biopsy
Nonproliferative	0.89	68.5	0.51	2
− Family history (FH)[b]	0.86		0.43	
+ FH	1.2		0.78	
Proliferative without atypia	1.6	26.2	<0.0001	4
− FH	1.5		0.002	
+ FH	2.1		0.009	
Atypical hyperplasia	4.4	3.6	<0.0001	
− FH	3.5		<0.0001	
+ FH	8.9		<0.0001	20

[a]Risk compared to incidence of breast cancer in Atlanta in Third National Cancer Survey.
[b]Family History of breast cancer in mother, sister, or daughter.
Source: Adapted from Dupont and Page [3].

of all the patients was 42 years (standard deviation, 10 years). All patients were older than 20 (Table 12-3). These investigators found that

1. Seventy percent of the women had a biopsy showing a nonproliferative breast lesion. These women had no increased risk of breast cancer. The lesions included cysts (without family history of breast cancer), fibroadenomas, and mild hyperplasia.
2. Approximately 27 percent of the women had a proliferative breast lesion but without atypia. They had a small but statistically significant (≤. 009) increased risk, up to twice that for women without proliferative lesions.
3. The remaining 3 percent of women with atypical hyperplasia had a markedly increased risk of breast cancer, especially if there was a mother, a sister, or a daughter with breast cancer.

The previously cited risk factors serve to delineate specific subgroups that are at higher risk of developing breast cancer. Yet despite the increased risk associated with these factors, only 2 to 8 percent of all women with breast cancer had a previous biopsy [2, 4]. Remember that

Table 12-4. Breast cancer at time of diagnosis

Size of lesion (cm)	% Palpable on physical examination	% In situ	Local invasion	% Positive lymph nodes
0–0.5	20	55	20	2
0.51–1	42	4	85	15
1.1 –2	53	3	95	20
2.1 –3	85	0	95	65
>3.1	98	0	100	78

Source: Adapted from Brunner [8].

the women with such risk factors are *not* the majority of those in whom breast cancer occurs. In fact, it should be noted that several other risk factors have been suggested for breast cancer, including dietary fat, age of menarche and first pregnancy, and alcohol [2, 5–7]. The fact remains that *for most women who develop breast cancer the important risk factor is age.* We can conclude, therefore, that the 50-year-old patient in your office— even if she does not have a family history of breast cancer, has never had a biopsy showing atypia, and has had children before she was 35 years old—is still in a high-risk group by virtue of her age.

Age identifies a subset of the population with high prevalence. In addition, those with a strong family history, or atypical hyperplasia from a biopsy specimen, or both represent a small group of women at particularly high risk. Will screening these groups facilitate early detection and thereby satisfy criterion 2?

Criterion 3. Improvement of Outcome
Now that you have received the data to help you decide who to screen, you need to decide whether screening will make a difference. Can we change the course of the disease if we detect it before it becomes symptomatic?

STUDY QUESTION 12-1

What conclusions can you draw from Tables 12-4 and 12-5?

From Table 12-5, we can see that breast cancer is an important cause of mortality [8]. We also know that there is a definable population in

Table 12-5. Percentage of survival after breast cancer detection

Interval from time of diagnosis (yr)	% Survival			
	Positive in situ lesions of <1 cm	Negative lymph nodes	Positive lymph nodes	Distant metastases
5	98	85	55	10
10	95	74	39	2
20	93	62	23	

Source: From Brunner [8].

which the disease is common and that if screening were effectively to detect breast cancer early, we might be able to decrease mortality. To fully satisfy criterion 2, we still must ask: Does our most important risk factor, age, facilitate early detection? To satisfy criterion 3, although the tables above suggest that early detection will improve the outcome, we still would like a controlled clinical trial showing a decrease in mortality with screening.

Criterion 4. Feasibility and Practicality

Criterion 4 requires us to ask: How effective are our tests for screening for breast cancer? How acceptable are they to patients? How feasible is it to implement a screening program? To answer these questions, let's review two major studies designed to investigate the impact on mortality and the feasibility of screening for breast cancer with annual mammography and physical examination.

THE HEALTH INSURANCE PLAN OF NEW YORK STUDY

The first major study to look at the impact of screening on mortality was conducted through the Health Insurance Plan of New York (HIP) from 1963 through 1970 [9, 10]. Sixty-two thousand women were randomly selected from the population of HIP members and randomized to a study or control group. The control group continued to receive the usual care. At that time, mammography was primarily used for evaluation of breast lumps but not for screening asymptomatic women. Women in the study group were offered four annual breast examinations and mam-

Table 12-6. Detection rates and mortality among
women in the Health Insurance Plan of New York Study

Mortality	Control group (N = 31,000)	Study group (N = 31,000)	Reduction in study group
Cancers at 5 years from entry (no. of women)	300	306	
Negative lymph nodes (%)	46	56	
Deaths at 5 years from breast cancer (no. of women)	63	39	
Decrease in mortality overall (%)			38 (p <.05)
Decrease in mortality among 50- to 59-year-olds (%)			54
Decrease in mortality among 40- to 49-year-olds (%)			Not statistically significant

Source: Data from Shapiro and colleagues [10].

mography in addition to their usual care. Of the 31,000 subjects in the study group, 20,000 came for one or more examinations. In this group, the detection of breast cancer by mammography and physical examination can be summarized as follows:

Method by which Cancer Detected	% of Cancers Detected	% Lymph Node–Positive
Mammography alone	33	21
Physical Examination alone	40	25
Both mammography and physical examination	27	50

Among the control group 54 percent of cases had positive lymph nodes at the time of detection [10].

Table 12-6 looks at detection and mortality from breast cancer in the study and control groups. The time of entry into the study group is the time of first screening.

_____ STUDY QUESTION 12-2

What conclusions can you draw from the data in Table 12-6?

Two additional points are worth noting: First, the majority of the patients were 50 to 60 years old. Since fewer women were in the 40- to 49-

Table 12-7. Deaths from breast cancers[a] within
5 and 14 years from date of entry into study

Age at entry	No. of deaths through 5-year follow-up			No. of deaths through 14-year follow-up		
	Study	Control	% Difference	Study	Control	% Difference
40–49	19	20	5[b]	46	61	24[b]
50–59	15	33	54[c]	53	68	22[c]
Total	39	63	38[d]	118	153	23[c]

[a]Breast cancers diagnosed during first 5 years after study.
[b]Not significant (p >.10).
[c]0.01 < p <.05.
[d]p <.01.
Source: From Shapiro and colleagues [11].

year-old age group, larger differences would have to be present to demonstrate statistical significance. Similarly, not enough women were in the older-than-60 age group to allow conclusions to be drawn. Second, both physical examination and mammography are technically more difficult in the premenopausal woman. The dense premenopausal breast is more opaque on mammography and can obscure the subtle signs of early cancer. The nodularity of the normal premenopausal breast can also obscure small lumps on physical examination. Postmenopausally, the breast becomes less dense and more homogenous in texture and is therefore easier to examine by both modalities.

Prospective studies of screening tests, if done over a short period of time, may reflect a lead-time bias. Long-term follow-up studies help reduce the importance of lead-time bias. Long-term follow-up data from the HIP study population show that although the differences in mortality are smaller at 14 years from the data of entry than at 5 years, statistically significant differences are maintained for the study group as a whole (Table 12-7) [11].

It is interesting that the mortality decreased more at 14 years than at 5 years among the 40- to 49-year-old group, although the decrease was not statistically significant. The authors express reservations, however, in concluding that their study results provide support for screening this age group, since the majority of the cancers in this group were actually detected after the subjects' fiftieth birthday.

Table 12-8. Breast cancers detected in
BCDDP and HIP studies by various modalities

Test	% Cancers detected in BCDDP study, by age		% Cancers detected in HIP study, by age	
	40–50 yr	50–60 yr	40–50 yr	50–60 yr
Mammography alone	35	42	19	41
Physical examination alone	13	7	61	40
Mammography and physical examination	50	50	19	18

BCDDP = Breast Cancer Detection Demonstration Project; HIP = Health Insurance
Plan of New York Study.
Source: From Baker [12].

BREAST CANCER DETECTION DEMONSTRATION PROJECT, 1973 THROUGH 1981

A decade after the HIP study, another major study was funded by the
National Cancer Institute and the American Cancer Society. In the
Breast Cancer Detection Demonstration Project (BCDDP), 280,000
women between the ages of 35 and 74 years (median, 49.5 years) were
offered physical examination and mammogram for 5 years [12]. This
study was different from the HIP study in at least two major ways: intent
and design. As a demonstration project, BCDDP was intended to show
the feasibility of screening a large number of women. It was not set up
specifically to show differences in mortality and detection rates compared to those not screened. In terms of design, there was no control
group, and participants were not randomly selected. Rather, subjects
were recruited from a variety of sources including advertisements and
word of mouth. The results of this project, compared to the HIP data,
are shown in Table 12-8.

_____ STUDY QUESTION 12-3

What differences do you see between the HIP study results and those of the
BCDDP (see Table 12-8)?

Table 12-9 demonstrates that mammography has become better than
physical examination at detecting early tumors. Eighty-eight and nine-
tenths percent of the total tumors were detected by mammography,

Table 12-9. Breast cancers stratified by lesion size and screening modality

Screening modality	% In situ breast cancer	% Infiltrating breast cancer lesions <1 cm	% Breast cancer lesions >1 cm	% Breast cancer lesion size unspecified	% Total breast cancers
Mammography alone	59	52.6	33.7	36.4	41.6
Physical examination alone	5.5	8.4	8.6	13.7	8.7
Mammography and physical examination	33	36.4	55.5	47.3	47.3
Unknown	2.6	2.7	2.2	2.6	2.4

Source: From Baker [12].

(41.6 percent by mammography alone, and 47.3 percent by physical examination as well). Although these data show improved detection rate of early lesions in the 40- to 50-year age group, actual mortality reduction cannot be calculated from this study since there was no control group [12].

Sensitivity and Specificity of Testing

To assess the BCDDP screening program, we need to estimate the sensitivity and specificity of mammography and physical examination in combination. To do this, we must make the following assumptions:

1. The biopsy rate reflects a positive test from the screening program as a whole, since those who came to biopsy had either a positive physical examination, a positive mammogram, or both.
2. The interval cancer rate (cancers *diagnosed* between screening tests) reflects in part the false negative rate (i.e., cancers missed by both screening tests). However, the interval cancer rate may slightly overestimate the false negatives since it also reflects those cancers that *developed* between screening tests.

Table 12-10 shows the biopsy rates, the cancers detected, and the interval cancer rates for the 5 years of the study.

————————————————————————— STUDY QUESTION 12-4
Why are the rates for the first year nearly double those for each of the following 4 years?

————————————————————————— STUDY QUESTION 12-5
(a) Using the first-year biopsy data to reflect a positive test in the screening program as a whole, and assuming the interval cancer rate reflects the false negatives, what is the sensitivity of the combined screening program? (b) What is the specificity of the combined screening program?

As a demonstration project, the BCDDP was designed to study the feasibility of implementing a cancer screening program in clinical practice. This is the advantage of a demonstration over a randomized trial since, in clinical practice, patients are self-selected and come by word of mouth and through advertising. Thus, the study population was designed to reflect patients who are generally encountered in the office setting. The prevalence and incidence of breast cancer in the BCDDP, therefore, can be used as an approximation of the prevalence and inci-

Table 12-10. Biopsy and cancer detection rates per 10,000 annual screenings in Breast Cancer Detection Demonstration Project

Rate	Year 1	Year 2	Year 3	Year 4	Year 5
Biopsy performance rates	358.1	187.6	173.4	145.9	117.8
Cancer detection rates	55.8	26.5	25.2	25.4	23.6
Interval cancer rates		8.0	7.7	8.0	7.5

Source: From Baker [12].

dence of cancer in actual clinical practice. This is an important aspect of the study since it allows us to use the BCDDP data to address the question of predictive value of the screening program.

Predictive Value of Testing

_____ STUDY QUESTION 12-6
(a) What is the probability that if a patient comes to biopsy because one or both screening tests are positive, the patient will have cancer (predictive value of a positive test)? (b) What is the probability that if both screening tests are negative, cancer will be detected in the patient within the year (predictive value of a negative test)?

_____ STUDY QUESTION 12-7
What factors affect the estimates of predictive value when applied in practice?

Making an Informed Decision About Screening

Having reviewed the data from the HIP and BCDDP studies [6–8], you now call your patient into your office to discuss your feelings about the effectiveness of mammography as a screening tool. "But what about the risk of radiation?" she asks. "Can't a mammogram *cause* cancer?"

The evidence that breast cancer can be caused by radiation appears in studies in which women have been exposed to high-dose radiation. Examples are those exposed to the atomic bomb, to radiation treatment for mastitis, and to multiple chest fluoroscopies. These studies show more risk of cancer the younger the women are at time of exposure and increased cancer rates with increased dose at exposure, especially more than 100 rads. In the HIP study, 8 rads were applied to each breast. BCDDP used 0.2 to 0.5 rads, which is consonant with current mammographic techniques. Risk of low-dose radiation from mammography can only be extrapolated from studies of high-dose radiation and animal studies. One such estimate is that 1 rad to the breast, given to 1 million women, may yield six breast cancers per year after a 6- to 10-year latency. Approximately 110,000 women develop breast cancer every year. If the mortality of these women is decreased by even a small percentage by screening, then the lives saved by screening are far in excess of those theoretically lost by radiation [10].

In summary, the data presented in this chapter suggest the following:

1. Screening with physical examination and mammography in women between the ages of 50 and 60 decreases the mortality from breast cancer by 30 percent.
2. New mammographic techniques with less radiation exposure are able to detect smaller cancers in younger women. Decreased mortality from screening 35- to 50-year olds has not been proved but is strongly suggested by present studies.
3. There is little data from the HIP and BCDDP studies to guide us in determining the frequency of screening for women older than 60 years. Other data show that the prevalence of breast cancer increases with age, and the risk of radiation decreases with age.

_____ STUDY QUESTION 12-8
How can you apply the studies just discussed to your 50-year-old patient? (b) Would you use mammography to screen asymptomatic women younger than 50 or older than 60?

References

1. Levin ML, Thomas DB. The epidemiology of breast cancer. In: Breast cancer (Progress in Clinical and Biological Research), Vol. 12. New York: Alan Liss, 1977:15.
2. Love SM, Gelman RS, Silen W. Fibrocystic disease of the breast—a non-disease? N Engl J Med 1982;307(16):1010.
3. Dupont WD, Page DL. Risk factors for breast cancer in women with proliferative breast disease. N Engl J Med 1985;312(3):146.
4. Seidman H, Stellman SD, Mushinski MH. A different perspective on breast cancer risk factors: some implications of nonattributable risk. CA 1982;32(5).
5. Lubin F, Wax Y, Modan B. Role of fat, animal protein, and dietary fiber in breast cancer: a case-control study. JNCI 1986;77(3):605–612.
6. Shatzkin AS, Jones I, Hoover RN, et al. Alcohol consumption and breast

cancer in the epidemiologic follow-up study of the first health and nutrition examination survey. N Engl J Med 1987;316:1169–1173.

7. Willmett WC, Stampfer MS, Golditz GA, et al. Moderate alcohol consumption and the risk of breast cancer. N Engl J Med 1987;316:1174–1180.

8. Brunner S. Early detection of breast cancer. Recent Results Cancer Res 1984;90:11–27.

9. Shapiro S, Strax P, Venet L, et al. Changes in 5 year breast cancer mortality in a breast cancer screening program. In: Proceedings of the 7th National Cancer Conference, 1973.

10. Strax P. Evaluation of screening programs for the early diagnosis of breast cancer. Surg Clin North Am 1978;58(1):667–679.

11. Shapiro S, Venet W, Strax P, et al. Ten-to-fourteen year effect of screening on breast cancer mortality. JNCI 1982;69(2):349.

12. Baker L. Breast cancer detection demonstration project: five year summary report. New York: American Cancer Society, 1982.

Screening for Colorectal Cancer

CHAPTER THIRTEEN

ALAN W. STONE
GENE A. H. KALLENBERG

Clinical Scenario

Georgianna Grady, M.D., having finished residency training, is planning to set up her medical practice. She expects to see middle-aged and older patients on a continuing basis as part of her practice. She has been wondering for which cancers she should screen and how to do it. Data brought to her attention by one of her teachers has convinced Dr. Grady that screening for breast cancer by physical examination, and especially mammography, is well founded and indeed recommended by several authoritative groups. She is, however, confused about whether and how to screen for colorectal cancer.

All of this comes to a head with Paul Callum, the first patient in her new office. Mr. Callum, a 50-year-old white man, has come in for a physical examination. His hidden agenda, quickly uncovered by Dr. Grady's skillful open-ended interview technique, is his fear of large bowel cancer. The patient has a friend who recently developed a colon cancer and wants to know whether screening tests for large bowel (i.e., colorectal) cancer are valuable in preventing or curing this disease. Mr. Callum has no family history of colon cancer or personal history of cancer or polyps. He is asymptomatic. Dr. Grady has read and received conflicting reports about screening for colorectal cancer. Hemoccult testing seems to have a widely varying reported sensitivity. The role of sigmoidoscopy is controversial. The report of the Canadian Task Force on the Periodic Health Examination, the most fully documented analysis of screening examinations in the last decade, recommended Hemoccult testing but not sigmoidoscopy [1]. The American Cancer Society recommends both [2]. Dr. Grady recently attended a course sponsored by the manufacturers of an excellent flexible sigmoidoscope and presented by respected gastroenterologists. The course had as its underlying premise the use of this instrument in periodic screening and cited references "demonstrating the value" of sigmoidoscopy in "improving mortality" from colorectal cancer.

What, then, should our up-to-date analytic physician, Dr. Grady, recommend to this anxious patient, and to her patients generally, regarding screening for colorectal cancer? That is the issue we explore in this chapter.

Principles of Screening Applied to Colorectal Cancer

Earlier, we reviewed principles of deciding for which conditions to screen and what tests to use. We will now apply these principles to colorectal cancer [1], in the following sequence:

1. Is there a substantial problem? Does the condition have a substantial morbidity or mortality, or a significant impact upon society? The section titled Epidemiology and Natural History of Colorectal Cancer will answer this affirmatively.
2. Is there a modifiable risk factor? In a section about polyps, we will look briefly at the evidence that polyps are a risk factor and contributory cause of colorectal cancer.
3. Does early detection improve outcome? We will critically examine representative evidence to try to answer this question.
4. Is screening feasible and practical? First, we will examine the data for Hemoccult testing. We will calculate sensitivity and specificity values from published data and apply them to screening populations. Secondly, we will discuss sigmoidoscopy as a test and compare the characteristics of rigid and flexible sigmoidoscopy.

Risk-Benefit Analysis, Cost Effectiveness, and Guidelines for Implementation of Screening for Colorectal Cancer

In this section, current published guidelines for screening for colorectal cancer promulgated by "expert groups" are cited. Then, risk benefit and cost-effectiveness analytic principles are reviewed and applied to colorectal cancer. Variables that can optimize screening yield are discussed.

Worth is a function of context: Thus, different scenarios may lead to different screening recommendations. A variety of scenarios are presented, and the reader is challenged to think through a screening policy for each.

Is There a Substantial Problem?

One of the criteria for deciding to screen for a disease is that it have a substantial impact on the individual or society. We all had the general impression this was true of colorectal cancer even before President Reagan's illness. In addition to documenting the total impact of this disease, knowledge of the epidemiology and natural history of a disease allows

Table 13-1. Dukes system of classification for
staging local lesions and associated 5-year survival rate

Dukes stage	Tumor extent	5-Year survival rate (%)
	In situ	100
A	Mucosa only	100
B	Penetration of muscularis	54–67
C	Local nodes involved	22–43
D	Distant spread	4

Source: Data from Astler and Coller [3].

us to better understand studies of the disease and to formulate a higher-yield screening program.

There are approximately 140,000 new cases of colorectal cancer yearly, second only to lung cancer. Colorectal cancer accounts for 16 percent of all new cancers in women and 15 percent of new cancers in men (excluding nonmelanoma skin cancer and carcinoma in situ). Colorectal cancer accounts for 60,000 deaths annually, again second only to lung cancer. The probability at birth of eventually developing colorectal cancer is 4 to 6 percent [3]. The case fatality rate is 55 to 60 percent. These facts proclaim clearly for whom the bell tolls.

Pathologically, colorectal cancer is an adenocarcinoma that arises in the mucosa. It spreads by piercing the bowel wall and then travels by lymph channels, contiguity, or hematogenous dissemination to mesentery, serosal surfaces, lymph nodes, liver, lung, bone, and brain. In patients with recurrent disease, repeated hospitalization for recurrent intestinal obstruction and other complications are common. Five-year survival rate is best correlated with anatomic extent at the time of resection. The Dukes system of classification is used to stage local lesions (Table 13-1) [4]. This correlation clearly implies that early discovery and resection will result in an improved prognosis.

Is There a Modifiable Risk Factor?
The Adenoma-Carcinoma Hypothesis

Risk factors for colorectal cancer are multiple. Common risk factors are age, current or past history of polyps or colorectal cancer, and family history of a first-degree relative with colorectal cancer. Less common risk factors include ulcerative colitis and multiple polyposis syndromes. The incidence doubles with each decade, starting at age 50. Rectal cancer is more common in men. These facts suggest high-risk groups for priority screening.

Many now believe that most colonic carcinomas arise in previously benign adenomatous polyps [5]. This relationship is called the adenoma-carcinoma sequence [6]. The rate of progression to cancer is relatively slow, on an average requiring at least 5 to 10 years. Said another way, most now believe that adenomatous polyps are a risk factor for colon cancer that may meet the criteria for being a *contributory cause* of colon cancer. Remember, however, that the causes of the appearance of the adenomas themselves and their malignant transformation are thought to be both hereditary and environmental factors [7].

One should note that only 20 to 30 percent of all colonic polyps are adenomas, the remainder being primarily inflammatory or hyperplastic polyps. Furthermore, only adenomas have a potential for malignant transformation, and of these, only approximately 5 to 10 percent actually become malignant.

The lines of evidence supporting the theory of the adenoma-carcinoma sequence are many. The scope of this chapter does not allow us a detailed discussion of the evidence, but some major points are listed below [6]:

1. Adenomatous polypoid tissue is commonly found contiguous to adenocarcinoma.
2. Adenocarcinoma is commonly found within polyps. This finding correlates positively with polyp size, histologic atypia, and villous structure.
3. Epidemiologic studies demonstrate a positive correlation between the presence of adenomas and colonic cancer in population studies.
4. It has been observed that patients with familial polyposis syndromes have virtually a 100-percent risk of eventually developing colon cancer in at least one of their many polyps and that the appearance of their polyps precedes the diagnosis of their cancers by approximately 12 years. This time lag is seen in the general population as well.
5. Finally, there is one followup study by Gilbertsen and Nelms [8] in which 21,150 patients in a cancer screening program were periodically endoscoped, with *removal of all polyps found.* Over a follow-up period of as long as 25 years, fewer than half of the expected number of cancers were discovered. Although the study was uncontrolled, the magnitude of the decrease in cancers and the length of the follow-up

are very impressive, suggesting that removal of the polyps prevented the expected number of cancers.

It should be noted that there is a persistent minority view that is not nearly as impressed with the relationship between adenomatous polyps and colorectal carcinoma. Best described by Castleman [9] as the "vulnerable mucosa theory," this minority view holds that the entire mucosa of a susceptible patient is vulnerable to the effects of the *direct* causes of both adenomas and colon cancers and that colon cancers frequently do not require the antecedent presence of a polyp before they appear. This view holds that polyps are really a "confounding variable" associated with both the direct contributory causes and with the effect (colon cancer) but playing no pathogenic role in the development of colon cancer. This minority view is mentioned not to confuse the reader but to emphasize the point that randomized controlled trials have not yet proved that adenomatous polyps are a contributory cause of colorectal cancer.

Nevertheless, many authorities do accept the adenoma-carcinoma sequence. If this is true, and the evidence does support it, then polyps are a modifiable risk factor for colorectal cancer. Therefore, it is very important throughout the discussion of screening and prevention of colon cancer that we maintain a dual approach in our minds. On the one hand, screening is directed toward the detection of already present cancers in their earliest and most curable stages. Second, there is possible benefit in the early detection, follow-up, and removal of adenomatous polyps, which could prevent colon cancers from occurring [10]. Some have predicted that 80 to 90 percent of all colon cancers could thus be prevented [7].

Does Early Detection Improve Outcome?
The answer to this pivotal question in large part determines the advisability of screening. If the answer is no, then one can rationally argue against screening at all. This is, in fact, the current state of affairs with screening for lung cancer, a disease whose outcome has not been improved by screening programs.

How shall we answer this question? We should *not* base the answer on our own anecdotal experience. Physicians have a tendency to overweight dramatic diagnostic pick-ups, misses, successes, and failures and generalize to their own practice population. Certainly, anecdotal evidence and personal experience influence how we practice medicine, but they are a poor substitute for determining screening policies when studies of large populations are available. For judging studies of the effectiveness of early detection, keep in mind the grading of evidence used by the Canadian and by the United States Task Forces [1].

DESCRIPTIVE STUDY OF THE NATURAL HISTORY OF THE DISEASE

Descriptive studies of the natural history of a particular disease generally are available. For colorectal cancer, as illustrated in Table 13-1, 5-year survival correlates very well with the degree of localization of the tumor at the time of diagnosis.

_____ STUDY QUESTION 13-1
What can we infer from this correlation about the value of early detection?

PROSPECTIVE UNCONTROLLED FOLLOW-UP STUDY

The study by Gilbertsen and Nelms [7] often is quoted as documenting the value of early detection in decreasing mortality from colorectal cancer. In this study, data was collected on persons screened at the Cancer Detection Center of the University of Minnesota. The group gradually grew larger as the data was collected, being composed of persons entering the screening program over a period of years (1948 through 1971). Eventually, 21,150 individuals underwent a total of 113,800 periodic examinations (i.e., general physical examination and annual rigid 25-cm proctosigmoidoscopy, as well as "pertinent examination procedures"). *All polyps found on proctosigmoidoscopy were removed.* Results are presented in Tables 13-2 and 13-3.

_____ STUDY QUESTION 13-2
(a) Examine Table 13-2. Compare the number of cancers found on initial examination with those expected. How do you explain the results? Now compare the number of cancers found on subsequent examinations with the number expected. How do you explain the difference? Are these results typical of screening programs? (b) Examine Table 13-3. How do you explain the expected and observed stages of tumor and 5-year survival rates?

As was discussed in an earlier chapter, a number of problems called biases may cloud the results of uncontrolled screening follow-up studies [2]:

Table 13-2. Number of cancers of distal 25 cm
of colon detected in uncontrolled cohort study

	Initial examination	Subsequent examinations
No. of examinations	21,150	92,650
No. of persons	21,150	21,150
No. of cancers found	27	13
Expected no. of cancers	<27	87–97*

*Estimated from epidemiologic data.
Source: Data from Gilbertsen and Nelms [8].

Table 13-3. Percentage of cancers of distal 25 cm of the colon at various stages

	Localized	Regional	Advanced	Overall survival
Expected percentage	45	29	26	31
Percentage at initial examination	78	11	11	64
Percentage at subsequent examination	100	—	—	85

Source: Data from Gilbertsen and Nelms [8].

Lead-time bias: Early detection may only move forward the time of detection of the disease without moving back the time of death.

Length bias: To understand length bias, we must first define the preclinical interval. As discussed in Chapter 3, the preclinical interval is the interval between the time a screening test could detect a cancer and the time the patient would seek a diagnosis because of symptoms or signs. In general, early detection screening programs diagnose tumors with longer preclinical intervals than tumors found in unscreened populations. That is to say, tumors picked up in screening programs may be slower growing and have a longer asymptomatic phase. This complicates the interpretation of screening studies.

Patient self-selection bias: The patient population that is screened is biologically or behaviorally different enough from an unscreened comparison group to affect their survival rate.

Overdiagnosis bias: Overdiagnosis (i.e., false positive diagnosis) of localized malignancy can lead to apparently higher incidence rates and give the appearence of a better 5-year survival rate.

_____ STUDY QUESTION 13-3
Review the follow-up study and consider the results with regard to the four biases listed. To what extent do you believe that these results show that early detection improves outcome?

RANDOMIZED CONTROLLED STUDY

The problems with uncontrolled follow-up studies can be overcome by a randomized controlled trial, in which the population is randomized to a screened study group or an unscreened control group. In such a study, the screened and unscreened populations should ideally have comparable cancers and host characteristics, eliminating most of the biases and patient selection problems enumerated previously. However, eliminating the lead-time bias still requires that the follow-up period be sufficiently long to demonstrate a difference in survival if one does exist.

One randomized controlled trial—the Kaiser-Permanente Multiphasic Checkup Evaluation Study [11–13]—is cited widely as evidence for the effectiveness of early screening for colorectal cancer. The setting for this study was a prepaid health maintenance organization. A group of approximately 5000 control and 5000 study subjects, aged 35 to 54 years, were randomly assigned from a subset of the subscribers to the health plan.

The study group was urged to receive periodic multiphasic checkups, including rigid sigmoidoscopy for persons older than 40. One of the outcome assessments was mortality from specific causes. In a 10-year follow-up report, comparison of more than 30 causes of death was made between the control and study group. There was a statistically significant decrease in mortality in the study group for one cause, colorectal cancer (p < .05). Follow-up data on patients with colorectal cancer [11] are summarized below.

	Study	Control
No. of deaths secondary to colorectal cancer	5	18
No. of cases of colorectal cancer	20	25
Percentage of cases in early stage	60	48–52
Percentage of sigmoidoscopies performed per patient-years of observation	8.1	5.2

In view of the large number of cases of mortality analyzed, how much importance does the finding of one statistically significant difference have? Looking at a large number of study outcomes weakens the statistical validity of the results. If we look at enough comparisons between a study and control group, we are likely to find some difference by chance alone. Statisticians refer to this as the multiple comparison problem. To have statistical validity, the hypotheses being tested must be stated explicitly at the start of the study and should be few in number. Thus, we would like to know whether the hypothesis that screening would improve outcome in colorectal cancer was stated prior to learning the results.

In fact, the following statement is found in the study reports [12]: "Before the results of the mortality comparisons became available, three physicians independently compiled lists of those causes of death they thought were most likely to be preventable or postponable" in the study group. The final agreed-upon "list includes: cancers of the large bowel, rectum, breast, cervix, uterus, kidney and prostate; hypertension and hypertensive cardiovascular disease; and intracranial hemorrhages." In light of this methodologic information, what conclusions can we draw from this study?

The authors have reduced the number of mortality comparisons hypothesized in advance to approximately eight [12]. This is still a large number of comparisons, and the possibility of a statistically significant difference owing to chance still exists (type I error). From the information available to us, we can say that this study is suggestive but not conclusive, primarily because of the multiple comparison problem. In fact, this study was not specifically designed to test the hypothesis that screening sigmoidoscopy reduces mortality from colon cancer.*

What can we say in summary about the benefit of screening sigmoidoscopy for early detection and improved survival in colorectal cancer? The improved prognosis for tumors resected at an early Dukes stage as well as the results of the Gilbertsen and Nelms study [8] point strongly toward substantial improvement in outcome. However, one must be cautious about drawing conclusions based on this information

---

*It is important to note that such a randomized controlled study of a screening test could demonstrate a *decreased mortality rate* from colon cancer for the screened group as compared with the control group. In assessing the usefulness of studies that evaluate screening tests, the demonstration of such a decreased cause-specific mortality rate for the screened group as a whole is a better measure of benefit than a reduced case-fatality rate among those individuals who are diagnosed as having the disease.

alone. Unfortunately, there has been no randomized controlled trial designed to test the utility of screening sigmoidoscopy. The Kaiser Multiphasic Health Checkup Trial [12–14] suffers from the multiple comparison problem and is inconclusive.† Clinicians are often faced with inconclusive data of this sort but nevertheless must make decisions based on the information at hand.

There are also two large ongoing prospective studies examining the role of Hemoccult testing in the early detection and outcome of colorectal cancer [15, 16]. Both are comparing control and study groups unscreened and screened by Hemoccult testing. More than 70,000 persons are involved in these studies. Preliminary results from both studies show a shift to earlier pathologic stages in the screened groups, confirming the results of the cohort studies. However, until a full follow-up period is completed and long-term survival rates are compared in the two groups, the lead-time bias cannot be discounted.

Is Screening Feasible and Practical?

How good are the screening tests for colorectal cancer? We will now examine in detail the two tests currently used for screening for colorectal carcinoma and polyps: guaiac occult blood testing and sigmoidoscopy. Remember that in choosing a screening test, we seek high sensitivity and specificity, reproducibility, low cost, and safety.

GUAIAC OCCULT BLOOD TESTING

Description of the Hemoccult Test

Guaiac occult blood testing using the Hemoccult test is currently the most widely used technique for screening for colorectal cancer. The test involves the application of a sample of feces on a card impregnated with guaiac. A drop of hydrogen peroxide in alcohol is then applied. If hemoglobin is present, a blue color quickly appears. The chemical mechanism

†Additional analysis of the Kaiser study data (JV Selby and GD Friedman, paper presented to the U.S. Preventive Services Task Force, April 1987) describes a lower incidence of cancer in the distal 20 cm of colon in the study group; this is the portion surveyed by rigid sigmoidoscopy. Moreover, only 250 more persons were exposed to this sigmoidoscopic screening in the study group than in the control group. Both of these facts suggest that the reduced mortality from colon cancer in the study group was primarily due to the chance occurrence of a lower incidence of cancer in this group and cannot be attributed to the screening sigmoidoscopies.

is the oxidation of guaiac to a blue product in the presence of hydrogen peroxide and peroxidase activity. Hemoglobin has peroxidase activity. Other substances that have peroxidase activity and can cause false positive reactions include many fresh fruits and vegetables and rare red meat. Rehydrating dry fecal smears with water prior to adding alcoholic hydrogen peroxide increases sensitivity. Iron tablets, aspirin, and nonsteroidal antiinflammatory drugs may also produce false positive reactions. Vitamin C ingestion may cause a false negative reaction. Hemoccult cards are inexpensive, and there are no risks of the test itself. The test can be performed by a nonmedical person with brief training.

Specificity of Hemoccult Testing
Specificity is defined as the ability of the test to be negative in the absence of disease (negative in health, or NIH). Thus, to determine specificity, one finds a population proved or presumed to be free of the disease and performs the screening test.

An example of such a study is that of McCrae and colleagues [17]. This study used 172 healthy subjects younger than 40 years of age (mean, 22 + 4.4 years). The subjects had no history of bleeding hemorrhoids, gastrointestinal disease, or ingestion of antiinflammatory or analgesic drugs. None of the subjects had any investigation for occult gastrointestinal bleeding. The subjects were given a specified diet for 6 days. On the last 3 days of the diet, they collected two stool specimens, each applied in duplicate on Hemoccult II cards. Some of the results are summarized in Table 13-4.

_____ STUDY QUESTION 13-4
(a) Which diet gives a higher false positive rate? (b) Given that rehydration increases the sensitivity of the test for cancer of the colon, what method would you choose, and what diet would you advise, for routine screening? Support your answer. (c) What is the specificity of the method and diet you would use?

Sensitivity of Hemoccult Testing
The sensitivity of a test for a specified disease is the ability of the test to be positive in the presence of that disease (positive in disease, or PID). Thus, to study sensitivity, one can take a study population all of whom have the disease, perform the screening test, and calculate the sensitivity.

The study of Crowley and co-workers [18] illustrates this approach. Colonoscopy was performed in 213 patients over a 10-month period. All patients had symptoms or signs suggesting colorectal pathology or were

Table 13-4. Summary of Hemoccult test results in normal subjects on a specified diet

| Diet | No. of subjects | No. of tests | Positive Hemoccult II test without rehydration | | | Positive rehydrated Hemoccult II test | |
			No. of tests	No. of subjects*		No. of tests	No. of subjects*
Rare red meat and high-peroxidase vegetables	52	306	0/306	0/52		13/306 (4.2%)	8/52
No red meat and no fresh fruit or vegetable	52	310	0/310	0/52		2/310 (0.6%)	2/52

*Individuals with one or more positive tests.
Source: Data from McCrae and Colleagues (17).

Table 13-5. Colonoscopic findings and Hemoccult test results in 198 patients

Colonoscopic findings	Hemoccult II positive	Hemoccult II negative	Total no. of patients
Carcinoma	14	13	27
Adenoma			
<1.0 cm in diameter	2	43	45
>1.0 cm in diameter	10	34	44
No lesions	6	60	66
Inflammatory bowel disease	2	9	11
Diverticulosis	0	5	5

Source: Data from Crowley and co-workers [18].

in a high-risk group. The procedure included a high-bulk, red meat–free, vitamin C–free diet and collection of two stool samples on each of 3 consecutive days, applied to Hemoccult II cards. All cards were read by the physician performing the colonoscopy within 5 days of collecting the first sample. The on-slide card monitors were used to ensure quality control. The cards were not rehydrated. A specimen was considered positive if any trace of blue appeared within 60 seconds. Hemoccult results for a patient were considered positive if one or more of the specimens tested positive. The results in patients who had cancer, polyps, or no lesions are summarized in Table 13-5.

_____ STUDY QUESTION 13-5
Calculate the sensitivity of (a) Hemoccult II for carcinoma, (b) adenomas of less than 1 cm, and (c) adenomas of more than 1 cm. (d) Calculate the specificity of Hemoccult II for patients in this study in whom no lesions were found in their intestines.

_____ STUDY QUESTION 13-6
For this group of 213 high-risk patients, calculate the predictive value of a positive Hemoccult test for colorectal cancer.

_____ STUDY QUESTION 13-7
Assuming a specificity of 96 percent and a sensitivity of 52 percent, calculate the predictive value positive and negative (i.e., the predictive value of a positive and a negative test) for colorectal cancer of a positive Hemoccult test applied to a screening population with a prevalence of colorectal cancer estimated to be 3 per 1000. Why is the predictive value positive so low? How can we improve it?

—————————————————————————— STUDY QUESTION 13-8
First-degree blood relatives of patients with known colorectal cancer have a 3-fold increased risk of developing colorectal cancer (9 per 1000). For this group, calculate the positive predictive value of a positive Hemoccult test, assuming the same specificity and sensitivity as in study question 13-7.

SIGMOIDOSCOPY
Rigid sigmoidoscopy has had a long heritage as a screening tool for the early detection and prevention of colorectal cancer. As discussed earlier, the follow-up study by Gilbertsen and Nelms [8] and the Kaiser randomized controlled study [12–14] used rigid sigmoidoscopy as their screening tool before guaiac occult blood testing was refined to the present status of Hemoccult II.

In one way, sigmoidoscopy is more like a gold standard than a screening test, because it is able to divide definitively a group of individuals into those with and those without adenomatous polyps or cancers. This accepts as a given the endoscopist's ability to recognize what he or she is seeing and a negligible rate of missed lesions. In another way, sigmoidoscopy is more like a screening test than a gold standard in that it is limited by its depth of insertion in its ability to determine whether a patient's entire colon is totally free of adenomatous polyps or cancer. Its sensitivity is less than 50 percent, since fewer than one-half of colorectal polyps and cancers are located in the distal 25 cm of bowel.

Most experts believe that sigmoidoscopy and guaiac testing are complementary [19]. Because of the sigmoidoscope's limited depth of insertion and the amount of colon surveyed, sigmoidoscopy alone cannot replace FOBT, which can pick up higher lesions that frequently bleed more. Similarly, for left-sided lesions that generally bleed less than right-sided ones, guaiac testing has a substantial false negative rate in the very region where sigmoidoscopy is more effective. Furthermore, many adenomas do not bleed substantially and will therefore not be picked up by FOBT. In one of the controlled trials currently in progress, as many as 76 percent of those adenomas larger than 0.5 cm in the distal or rectal sigmoid were missed by guaiac testing and picked up by rigid sigmoidoscopy [15]. Further preliminary data from this ongoing trial indicate that of 59 study group cancers detected, 36 (61 percent) were detected by guaiac testing alone, 7 (12 percent) by both methods, and 8 (13 percent) by proctosigmoidoscopy alone. The remaining 8 (13 percent) were discovered by "further diagnostic evaluation" undertaken secondary to symptoms.

Clearly, one of the major limitations of rigid sigmoidoscopy is the limited depth of insertion of the scope. Studies have demonstrated that only
the distal 16 to 19.5 cm of colon is reliably examined [20]. Also of concern is that more modern assessments of the distribution of colonic neo-
plasias undertaken by pathologists and colonoscopists reveal a "proximal
or rightward progression" of such neoplasia. This discovery in effect reduced the expected yield from both rigid sigmoidoscopy and digital rectal examination [21].

In 1969, the first fiberoptic colonscopes were invented. Shortly thereafter, several investigators developed the technique of using flexible fiberoptic scopes of various lengths (so-called short colonoscopes) in place
of the rigid sigmoidoscope to perform sigmoidoscopy. Greater length
provided greater yield, and the flexible scopes provided greater patient
comfort as well.

After settling on a 60- to 65-cm length (because of ease of preparation
and patient tolerance without anesthesia), several technical modifica-
tions and advances in scope construction were made over the ensuing
years. The most recent innovation is again related to length—the appearance of a 30- to 35-cm scope that is advertised as being easier for
nonendoscopists to learn to use [22]. Table 13-6 compares the various
sigmoidoscopic technologies available today [15, 23]. Current expert recommendations for guaiac testing and sigmoidoscopic screening for colorectal cancer are outlined in Appendixes A, B, and C.

Risk-Benefit and Cost-Effectiveness Issues
In the previous section, we explored many characteristics of the screening tests for colorectal cancer. The question remains: Are these tests safe
and affordable enough to recommend for large groups of people? To
approach an answer to this question, we will perform some simplified
analyses that apply the principles of risk-benefit and cost effectiveness
to the problem of screening for colorectal cancer.

RISK-BENEFIT ANALYSIS
In risk-benefit analysis, the risks and benefits of the therapy, screening
test, or preventive maneuver are weighed without considerations of cost,
and if found favorable in terms of lives saved and disability prevented,
the maneuver can be recommended. Typically, results are in terms of
patient-years of life saved for a given intervention.

The risks of the screening tests in question have already been outlined.

Table 13-6. Comparison of sigmoidoscopic technologies

Characteristic	Rigid sigmoidoscopy	Flexible sigmoidoscopy	
Perforations	0.2–7/10,000 cases	1/10,000 cases	
Safety	Mortality near 0	Complications 1/1000	

Detection rate
  Usually published
    screening rate
	Cancer: 0.15–0.3%
	Polyps: 6.0%
		—
		—	

Maximum potential yield
  compared with
  colonoscopy (100%)
	Cancer: 28%
	Polyps: 5%
		Cancer: 64% (60-cm scope)
		Polyps: 66% (60-cm scope)	

		30-CM FFS	60-CM FFS

Relative total diagnostic
  yield compared with
  rigid sigmoidoscopy
	1	2 : 1	3.2 : 1

Depth of reliable insertion	16–19.5 cm	27–29 cm	45–55 cm
Minutes required for procedure	2–5	5–6	8–10
Discomfort index*	0.8	0.3	0.4
Cost of equipment	$400	$1200–$1500	$3000–$4000

FFS = flexible fiberoptic sigmoidoscope.
*0 = no pain; 1 = mild to moderate pain; 2 = severe pain.
Source: Data from Crespi and Weissman [19]; Tedesco et al. [21]; Bolt [23]; and W Steinberg, unpublished research on screening for colon cancer.

For sigmoidoscopy, see Table 13-6. There are essentially no risks of guaiac testing. What, then, are the putative benefits from screening?

The most direct benefit is early detection of cancers in asymptomatic individuals. The Gilbertsen and Nelms cohort study [8] and other published data imply an improved 5-year survival of 80 to 90 percent for patients with lesions detected on screening in asymptomatic individuals, as compared to 40 to 50 percent survival for patients in whom lesions are diagnosed after symptoms occur. This improved survival is attributable to the earlier stage at which the cancers are detected on screening. The rate at which such cancers are detected by sigmoidoscopy or guaiac testing at screening is estimated to vary from 1.5 to 3 per 1000 examinations.

When the two screening methods are together, there is an appreciable amount of overlap, as evidenced by the data from one of the modern controlled trials currently in progress [15]. This overlap will no doubt be even greater with the use of a flexible sigmoidoscope, which can see farther and detect more neoplasia than the rigid sigmoidoscopes used in this trial. Even if the tests are found to be totally additive (i.e., little overlap), we must remember that this represents only a percentage of the cancers expected to occur in the screened group because neither test is 100-percent sensitive.

Sample Case

For every 10,000 screening examinations (both guaiac testing and sigmoidoscopy), let us see how many patient-years of life can be saved. With an additive detection of 3.0 per 1000 (allowing for a substantial degree of overlap when both tests are used together), 30 cancers would be detected per 10,000 patients. Using a 90-percent survival rate (*survival rate* meaning a 5-year disease-free period*) and assuming cancers are detected by screening in asymptomatic individuals, 90 percent of 30 patients would live an extra 5 years each; thus, 135 patient-years would be saved. If these same cancers are not detected until symptoms appear, only a 50-percent survival rate is operating, and only 75 patient-years will be saved. Screening results in 60 *additional* years of life saved.

What about the potential benefits derived from detecting and remov-

---

*This simplified analysis does not take into account years of life saved beyond 5 years nor the years gained by those who die within 5 years. These simplifications probably underestimate the benefit.

ing adenomatous polyps before they become malignant? Recall that one of the most powerful possible interpretations of the Gilbertsen and Nelms data [8] (biases notwithstanding) was that the less-than-expected incidence of lower bowel cancers detected after initial screening could well have been caused in part by the removal of adenomas with malignant potential. Because adenomas are much more common, the rate at which they are detected by screening is substantially higher than that for cancer—perhaps 10-fold higher. Because patients are at increased risk for cancer if adenomas are present (approximately 5 percent versus 0.2 percent, with a relative risk of 25 : 1) and the risk increases as the number, size, and degree of atypia of the adenomas increases, the potential benefits of finding an adenoma are really 2-fold: First, the discovery places the patient in a higher-risk category, which requires, according to present recommendations, surveillance of the entire colon. The reason for this is the increased risk of cancer and a 20 to 30 percent chance of having a second synchronous (i.e., concurrent) adenoma. There is also a 20 to 30 percent chance of having a metachronous (i.e., subsequent) adenoma after all initial ones are detected. Thus, there is an additional requirement of follow-up surveillance of the *entire colon* [8]. Second, there is the potential benefit, as discussed earlier, of preventing the development of all future colorectal cancers if all adenomas are removed.

_____ STUDY QUESTION 13-9
Would this more aggressive approach to cancer detection and prevention affect our risk-benefit assessment of screening?

Because of the exceedingly low risks of sigmoidoscopy (even with polypectomy) and of guaiac testing, the risk-benefit assessment for screening for colorectal cancer appears favorable even if only a relatively modest benefit is eventually proved.

COST EFFECTIVENESS
In today's world of ever-increasing constraints on health care resources, more and more of what we do in medicine is being subjected to question and analysis from an economic point of view. It is no longer adequate to show that benefits are tangible and risks are negligible. Because the pie of health care resources is finite and because resources spent on one program are no longer available for another (opportunity cost), society is increasingly concerned with maximizing benefit for each health care dollar.

Hence, cost-effectiveness analyses are undertaken to ensure that the greatest benefits are obtained within the limits of resources that exist. It is the final, qualifying phrase that is most important. Another way of saying this is that a particular health benefit achieved must be viewed as worth the additional cost. Cost-effectiveness analyses do not provide a magic ratio or number that indicates whether something should or should not be done. Rather, they provide data that allow one to make choices about how to spend health care dollars. Usually, the benefits have already been proved to be greater than the risks. The question then becomes: How much are we willing to pay for the benefits? [24].

Doubilet and colleagues [24] in a recent article point out the caution we must use in posing and interpreting cost-effectiveness questions. Though used frequently today, the term *cost effectiveness* does not always appear in the same context. At times, the issue is a comparison of doing something and doing nothing (such as screening for or not screening for lung cancer). More frequently, though, the choice is between two different strategies of care with a common goal, such as surgical and medical approaches to a given problem or, in our case, screening for colonic cancer with guaiac testing, flexible sigmoidoscopy, or both. In such cases, it may be possible to demonstrate a clear preference within a certain limit of resources, but it may also be possible to achieve even greater benefit with greater resources. Such alternatives raise the large social and political questions of values and opportunity cost, issues that will be debated into the future.

Cost-Effectiveness Calculations

SIMPLIFIED ANALYSIS.   We will discuss a simplified cost-effectiveness analysis of screening for colorectal cancer in order to illustrate how such an analysis works. The actual methods of accounting for all the costs and benefits of screening for colorectal cancer are beyond the scope of this chapter. They include methods for calculating exact direct cost (the cost of production of materials and manpower used), indirect costs (overhead and shared support), and induced costs (those costs or savings that result from further evaluations either undertaken or avoided because of the results of the screening tests). Such methods also take into account the differences that are believed to exist between costs and benefits that are available today and those that are projected to occur in the future. Depreciation and discounting are used for such an analysis. There are also methods for adjusting benefits from the mixed health outcomes achieved in the real world (i.e., the effects of morbidity as well as mortality) by calculating quality-adjusted life years rather than just assigning equal value to all years of life gained or lost regardless of their quality as a result of a particular intervention.

These complexities are beyond the scope of our discussion, but Weinstein and Fineberg [25] have elaborated on them. Let us begin with a rather streamlined definition of cost effectiveness, which we will further simplify to demonstrate such an analysis for colorectal cancer screening. Cost effectiveness is a calculation of the cost of providing additional years of life, represented most simply by the formula: net cost/net effectiveness (C/E). It is usually expressed in terms of dollars per year of life saved. Net *cost* equals the cost of screening (Cp) plus the (induced) cost of treating side effects of screening (Cse) minus the (induced) cost that would have been required to treat those "saved" by screening (Ct). Net *effectiveness* equals the years of life gained (Eli) and disability avoided (Em) by screening minus the years of life lost owing to death or disability caused by the screening process itself (Ese). Thus, the formula is:

$$C/E = \frac{net\ cost}{net\ effectiveness} = \frac{Cp + Cse - Ct}{Eli + Em - Ese}$$

Using a simplified version of this formula, one can determine a first approximation of the cost effectiveness of screening for colorectal cancer. One first considers only the cost of screening and assumes a zero rate of side effects; that is, Cse and Ct are set to equal zero. Next, if one considers only cures or years of disease-free life gained by screening and leaves aside the issues of disability and quality of life, Em and Ese (zero side effects) are also set to equal zero. The simplified formula now reads C/E = Cp/Eli.

_____ STUDY QUESTION 13-10

Given the following, what would the cost effectiveness of such a screening program be in dollars per year of life preserved?

A 50-percent year survival rate for cancers detected at appearance of symptoms

A 90-percent-year survival rate for cancers detected at screening

A screening including 10,000 asymptomatic individuals that detects 30 cancers

A cost of $50 per screening examination

An interpretation of survival rate as 5-years of disease-free life

Now, if we did indeed save an additional 12 people, we would really be able to calculate into our net cost the saving accrued from not having to treat 12 ultimately fatal cases of colorectal cancer (a negative induced cost). Because this is an expensive disease to treat, our savings could be substantial. For instance, if it cost $40,000 to treat a patient with metastatic (late) colon cancer before he or she succumbs, the calculations would change as follows: $500,000.00 − (12 × $40,000.00) = $20,000.00/60 years = $333 per year of life preserved.

In reality, patients who are "saved" may need surgery to remove the early cancer and because an early cancer was found, may need high-risk surveillance for at least 5 years because they are at risk of developing a metachronous lesion. These positive induced costs would need to be added as well, thereby reducing the favorability of our cost-effectiveness ratio. Nonetheless, the point here is that because colorectal cancer is such an expensive disease to palliate before the patient's ultimate demise, there is an overall good chance that the cost-effectiveness ratio will be reasonable regardless of whether the difference in survival is shown in controlled randomized trials to be as favorable as the 80 to 90 percent predicted. The favorable ratio should remain even after the cost of future surveillance of such high-risk patients is added in.

COMPARING DIFFERENT APPROACHES TO THE SAME PROBLEM.   Now, as we indicated earlier, another way of using cost-effectiveness analysis is in comparing different approaches to the same problem. One of the currently relevant questions facing those screening for colorectal cancer is whether to perform flexible sigmoidoscopies. Guaiac testing is certainly cheap and easy, and the question many are asking is whether the additional cancers discovered with flexible sigmoidoscopy are worth the cost. (We will ignore the issue of polyps for the present discussion.) Let us perform an *incremental cost-effectiveness analysis* on screening for colorectal cancer, comparing guaiac testing alone (approach A)with combined guaiac testing and flexible sigmoidoscopy (approach B), to determine the utility of adding flexible sigmoidoscopy to the screening package [25].

1. Consider the same survival rates as were noted in study question 13-10.

2. Consider a screening of 10,000 asymptomatic individuals in which 30 cancers are discovered.
3. Consider that 65 percent of the cancers are detected by guaiac testing and 35 percent are detected by flexible sigmoidoscopy. (These numbers are derived in part from the data on page 216 and were adjusted for the fact that we are using flexible rather than rigid sigmoidoscopy.)
4. Consider that of our previously quoted $50 charge, $5 is for guaiac testing and $45 is for sigmoidoscopy.

	Cancers Found	Total Cost	Additional Cancers	Incremental Cost	Incremental Cost per Additional Cancer
Approach A Guaiac testing	19.5	$50,000	19.5	$50,000	$2564
Approach B Guaiac testing and flexible sigmoidoscopy	30	$500,000	10.5	$450,000	$42,857

Translating this into cost per year of life saved (using the method from our first example), we would obtain the following (excluding the large costs avoided by *not* treating those saved by screening):

Approach A $50,000/39 patient-years = $1282/per patient-year

Approach B $500,000/60 patient-years = $8333/per patient-year

$$\text{Incremental Cost-effectiveness ratio} = \frac{\text{cost of B} - \text{cost of A}}{\text{years of life saved by B} - \text{years of life saved by A}}$$

$$= \$21,429 \text{ per additional patient-year saved}$$

As you can see, the additional lives saved by the inclusion of flexible sigmoidoscopy in the screening regimen are very costly. Whether it is appropriate to pay for this additional health benefit is a matter of values, choice, and opportunity costs.

Variables Affecting Cost Effectiveness

We still need to demonstrate the improved survival of patients with earlier-stage lesions detected by screening and assumed in the preceding example. That notwithstanding, the issue of cost effectiveness of screening for colorectal cancer is actually far more complicated. The goal is one of maximizing effectiveness: to pick up or prevent more early cancers per number of patients screened or number of screenings done per patient [26]. The specific issues include:

The sensitivity and specificity of the screening test

The frequency of the screening maneuver

The risk level of the group screened

The costs of the screening tests

Whether detection and removal of polyps should be part of the screening maneuver.

SENSITIVITY AND SPECIFICITY OF THE SCREENING TESTS.   If the sensitivity of one's screening tests is too low, there is a likelihood that too many cases will be missed on screening and that the overall group mortality from colorectal cancer among those screened will not be substantially affected. This would be true even if the survival were substantially prolonged for those in whom cancers were detected by screening. In such a case, the costs of screening the whole population would not be justified for the benefit shown in just a few individuals.

If the specificity is too low (i.e., if we have too high a false positive rate), and we waste many dollars in evaluating false positive individuals who are healthy, our cost per patient-year of life preserved can quickly become exorbitant.

FREQUENCY OF THE SCREENING MANEUVER.   As exemplified by the Gilbertsen and Nelms study [8], the number of subsequent (or incidence) cancers detected by follow-up screening is less than the number of initial (or prevalence) cancers detected at the first screening. The obvious reason for this is that prevalence is much higher than incidence. Additionally, this may be attributable to the decrease in premalignant lesions, because in several studies all polyps discovered were removed. Another explanation is the proposed slow pace of the adenoma-carcinoma sequence. Remember, it is believed to take 5 to 10 years or longer for an adenoma to transform into colonic cancer. Recognition of this fact is

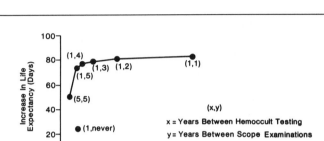

Fig. 13-1. Effect of sigmoidoscopy and occult blood test on life expectancy and financial costs of screening an average-risk woman for colon cancer. Main assumptions are: (1) screening is begun at age 50; (2) statistics for the occult blood test are estimated from an ongoing randomized controlled trial of the Hemoccult test; (3) Hemoccult testing costs $2 and is mailed to a laboratory or a physician's office; (4) sigmoidoscopy costs $35; (5) the false positive rate of Hemoccult testing is 1 percent; (6) 85 percent of cancers come from adenomatous polyps, and polyps in the sigmoid region are detectable by a sigmoidoscope an average of 7 years before causing signs or symptoms; (7) 60 percent of cancers are within reach of a sigmoidoscopic examination. (From Eddy [26].)

responsible for the current recommendation for sigmoidoscopy every 3 to 5 years rather than annually, as was previously recommended. It has been estimated that annual screening of all people in the United States who are older than 40 would cost $2.75 billion! As Eddy [26] has illustrated in Figure 13-1, the improvement in survival is only minimally affected by this degree of lengthening of the screening interval. The money saved could be used to reach more people for screening (or to help balance the federal, health maintenance organization, or family budget, depending on who is paying).

RISK LEVEL OF THE GROUP SCREENED.   If we screen patients at greater risk for cancer, we will increase the pick-up rates for screening tests performed and improve our cost-effectiveness ratio. This is true because if we increase the pretest probability of disease or prevalence (as exists in a high-risk group), the predictive value of a positive screening increases (i.e., a positive screening test is more likely to represent a true positive than a false positive). Hence, we will be less likely to waste money working up a false positive test.

The decision about whom to screen is a central one to all cancer detection and prevention programs. Exactly where to draw the line in average-risk patients is a judgment call, but costs can be calculated for each point chosen. The general recommendation for colorectal cancer screening is to start screening individuals between the ages of 40 and 50 years. This is in recognition of the fact that the incidence doubles with each decade beyond age 40.

COSTS OF SCREENING TESTS.   Clearly, if the costs of the screening tests increase substantially, the cost-effectiveness ratio for large-scale screening programs will be seriously affected. With regard to sigmoidoscopy, the major issue is the increased costs of flexible sigmoidoscopy compared to rigid sigmoidoscopy. The flexible instruments are more expensive to purchase and maintain, but over many examinations, these differences in cost outlays diminish. The more important component is the physician cost. If this is closer to the fee charged for rigid sigmoidoscopy, then the cost-effectiveness ratio will definitely be improved by the increased detection rates of which the flexible method is capable. If, however, the physician cost is substantially higher, such cost-effectiveness benefits could easily be nullified. With regard to guaiac testing some of the newer methods offer potential benefits in both increased sensitivity and specificity, which would increase the pick-up rate and lower the false positive rate. The problem is that these new tests presently cost 10 times more than Hemoccult testing and are not generally available. Their costliness currently prohibits their use in large-scale screening programs.

SHOULD DETECTION AND REMOVAL OF POLYPS BE A PART OF THE SCREENING MANEUVER?   We have indicated that in as many as 10 to 20 percent of patients screened polyps will be discovered, and these patients are at increased risk for further development of polyps and for cancer. Such patients are currently recommended for high-risk screening and periodic surveillance (the exact protocol may depend on the characteristics of their polyps) until a cancer is found or until their risk returns to average. This could produce an even higher level of effectiveness by eliminating additional cancer deaths not prevented by usual or single first-line screening for cancer alone. However, effectiveness may be decreased if the side effects of colonoscopy plus polypectomy result in a substantially higher rate of morbidity and mortality than the negligible rate with sigmoidoscopy alone.

Also, the cost of this approach—polyps detection and removal—would certainly increase because of the attendant positive induced costs of the high-risk surveillance protocol that would be applied to *all* patients with adenomas even though only a minority of them would ultimately develop cancer. Ultimately false positive patients would undergo a high-cost work-up. These added induced costs would result in a less favorable cost-effectiveness ratio.

Alternatively, as more information about polyps is learned, patients in whom no polyps have been detected over several screenings may be found to be at a substantially below-average risk, and their surveillance interval could be lengthened, which could result in a decrease in net cost.

The question of the effect of polyp removal on colorectal cancer mortality is one of great interest and considerable activity. While the randomized controlled trials in progress now may provide some answers to this question, there are other studies in progress to assess the outcomes of high-risk surveillance protocols once an adenoma is detected [27]. The goal of these latter studies is to further define the risk of subgroups and the prognosis for the ultimate development of colorectal cancer. With this information, a better assessment will be possible for the cost effectiveness of screening in which adenomas are considered a positive finding and patients are followed up with colonoscopy and prophylactic removal of such polyps.

Worth Is a Function of Context

Given different scenarios and points of view, we would like you to list the factors that would enter into a decision regarding a policy for screening for colorectal cancer on the basis of current evidence. Consider the following:

1. You are an asymptomatic 50-year-old patient without any risk factors for cancer of the colon. You are insured by a commercial carrier who does not cover preventive services.
2. You are an asymptomatic 50-year-old patient with the same insurance as in item 1. Your father died of colonic cancer.
3. You are an internist or family practitioner in private practice (i.e., fee for service). You can bill $35 for a 25-cm rigid sigmoidoscopy and

$100 for a flexible sigmoidoscopy. Most patients who are asymptomatic will not be covered for preventive screening for sigmoidoscopy or Hemoccult testing.
4. You are a salaried general internist. You work for a health maintenance organization. Your income does not vary with the specific procedures that you perform.
5. You are the medical director of a health maintenance organization. You are asked to formulate for the organization a screening policy regarding colorectal cancer, taking into account the cost benefit aspects of this policy to the patients and to the health maintenance organization.
6. You are a physician-administrator for a major commercial insurance carrier (e.g., Blue Shield). You are asked to develop a policy regarding coverage or noncoverage for screening for colorectal cancer.

What Will You Do, Dr. Grady, in regard to this and many other complex issues of clinical prevention? Apply the concepts outlined in this chapter, analyze the relevant studies, and make an informed and rational decision.

References

1. Report of the Canadian Task Force on the periodic health examination. Hull, Quebec: Canadian Government Publishing Center, Supply and Services Canada, 1980.
2. American Cancer Society. Guidelines for the cancer-related checkup: recommendations and rationale. 1980;198:44–46.
3. American Cancer Society. CA: Cancer J Clinicians Cancer Statistics, 1985;35:19–56.
4. Astler VB, Coller FA. The prognostic significance of direct extension of carcinoma of the colon and rectum. Ann Surg 1951;139:846–851.
5. Winawer SJ, Fleisher M, Sherlock P. Sensitivity of fecal occult blood testing for adenomas (editorial). Gastroenterology 1982;83:1136–1141.
6. Morson BC. Genesis of colorectal cancer. Clin Gastroenterol 1976;5:505–55.
7. Sherlock P, Lipkin M. The prevention of invasive cancer. Am J Med 1980;68:917–931.
8. Gilbertsen VA, Nelms JM. The prevention of colon cancer of the rectum. Cancer 1978;41:1137–1139.
9. Castleman B. The colonic adenoma-carcinoma sequence: the evidence against the relationship. Bethesda, Md.: National Institutes of Health,

1979. (NIH publication no. 80–2075; screening and early detection of colorectal cancer.).

10. Lambert R, Sobin LH, Waye JD et al. The management of patients with colorectal adenomas. CA: Cancer J Clinicians 1984;31:167–176.

11. Dales G, Friedman GD, Collen MF. Evaluating periodic multiphasic checkups: a controlled trial. J Chronic Dis 1979;32:385–404.

12. Dales LG, Friedman GD, Ramcharan S, et al. Multiphasic checkup evaluation study 3. Outpatient clinic utilization, hospitalization and mortality experience after seven years. Prev Med 1973;2:221–235.

13. Cutler JL, Ramcharan S, Feldman R, et al. Multiphasic checkup evaluation study 1. Methods and populations. Prev Med 1973;2:197–206.

14. Ramcharan S, Cutler JL, Feldman R, et al. Multiphasic checkup evaluation study 2. Disability and chronic disease after seven years of multiphasic health checkups. Prev Med 1973;2:207–22.

15. Winawer SJ, Andrews M, Flehinger B, et al. Progress report on controlled trial of fecal occult blood testing for the detection of colorectal neoplasia. Cancer 1980;45:2959–2964.

16. Gilbertsen VA, McHugh R, Schuman L, et al. The earlier detection of colorectal cancers: a preliminary report of the results of the occult blood study. Cancer 1980;45:2899–2901.

17. McCrae FA, St. John JB, Caligiore P, et al. Optimal dietary conditions for hemoccult testing. Gastroenterology 1982;82:899–903.

18. Crowley ML, Freeman LD, Motlet MD, et al. Sensitivity of guaiac-impregnated cards for the detection of colorectal neoplasia. J Clin Gastroenterol 1983;5:127–130.

19. Crespi M, Weissman GS. The role of proctosigmoidoscopy in screening for colorectal neoplasia. CA: Cancer J Clinicians 1984;34:158–165.

20. Winnan G, Berci G, Parish J, et al. Superiority of the flexible to the rigid sigmoidoscope in routine proctosigmoidoscopy. N Engl J Med 1980;302:1011–1012.

21. Tedesco FJ, Wayne JD, Avella JR, et al. Diagnostic implications of the spatial distribution of colonic mass lesions (polyps and cancers). Gastrointest Endosc 1980;26:95–97.

22. Winawer SJ, Cummins R, Baldwin MP, et al. A new flexible sigmoidoscope for the generalist. Gastrointest Endosc 1982;28:233–236.

23. Bolt RJ. Sigmoidoscopy in detection and diagnosis in the asymptomatic individual. Cancer 1971;28:121–122.

24. Doubilet P, Weinstein MC, McNeil BJ. Use and misuse of the term "cost-effective" in medicine. N Engl J Med 1986;314:253–255.

25. Weinstein MC, Fineberg HV. Clinical decision analyses. Philadelphia: Saunders, 1980:228–263.

26. Eddy DM. The economics of cancer prevention and detection. Getting more for less. Cancer 1981;47:1200–1209.

27. Winawer SJ, Gottlieb, Stewart EJ, et al. National polyp study progress report. Gastrointest Endosc 1984;30:147.
28. Recommendations of the Third International Symposium on Colorectal Cancer. CA: Cancer J Clinicians 1984;34:145, 164.

Appendix A. Current Recommendations for Fecal [Guaiac] Occult Blood Testing and Further Research [28]

RECOMMENDATIONS

Although we do not endorse fecal [guaiac] occult blood test (FOBT) screening outside the health care system without further information on reduction in mortality as a result of screening, we do consider it desirable to standardize test recommendations with conditions in ongoing and evaluable controlled screening trials. The following recommendations for the proper use of the FOBT in screening asymptomatic, average-risk adults may not be applicable to tests other than Hemoccult II:

Testing should be done annually beginning between the ages of 40 and 50.

The patient should avoid rare red meat and high-peroxidase foods for 3 days before and during testing.

Vitamin C, iron tablets, and nonsteroidal antiinflammatory drugs should be avoided.

Two samples of each of three consecutive stools should be tested, following the collection procedure as recommended by the manufacturer.

The delay between preparation and laboratory testing should not exceed 6 days.

Slides should not be rehydrated.

A single positive smear should be considered as a positive test and lead to appropriate investigation, even in the absence of dietary restriction.

A positive result need not be repeated before diagnostic workup.

Quality control and proficiency testing should be established prior to use of FOBTs in clinical screening programs. This necessitates appropriate training of personnel who perform the tests.

FUTURE RESEARCH
Further research should focus on:

Improved methods of specimen collection.

Test conditions and methods to improve sensitivity and specificity.

Evaluation in clinical trials of rehydration of slides in patients taking a low-peroxidase diet; extending the test period; consecutive stool versus consecutive day testing; food peroxidase inhibitors; and immunochemical tests

Consideration of different testing techniques and strategies according to subject risk

Proficiency testing

Appendix B. Recommendations for Sigmoidoscopy and Further Research [28]

RECOMMENDATIONS
Screening should include proctosigmoidoscopy once every 3 to 5 years beginning between the ages of 40 and 50.

Flexible fiberoptic sigmoidoscopy (FFS) should replace rigid sigmoidoscopy whenever possible. FFS, using a 60-cm scope by a trained endoscopist, or a 35-cm scope by a nonendoscopist, is strongly advised.

FFS should be introduced in medical student programs utilizing colon models; audiovisual programs and brochures should be developed.

FFS should be incorporated into residency training programs in family practice, internal medicine, and general surgery.

FFS training programs should be established for physicians who are either currently using the rigid sigmoidoscope or not doing sigmoidoscopy at all.

Centers or institutions with planning programs for screening or case finding for colorectal cancer should implement the use of the FFS whenever possible.

National and international organizations (WHO, cancer societies) should disseminate the principles of colorectal cancer prevention, with emphasis on the safety and acceptability of FFS, to the public, physicians, and public health officials.

The fee structure for FFS should be in the same range as for rigid proctosigmoidoscopy when the procedure is used for screening.

Manufacturers must be urged to develop flexible sigmoidoscopes (both 35 cm and 60 cm) at a decreased cost.

RESEARCH PRIORITIES
Determine the difference in detection of lesions when nonendoscopists use the 35-cm and the 60-cm scopes

Determine the difference in time required for nonendoscopists to learn to use the 35-cm and the 60-cm flexible instruments.

Determine the complication rate when nonendoscopists use the 35-cm and the 60-cm scopes.

Institute studies on colonic cancer mortality and incidence changes when utilizing FFS as a screening procedure.

Determine the rate of neoplastic lesions beyond the reach of FFS scopes.

Consider the cost effectiveness of screening programs with FFS in various settings (centers versus individual physicians' offices).

Appendix C. American Cancer Society [2]

RECOMMENDATION
All persons age 40 and over should have a digital rectal examination annually; a stool guaiac slide test should be added at age 50 on an annual basis and sigmoidoscopy should be performed every 3 to 5 years after two initial negative sigmoidoscopies 1 year apart.

Persons who are at a high risk of developing colorectal cancer should receive more frequent and intensive examinations beginning at an earlier age. This includes persons with familial polyposis, Gardner's syndrome, ulcerative colitis, a history of polyps or prior colon cancer, and a family history of cancer of the colon or rectum.

Screening for Syphilis

CHAPTER FOURTEEN

MARIANA KASTRINAKIS

John is in love. He and his fiancée are about to get married. You have been John's doctor since he was an infant. As required by law in your state, you test John for syphilis prior to their marriage. John has never been tested before. To your surprise, John's test comes back positive.

Does John have syphilis? What do you need to do to decide? Should you treat him? What about his fiancée? Although this case seems routine in medical practice, it raises important questions that are incompletely answered in the medical literature. To decide on a further course of action, you must know some properties about the tests used for detecting syphilis as well as some information about the population of patients being tested. The purpose of this chapter is to help you understand properties of screening tests and to use them in the context of clinical decision making.

Natural History of Syphilis

Before we discuss the use of syphilis tests, we should review some basic concepts about the disease itself [1–12]. Syphilis is a venereally transmitted disease caused by a spirochete, *Treponoma pallidum*. This is one in a family of spirochetes known to cause other illnesses such as yaws, pinta, and nonvenereal syphilis. Only venereal syphilis, which occurs in several stages, will be considered here.

PRIMARY STAGE

The primary stage affects the skin, most commonly in a venereal or mucosal location. The lesion, usually located at the site of contact, is a chancre and lasts days to months after exposure. The chancre often is painless and thus can go unnoticed when it is intravaginal or perianal in location. Although the lesions heal spontaneously in an average of 3 weeks, the disease, if untreated, can progress to later stages.

SECONDARY STAGE

The secondary stage is characterized by a systemic illness that usually develops after the primary stage and reflects hematogenous spread of the spirochete. It often produces fever, diffuse adenopathy, and skin rash. The disease also can affect specific organs, causing hepatitis, glomerulonephritis, and a widespread variety of other inflammatory manifestations. The symptoms often spontaneously resolve and then recur if this stage is untreated.

LATENT STAGE

Prior to a so-called tertiary stage and after the secondary stage, the disease may be quiescent for months to usually years. During this latent stage, the untreated individual is infected but mostly asymptomatic. With the advent of serologic testing for the spirochete *T. pallidum* after the turn of the twentieth century, this stage was defined by positive syphilis serology and no symptoms, as well as a normal physical examination. There is an early latent and a late latent phase, depending on the duration of this stage.

TERTIARY STAGE

The tertiary stage is probably the most serious and potentially fatal stage of the illness, and it follows the earlier stages if untreated. The disease affects one or more organ systems in several possible ways, and at least two major disabling syndromes are described: cardiovascular syphilis and neurosyphilis. Cardiovascular syphilis primarily involves the heart and ascending aorta, causing aortic insufficiency and aortic aneurysm. It is attributable to an infectious vasculitis of the vasa vasorum in those vessels. Neurosyphilis can manifest itself as meningitis, brain abscess, or the more common syndromes of slowly progressing tabes dorsalis (posterior column spinal cord syphilis) or general paresis (a diffuse meningoencephalitis). Finally, a nonfatal spectrum of disease can be caused by gummas, an inflammatory response to *T. pallidum* organisms. For unknown reasons, these lesions tend to affect nonvital organs and so they are part of a syndrome known as late benign syphilis. Organs most commonly affected are bones, skin (nodular or ulcerative), upper respiratory tract, esophagus, eyes, and breast. This tertiary stage can last many years.

CONGENITAL SYPHILIS

Since the fifteenth century, it was recognized that there could be vertical transmission of syphilis from mother to child. Syphilis in the untreated mother can cause intrauterine growth retardation, spontaneous abortions, and prematurity. The first clinical manifestations in the newborn child can be absent until after the first few weeks of life. The full-blown syndrome of congenital syphilis involves, at one time, the histopathologic features of all stages of syphilis in the adult. Organs affected include bones, as in tibial thickening or "saber shin deformity," teeth (Hutchinson's incisors), skin, bone marrow, and the central nervous system. The cardiovascular organs may be spared. Inadvertent partial treatment (for intercurrent illness other than congenital syphilis) with penicillin can cause delay of the clinical presentations until later years of childhood or adolescence. In this case, a syndrome of late congenital syphilis akin to adult tertiary disease occurs.

Of note is the fact that the incidence of congenital syphilis declines when the mother is affected with more advanced states of syphilis. The chances of vertical transmission are greatest when the mother acquires primary or secondary syphilis during the pregnancy. Thus, it is especially important to detect and treat syphilis in its early stages among pregnant women. The primary and secondary treatment of syphilis is determined by the duration, not the stage, of the disease. Disease of less than 1 year's duration is treated with low-dose antibiotics, such as 2,400,000 units of penicillin G benzathine. Disease of more than 1 year's duration or of undetermined duration is treated with high-dose antibiotic treatments, such as three doses of 2,400,000 units of penicillin G benzathine at 1-week intervals.

UNTREATED SYPHILIS

The impact of untreated syphilis in affected individuals is shown by the Oslo study [13], which was conducted because of the suspicion that the early treatment of syphilis with mercurials was more harmful than the disease itself. The study was a massive project involving prospective and retrospective follow-up of 1904 Oslo residents between the years 1948 and 1951. This group of patients was part of a larger study population identified by Boeck 50 years earlier and followed prospectively and retrospectively since then. The criteria for diagnosis were mostly clinical. Since serology did not yet exist, the study will not be presented in detail. Instead, we will use Table 14-1 to summarize its findings. The table outlines the percentage of cases that went on to develop progressive disease at each stage, giving us an idea of the natural history of untreated syphilis.

The Oslo study underestimates the total morbidity and mortality of untreated syphilis because of the numbers of patients lost to follow-up. Even so, the percentages of cases progressing to more severe stages are substantial when the disease is untreated.

Currently, we do not have an accurate estimate of the morbidity and mortality of untreated syphilis. The advent of penicillin has made repeating such a study unethical. In addition, inadvertent use of penicillin to treat infections other than syphilis may have dramatically altered the

Table 14-1. Percentage[a] of cases in progressive stages of syphilis after initial infection that was not treated

	Secondary early relapsing stage[b]	Latent stage	Tertiary cardiovascular stage[c]	Neurosyphilis[d]	Death[e]
Affected women (N = 620)	24.0	16.7	7.6	5.0	8.0
Affected men (N = 331)	22.7	14.4	13.6	9.4	17.1
Estimated time since primary infection (years)	2–5	1–46	30–40[f]	1–30[f]	40+

[a]Numbers do not add up to 100 percent since cases in primary stage and many patients lost to follow-up were not accounted for in the study.

[b]Multiple relapses in 22.5 percent of these cases.

[c]No patients infected *after* age 15 developed cardiovascular syphilis.

[d]Only a rare patient affected after 40 years of age in this group.

[e]Cumulative probability of dying *directly* as a result of syphilis after 40 years of infection.

[f]These are consensus figures and not solely from the Oslo study.

Source: Adapted from Clark and Danbolt [13].

natural history of syphilis. Our best estimates of the prevalence of syphilis in populations come from serologic surveys, as we shall soon see.

Testing for Syphilis

To understand syphilis testing, it is necessary to have an idea of what tests are available and how they are evaluated. This discussion will focus solely on tests specific for venereal syphilis and not on tests for other treponemal illnesses [14–24]. Testing for syphilis is limited by the fact that reliable methods do not exist for culturing the organism.

TYPES OF DIAGNOSTIC TESTS AVAILABLE

There are three types of tests used to diagnose syphilis: one based on direct visualization of the spirochete and two types of serologic assays. These will be briefly described.

Dark-field Microscopy

Dark-field microscopy depends on direct visualization of spirochetes using dark-field microscopic techniques. This test allows rapid confirmation of the diagnosis if it is positive and read by an expert. However, it is costly and requires expert technique. (The examiner must be careful to exclude possible commensal spirochetes of the oropharynx.) Also, it is useful only where there are infected lesions (skin, mucous membranes) or aspirated material from lymph nodes. Thus, it is useful only in the primary and secondary stages of disease in vivo. False negative results can occur if there is poor specimen preparation (e.g., the lesion is superinfected or topical ointments have been used). Finally, dark-field microscopy is not easily or widely available.

Nontreponemal Serology

Nontreponemal serology tests the presence of a heterogeneous, nonspecific human antibody. Many names are available for this kind of test, but the procedures differ only slightly. Some of the names are: the VDRL (Venereal Disease Research Laboratory) test, the RPR (rapid plasma reagin) test, or the STS (serologic test for syphilis). Nontreponemal serology is *not* 100 percent sensitive or specific for syphilis. At high titers, these properties improve.

Some advantages of nontreponemal serology are that it is an easy, inexpensive, and rapid test to perform and titer correlates roughly with disease activity. Therefore, it can be used serially to monitor disease activity and as a test of cure.

Among the disadvantages is the fact that it is not 100-percent sensitive or specific for syphilis. In addition, many false positive results are obtained, especially at low titers. These so-called biologic false positives (BFPs) can be caused by multiple conditions, such as connective tissue diseases, normal pregnancy, viral illness, immunizations, narcotic addiction, malaria, and leprosy. The BFP rate decreases at titers greater than 1 : 8. Also, the test "burns out" in late syphilis and often in cardiovascular and neurosyphilis, so it loses sensitivity with late stages of illness. Finally, there is a prozone effect: That is, undiluted serum can cause a weakly positive or even negative test that becomes strongly positive when the serum is diluted. Testing of serial dilutions of the serum circumvents this problem.

Treponemal Testing
Treponemal testing detects antibody specific to *T. pallidum* in serum. The most commonly used and accepted test of this type is the fluorescent treponemal antibody absorption (FTA-ABS) test.* It is predominantly a qualitative test.

The FTA-ABS test is the most accurate test known for syphilis. It gives very few false positive results. Thus, if positive, it serves as the best available gold standard for the current or previous existence of syphilis.

It is however, technically difficult to perform, and therefore is expensive and potentially inaccurate owing to poor technique [25]. The FTA-ABS test is not a gold standard for ruling out disease; false negative results can occur in early disease. Also, it can take a few weeks for the test to become positive at the onset of illness, so it is not a very good test for early primary syphilis. Finally, it usually remains positive for life after one infection, making it difficult to interpret when subsequent episodes are suspected.

_____ STUDY QUESTION 14-1
Which type of test is most appropriate for initial screening?

---

*A series of treponemal testing techniques are currently being used. Some of these are technically more reliable or more suitable to automated large-scale use. When properly done, all these tests provide the same type of data and are currently employed to address the same questions.

SELECTING THE APPROPRIATE TEST AND
INTERPRETING THE RESULTS

Prevalence data are difficult to assess in syphilis. Part of the problem is the long, clinically silent (latent, for some) stages. Although serology is an excellent diagnostic aid, as we shall see later, it does not constitute proof of the disease. Proof of the diagnosis, or what is known as a gold standard test (one that is 100 percent sensitive and 100 percent specific) is absent for most stages of syphilis. The advent of serologic testing has greatly improved the detection of disease in syphilis, and other than the direct demonstration of spirochetes by dark-field examination in a primary or secondary lesion, treponemal testing serves as the closest approximation to a gold standard test.

How do we know *which* test to use in each clinical situation and what its results represent? Let us see how we evaluate tests for syphilis. Usually, to evaluate the performance of any test, we would perform the test in question and the gold standard test and compare their results. Thus, the sensitivity and specificity of the test can be calculated. In syphilis, since a true gold standard test is absent, the performance of any *single* serologic test is compared with a combination of clinical and serologic criteria that define the presence or absence of disease. The latter combination is an approximation of the gold standard. The shortcomings of method are that clinical criteria can vary and that serologic tests are also variable depending on the stage of disease and the laboratory where the test is performed.

This accounts for part of the variability in estimates of sensitivity and specificity of syphilis serologic tests as it appears in the scientific literature. Despite the problems, it is important for us to review the data of the sensitivity and specificity to tests for syphilis.

Sensitivity and Specificity of Syphilis Serology

How are estimates of sensitivity and specificity arrived at in syphilis? How do they help us to use the tests for screening and diagnosis? To see how one such estimate was obtained, we shall review a report by Jaffe and colleagues [26]. In 1978, Jaffe and his co-workers surveyed a population of 1003 individuals pooled from a student and employee health clinic, a venereal disease clinic, and a hospital inpatient population to assess the performance of syphilis serology. They compared the percentages of positive treponemal (VDRL) and nontreponemal (FTA-ABS) serologic tests to a gold standard. The gold standard was determined by clinical, serologic, and dark-field criteria that are explicitly stated in the paper. This gold standard is subject to error, but it was the best available approximation of the presence of syphilis.

Of the 1003 subjects in the study, 68 were considered to have syphilis by the gold standard and 935 were unaffected. All subjects underwent a VDRL and an FTA-ABS test. The calculations and results for the VDRL test are as follows:

	Gold standard diseased (N=68)	Gold standard disease-free (N=935)
Positive VDRL test	(true positives) 50	(false positives) 11
Negative VDRL test	(false negatives) 18	(true negatives) 924

From these data, sensitivity and specificity for the VDRL test can be calculated:

$$\text{Sensitivity} = \frac{\text{true positives}}{\text{true positives} + \text{false negatives}} = \frac{50}{50 + 18} = \frac{50}{68} = 74\%$$

$$\text{Specificity} = \frac{\text{true negatives}}{\text{true negatives} + \text{false positives}} = \frac{924}{924 + 11} = \frac{924}{935} = 99\%$$

These results underestimate sensitivity and overestimate specificity since the study does not consider borderline positive findings as positive tests.

The results for the FTA-ABS test were as follows:

	Gold standard diseased (N = 68)	Gold standard disease-free (N = 935)
Positive FTA-ABS test	(true positives) 57	(false positives) 31
Negative FTA-ABS test	(false negatives) 11	(true negatives) 904

STUDY QUESTION 14-2
Calculate the sensitivity and specificity of the FTA-ABS test based on the data just cited.

Other investigators have done surveys similar to the one by Jaffe and colleagues [26] and have looked at the different stages of syphilis to assess the performance of these tests. More or less widely accepted ranges of results for sensitivity and specificity of the commonly used serologic tests for syphilis are now published in the literature. Some are stage-specific and others combine stages and are designated as screening values. An adaptation of accepted values for syphilis test sensitivity and specificity at different stages of disease is shown in Table 14-2 [27, 28].

We can use these numbers to calculate the performance of each test in our office for different populations and to determine which test best fits each clinical situation. For our calculations, we shall use the numbers given by Griner and co-workers [28] for screening sensitivity and specificity, since we are interested in screening or case finding asymptomatic syphilis cases. The evaluation of the performance of these tests in specific clinical applications depends on the concept of predictive value of a test.

Predictive Value of Tests in Syphilis
Sensitivity and specificity alone do not tell us what the chances are that a patient has a certain condition regardless of the outcome of the test. A concept that incorporates the *prevalence* of the disease in the population from which the patient is drawn will give us that information. This is the predictive value of a test, and it helps us to know how likely it is that a patient has syphilis after the test results are obtained.

CALCULATING PREDICTIVE VALUES. To understand this concept better, let us calculate the predictive values of a positive and negative test for syphilis in screening a population of 10,000 individuals. Use an estimated disease prevalence of 1 percent. Assume a sensitivity of 86 percent and a screening specificity of 97 percent, as indicated for the VDRL test in Table 14-2. Remember our 2 × 2 tables and formulas for sensitivity and specificity.

Table 14-2. Sensitivity and specificity of serologic tests for syphilis at various stages of disease

Test	Sensitivity (%) at specific stages of syphilis					Specificity (%) in screening
	Primary	Secondary	Latent	Late	Screening	
VDRL	59–87	100	73–91	37–94	86	97
FTA-ABS	86–100	100	96–99	96–100	99	99

Source: Adapted from Jaffe and Holmes [27] and Griner and colleagues [28].

	Disease present	Disease absent
Positive test	TP	FP
Negative test	FN	TN

Recalling our formulas:

$$\text{Sensitivity} = \frac{TP}{TP + FN}$$

$$\text{Specificity} = \frac{TN}{TN + FP}$$

The predictive value formulas are:

$$\text{Predictive value positive} = \frac{\text{true positives}}{\text{true positives} + \text{false positives}}$$

$$\text{Predictive value negative*} = \frac{\text{false negatives}}{\text{false negatives} + \text{true negatives}}$$

If the true prevalence of disease is 1 percent, and we are applying the test to 10,000 individuals, then the total number of cases of syphilis is $0.01 \times 10,000 = 100$.

Thus, we can begin to construct our 2 × 2 table as follows:

	Syphilis present (N = 100)	Syphilis absent (N = 9900)
Positive VDRL test		
Negative VDRL test		

*We have arbitrarily picked this definition of the predictive value negative of a test. It can also be expressed as:

$$PV \text{ (-) test} = \frac{TN}{FN + TN} =$$

We now know that in the population of 10,000, only 100 individuals actually have syphilis. We also know the sensitivity and specificity of the VDRL test. Since the sensitivity is 86 percent, 86 of the 100 individuals with syphilis will have a positive VDRL test. Since the specificity is 97 percent, 9603 of the 9900 individuals without syphilis will have a negative VDRL test. Thus, we can complete the 2 × 2 table as follows:

	Syphilis present (N = 100)	Syphilis absent (N = 9900)
Positive VDRL test	(true positives) 86	(false positives) 297
Negative VDRL test	(false negatives) 14	(true negative) 9603

Now we can directly apply our formulas for predictive value of a positive and negative test.

$$\text{Predictive value positive} = \frac{TP}{TP + FP} = \frac{86}{86 + 297} = \frac{86}{383} = 22\%$$

$$\text{Predictive value negative} = \frac{FN}{FN + TN} = \frac{14}{14 + 9603} = \frac{14}{9617} = 0.15\%$$

This predictive value positive of a VDRL test means that there is a 22 percent chance that a patient has the disease if the patient's test is positive in a population with a prevalence of disease of 1 percent. This might be an estimate of the prevalence in a general population of people who are sexually active. The predictive value negative in this same population is 0.1 percent, meaning that there is approximately 1 chance in 1000 that the patient with a negative VDRL test has syphilis.

_____ STUDY QUESTION 14-3
Repeat the previous exercise for the FTA-ABS test assuming a 99-percent sensitivity, 99-percent specificity, and a 10-percent prevalence for screening a population of 1000 individuals.

Table 14-3 reflects the predictive values of positive and negative VDRL and FTA-ABS tests, assuming various pretest probabilities that roughly approximate those in specific populations, as follows:

Table 14-3. Predictive values of serologic tests
for syphilis given various pretest probabilities

Serologic test	Pretest probability or prevalence (%)				
	0.1	1	10	50	90
VDRL					
Predictive value positive	2.8	22	76	96	99
Predictive value negative*	0.1	1	2	13	57
FTA-ABS					
Predictive value positive	9	49	91	99	99.8
Predictive value negative*	1	1	1	2	8

*Predictive value negative here has been calculated as false negatives/(false negatives
+ true negatives).

0.1%	Approximate prevalence of syphilis in a general population
1%	Approximate prevalence of syphilis in a young sexually active general population
10%	Approximate prevalence of syphilis in a sexually active group with coexistent sexually transmitted disease
50%	Approximate pretest probability in a patient presenting with a genital lesion without classic features of syphilis
90%	Approximate pretest probability in an individual presenting with clinical features strongly suggestive of syphilis

_____ STUDY QUESTION 14-4
What happens to the predictive value of positive and negative tests as the prevalence increases?

As you can see, the degree to which a test is helpful to the clinician depends on the prevalence of the disease in the population tested. This concept is very important because it emphasizes that a knowledge of the epidemiology of the disease is required for the clinician to make educated guesses about his or her patients as individuals. Table 14-3 also illustrates that in groups with a very low prevalence of disease, a negative test is more definitive diagnostically than a positive one. For example, in a young heterosexual individual (prevalence of syphilis of approximately 1 percent), a negative VDRL test gives us 99 percent confidence that he does not have syphilis, and the disease can be effectively ruled out. Note that when using the formula predictive value negative = true negatives/(true negatives + false negatives), we obtain a result of 1 percent, meaning that there is only a 1-percent chance that the patient has syphilis. This is another way of saying the same thing. A positive test in this same individual indicates that there is only a 22-percent chance that he or she has the disease. This may not be enough to rule in or rule out the disease, and further confirmatory tests may be needed. Notice that as the pretest probability (prevalence) increases (e.g., prevalence of 90 percent in the preceding example), a positive test gives us a more definitive diagnosis than a negative test: The predictive value positive is 99 percent, whereas the predictive value negative is 43 percent.

SEQUENTIAL TESTING.   Clinicians may know the prevalence of a given disease based on clinical or epidemiologic studies, or they may make best-guess estimates from their own experience. When such estimates are applied to a patient, the clinician must also take into account the presence or absence of other features in the history and physical examination that alter the likelihood of an individual patient having the disease.

Once the prevalence is known or estimated, the clinician might be tempted to select the test directly from Table 14-3. Using this table, it would seem, at first glance, that for the midrange probabilities (prevalence of 1, 10, or 50 percent) the FTA-ABS test performs best in ruling the disease in or out. However, we must consider other factors that may affect this choice.

1. The FTA-ABS test is technically more difficult and expensive than other tests for syphilis and thus is not a good test for screening large populations.
2. Because of the technical difficulties, if used widely the FTA-ABS test may become less accurate.
3. If we use FTA-ABS or similar tests for screening, we do not have other types of tests to confirm our results.
4. The FTA-ABS test remains positive even in cases of old disease, so the results are difficult to interpret in a person who had syphilis and was appropriately treated in the past.

Suppose we first applied an easier, more available test and then used the posttest probability as the pretest probability of a subsequent test. We would be using the two tests *sequentially,* which is a powerful aid in decision making. In using this approach, we have to assume that the false positives and false negatives of the two tests occur independently

Table 14-4. Predictive values positive of
serologic tests for syphilis when used sequentially

Serologic test	Pretest prevalence (%)				
	0.1	1	10	50	90
VDRL	2.8	22	76	96	99
FTA-ABS	9	49	91	99	99.8
VDRL and FTA-ABS sequentially	74.0	96.5	99.6	99.9	99.9

of each other. It is standard procedure to obtain an FTA-ABS test after obtaining a positive VDRL test, regardless of the pretest probabilities of syphilis.

In using the VDRL and FTA-ABS tests sequentially, one makes the same calculations as were made previously but uses the posttest probability of the VDRL test as the pretest probability of disease for the FTA-ABS test. Table 14-4 lists the predictive values of the VDRL and FTA-ABS tests independently for various pretest probabilities. It then shows the predictive value of a positive FTA-ABS test done in sequence *after* the finding of a positive VDRL test.

Let us return to John's case as an example. Assume John is sexually active, and there is a pretest probability of 1 percent that he may have syphilis (a clinician's estimate before any test is performed). Using Table 14-4, we can determine his probability of having syphilis if we obtain a positive VDRL test: The predictive value of a positive test in this situation is 22 percent. In contrast, if John were screened solely with an FTA-ABS test and the results were positive, he would have a 49-percent chance of having syphilis. Neither of these two probabilities is completely diagnostic of syphilis.

If we first perform a VDRL test and it is positive, we can use the posttest probability (22 percent) as the pretest probability for the FTA-ABS test. Thus, if John also has a positive FTA-ABS test, his posttest probability after the sequence of tests is 96.5 percent. This result gives us a greater degree of confidence in a positive test than if we consider either test alone.

———————————————————————— STUDY QUESTION 14-5
On the basis of positive VDRL and FTA-ABS tests, would you diagnose and treat John as having syphilis?

The diagnosis and treatment of syphilis carries a special implication. One is required to report to the local Health Department as a communicable disease every diagnosis of syphilis [29]. Even when physicians fail to report syphilis, the diagnostic test results are available through the laboratory. The local Health Department has a legal right to follow up these results and locate and inform sexual contacts of diseased patients. The Centers for Disease Control (CDC) recommend treatment of sexual contacts of those with syphilis even if the contacts have a negative test.

_____ STUDY QUESTION 14-6
(a) What assumptions underly these recommendations? (b) How would you apply the recommendations in the case of John and his fiancée?

Deciding Whom to Screen

Thus far we have seen what tools are available to screen for syphilis. We have concentrated on case finding, as clinicians do in their office. But how do we decide whether or not to screen? Should we be doing a serologic test for syphilis on all patients that come to us? If not, whom should we screen? In other words, which risk groups would benefit from screening and intervention?

Expert sources have critically evaluated the periodic health examination. Several authorities recommend periodic screening with a VDRL test for all pregnant women and sexually active individuals at least once at first presentation to the physician [31, 32]. Nonetheless, how do we decide whether or not to screen a group of individuals on a large-scale basis? Any program designed to screen for a disease or risk factor must meet certain screening criteria. Let's review these criteria here:

1. The disease must cause a substantial morbidity or mortality leading to a substantial impact on society as a whole or on an identifiable subgroup of individuals in society.
2. There are risk factors that can be identified before the development of symptoms which can serve to identify high-risk groups and to facilitate the early detection of disease.
3. Treatment begun during the asymptomatic preclinical phase results in a better outcome than treatment that awaits the appearance of symptoms.
4. There is a testing approach that makes it feasible to detect or rule out

disease effectively at the asymptomatic (preclinical) stage; and that is satisfactory in terms of safety, patient acceptability, and affordability.

_____ STUDY QUESTION 14-7
Which of these criteria are fulfilled by syphilis screening?

If we conclude that syphilis screening is desirable for high-risk groups, we need to consider who these groups are and how screening should be done. We know from many epidemiologic surveys that primary and secondary disease are definitely clustered in the young, sexually active population. CDC reports show that more than 95 percent of all cases of syphilis occur in the 15 to 49-year-old group [5, 6]. There is a considerable male predominance, with a high incidence of syphilis among homosexual men. This evidence then seems to target as high-risk groups the young, sexually active (especially if promiscuous), child-bearing-age population as well as male homosexuals.

After the advent of syphilis serology in the 1930s and of penicillin in the 1950s, the United States government instituted widespread programs of detection and treatment for syphilis that fulfilled most, if not all, of the criteria for screening cited earlier. Since then, changes in funding policies have led to the elimination of most such programs. As a result, few concerted effective screening programs exist outside of the clinician's office. Two programs still in existence are prenatal and premarital screening. The justification for state-mandated prenatal screening is the prevention of congenital syphilis. Congenital syphilis occurs by vertical transmission, especially if the mother acquires syphilis during pregnancy. The rates of congenital syphilis parallel the rates of primary and secondary syphilis among people of child-bearing age [5, 6]. First-trimester screening of pregnant women is aimed mostly at detecting primary and secondary syphilis and at the prevention of vertical transmission to the fetus. Some states also mandate third-trimester and cord blood screening. Insofar as screening is conducted in the context of prenatal care, this form of disease detection meets our criteria for screening as stated previously. However, populationwide prenatal screening is difficult to implement since not everyone receives prenatal care, and often it may be the groups most at risk for infection who may not seek care. Even so, since large-scale efforts to control syphilis began, reported cases of congenital syphilis dropped by 98 percent between 1941 and 1982, with a parallel decline in infant mortality [6]. Recent trends have shown an increase in the rates of primary and secondary syphilis without a similar increase in the number of reported prenatal cases [5].

Premarital syphilis screening laws have been in effect in some states from as early as 1935. Such programs involved not only premarital screening with available serologic tests, but also free and easy access to medical follow-up. It was part of a widespread effort at many levels to eradicate syphilis, and it paralleled premarital syphilis screening. Premarital syphilis screening was viewed as a way to reach the young, sexually active population at an age when most new cases of syphilis were known to occur [33]. Screening was offered at the state level, with state-run clinics to provide treatment and follow-up. The latter have largely disappeared, and nowadays, most screening occurs privately. Thus, state agencies have diminishing control of appropriate treatment and follow-up of syphilis cases and contacts. Modern trends also show that only a small percentage of the population at risk may marry at any one time. Consequently, many sexually active homosexual and heterosexual unmarried groups, with a variably high incidence of syphilis, are excluded from premarital screening programs. All these factors raise legitimate questions about the continued existence of these syphilis programs.

_____ STUDY QUESTION 14-8
What are the advantages and disadvantages of maintaining premarital screening programs?

As with most issues in medicine, science can provide wonderful tools for the detection and cure of disease, but scientific methods alone are no substitute for the clinician's judicious use of these tools in medical practice and in determining health care policies.

References

1. Holmes KK, Per Anders M, Sparlins PF, Wiesner PJ. Sexually transmitted diseases. New York: McGraw-Hill, 1984.
2. Fiumara NJ, Fleming WL, Downing JG, et al. The incidence of prenatal syphilis at the Boston City Hospital. N Engl J Med 1952;247:48–52.
3. Aho K, Sievers K, Salo OP. Late complications of syphilis. Acta Derm Venereol (Stokh) 1969;49:336–342.
4. Lucas JB. The national venereal disease problem. Med Clin North Am 1972;56:1073–1086.

5. Centers for Disease Control. Leads from the MMWR. Syphilis—United States, 1983. JAMA 1984;252:992–993.

6. Centers for Disease Control. Annual summary 1982: reported morbidity and mortality in the United States. MMWR 1983;31(54):77–82.

7. Wiesner PM. Syphilis. In: Gellis SS, Kagan BM, eds. Current pediatric therapy. Philadelphia: Saunders, 1973, pp. 625–627.

8. Parran T. The public health aspects of syphilis as it concerns the general practitioner. N Engl J Med 1940;223:450–454.

9. Hooshmand H, Escobar MR, Kopf SW. Neurosyphilis, A study of 241 patients. JAMA 1972;219;726–729.

10. Holder WR, Knox JM. Syphilis in pregnancy. Med Clin North Am 1972;56:1151–1160.

11. Mascola L, Pelosi R, Blount JH, et al. Congenital syphilis. JAMA 1984;252;1719–1722.

12. Lundberg GD. Prevention of congenital syphilis (editorial). JAMA 1984;252:1750–1751.

13. Clark GE, Danbolt N. The Oslo study of the natural course of untreated syphilis. Med Clin North Am 1964;48:613–623.

14. The laboratory aspects of syphilis. Dept. of Health, Education and Welfare/ PHS, Centers for Disease Control, Venereal Disease Control Division, Atlanta, Ga, 1971.

15. Criteria and techniques for the diagnosis of early syphilis. Dept. of Health, Education and Welfare/PHS, Centers for Disease Control, Venereal Disease Control Division, Atlanta, Ga, 1976.

16. Olansky S. Serodiagnosis of syphilis. Med Clin North Am 1972;56:1145–1150.

17. Sparling PF. Diagnosis and treatment of syphilis. N Engl J Med 1971;284;642–653.

18. Hart G. Syphilis tests in diagnostic and therapeutic decision making. Ann Intern Med 1986;104:368–375.

19. Jaffe HW. The laboratory diagnosis of syphilis. Ann Intern Med 1975;83:846–850.

20. Goldman JN, Lantz MA. FTA-Abs and VDRL slide test reactivity in a population of nuns. JAMA 1971;217:53–55.

21. Duncan WC, Knox JM, Wende RD. The FTA-Abs test in dark field positive syphilis. JAMA 1974;228:859–860.

22. Deacon WE. Fluorescent treponemal antibody-absorption (FTA-Abs) test for syphilis. JAMA 1966;198:156–160.

23. Harner RE, Smith JL, Israel, CW. The FTA-Abs testing in treated late syphilis. JAMA 1968;203:103–106.

24. Atwood WG, Miller JL, Stout GW, et al. The TPI and FTA-Abs tests in treated late syphilis. JAMA 1968;203:107–109.

25. Dans PE, Judson FN, Larsen SA, et al. The FTA-Abs tests: a diagnostic help or hindrance? South Med J 1977;70:312–315.
26. Jaffe HW, Larsen SA, Jones OG, et al. Hemagglutination test for syphilis antibody. Am J Clin Pathol 1978;70:230–233.
27. Jaffe HW, Holmes KK. Management of the reactive serology in sexually transmitted diseases. New York: McGraw-Hill, 1984.
28. Griner PF, Mayewski RJ, Mushlin AI, et al. Selection and interpretation of diagnostic tests and procedures. Ann Intern Med 1981;94:553–600.
29. Frye WW. The importance of contact investigation in the control of syphilis. Med Clin North Am 1964;48:637–651.
30. Centers for Disease Control. Sexually transmitted diseases: 1985 treatment guidelines. 1985;(suppl):334.
31. Spritzer WO, Bayne RD, Chorron KC, et al. Task force report: the periodic health examination. Can Med Assoc J 1979;121:1193–1254.
32. Council Report. Medical evaluation of healthy persons. JAMA 1983; 249:1626–1633.
33. Kingon RJ, Wiesner PJ. Premarital syphilis screening: weighing the benefits. Am J Public Health 1981;71:160–162.

Tuberculosis

CHAPTER FIFTEEN

LILA T. MCCONNELL
RICHARD K. RIEGELMAN

Clinical Scenarios

CASE A.   Let us assume we are annually testing patients in a nursing home with purified protein derivative of tuberculin (PPD). Most patients seem to have negative skin tests. However, on one of the floors one patient reacts to PPD with a skin test that measures 15 mm of induration. This 82-year-old male patient has been a resident of the nursing home for 5 years. His problem list is as follows; status post cerebrovascular accident with expressive aphasia; dementia, probably multiinfarct type predominating; high blood pressure; and mild renal insufficiency. His medications include furosemide, laxatives, atenolol, nitroglycerine, and hydralazine. He is not ambulatory and has no symptoms that might suggest he has active tuberculosis. He has been cared for by the nursing home staff, which is relatively constant but from time to time includes temporary nursing staff and nursing home volunteers. His family, who lives in Washington, D.C., visits him from time to time. The patient has had negative PPD tests in the 2 years preceding this positive test.

CASE B.   A 1-year-old son of one of your patients who has newly diagnosed active tuberculosis is tested with PPD for evidence of infection with tuberculosis. The child's PPD test is negative.

CASE C.   A 35-year-old white man who lives in the inner city has an infiltrate on his chest roentgenogram. A positive PPD test is obtained during the course of evaluating the etiology of the infiltrate, which then completely clears with antibiotic therapy. This patient is an alcoholic who says he has stopped drinking and who has a hard time holding a job.

What issues must you consider when deciding whether or not to use isoniazid prophylaxis in these individuals? Would you go ahead and treat? These are the types of questions we will be addressing in this chapter. Before attempting to answer, let us take a look at what has been and can be done to prevent tuberculosis. Then we will examine the role of isoniazid prophylaxis and return to our cases.

Social History of Tuberculosis

Before the turn of the century, tuberculosis was a very prevalent disease. It was a scourge that at its peak accounted for an estimated 25 percent

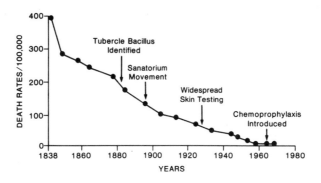

Fig. 15-1. Declining death rate from respiratory tuberculosis. (Adapted from McKeown T. The role of medicine: dream, mirage or nemesis. London: Nuffield Provincial Hospitals Trust, 1976.)

of adult deaths in Europe. Early in the twentieth century, a huge percentage of the population (an estimated 80 percent) were infected with tuberculosis before reaching the age of 20.

By 1980, the incidence of tuberculosis was approximately 13 cases per 100,000, and it accounted for only 2800 deaths per year in the United States. Clearly, the impact of tuberculosis in the United States has decreased. However, as we shall see later, it is still an important infectious disease.

Figure 15-1 illustrates the decline in the death rate secondary to tuberculosis along with the times of occurrence of events that were directed at controlling the disease. Beginning just before the turn of the century and extending into the early 1940s, control measures were instituted in the United States that began to hasten the eradication of the tuberculosis organism from the population at large. For example, in 1917 and on through 1967, more than 470 million cattle were tested for bovine tuberculosis, which can infect humans and other animals. As a result of such testing, more than 4 million cattle with positive tests were removed from herds across the country so that by 1940 most states had only 0.5 to 1 percent or fewer infected cattle. Also instituted was the establishment of sanitoriums and wards in general hospitals where patients with active tuberculous disease were isolated. Other measures included the establishment of committees, through medical associations and other interested groups, that began to educate physicians about the principles of tuberculosis control. In 1934, school personnel all over the United States began to be tested for the presence of tuberculosis, and many cases of the disease were identified [1].

Chemotherapy for active tuberculosis began in 1944 with the recognition that streptomycin is effective against the disease. Streptomycin's tendency to produce resistant strains was quickly recognized and then lessened with the addition to it in 1949 of para-aminosalicylic acid (PAS). The introduction of isoniazid (INH) in 1952 led to the development of two- and three-drug regimens that, when given over 18 to 24 months, were curative. INH was recognized as efficacious in providing chemoprophylaxis in large-scale controlled clinical trials that began in the late 1950s and was widely administered as a preventive measure beginning in the 1960s.

_____ STUDY QUESTION 15-1

Examine Figure 15-1. What do you think was the relative importance of preventive and curative approaches in bringing tuberculosis under control? Are you surprised to see the decline that occurred even before bacteriologic identification of *Mycobacterium tuberculosis*?

Natural History of Tuberculosis

Tuberculosis infection starts when a susceptible host inhales fresh droplets that contain the bacillus and are less than 10 μm in size, which are produced when a person with active tuberculosis coughs, sneezes, or speaks. Tuberculosis is not transmitted through inhalation of dust or fomites and is not spread by the hands. These very tiny droplets are not cleared easily by the ciliary system in the lungs and so reach the respiratory bronchioles and are deposited in lung tissue. The bacilli contained in the droplets are then phagocytosed and protected from destruction by macrophages. At this stage, the host is said to be infected with the tuberculosis organism but has not yet developed active disease.

When an individual is infected with the organism, an area of bronchopneumonia is always produced. In most cases, this bronchopneumonia is subclinical and therefore asymptomatic. Nonetheless, it will herald the appearance of a positive test for tuberculosis should the patient receive such a test. In a very few instances, the immune system may overwhelm the organisms present in the area of lung involvement, and the body will completely rid itself of the organism. However, in most cases, there is spread of the tubercle bacillus through the lymphatic system and the bloodstream. Most individuals react with an optimal immune response to the organism, and progression of the infection is halted. This response consists of caseous necrosis, granuloma formation, and the elaboration by sensitized T-lymphocytes of lymphokines that destroy the bacilli. Healing of the lesion then occurs by resolution, fibrosis, and calcification. If the individual has a suboptimal immune response and the organism is not contained, active disease will occur, resulting in chronic cavitary tuberculosis. If there is minimal or no immune response, then the host may develop disseminated or miliary tuberculosis.

In many cases, the individual will live with the granuloma and thus remain infected with *M. tuberculosis* but will not develop active disease. The probability of developing active disease is the greatest within the first 2 years after becoming infected. In most studies, the risk of active tuberculosis for patients whose PPD tests have recently converted from negative to positive has been greater than 5 percent during the initial year of follow-up after conversion. Therefore, it is important to consider chemoprophylaxis in all recent converters, regardless of age. It must be remembered, however, that once infection occurs an individual is always susceptible to developing active disease even if this occurs 40 to 50 years after infection. Tuberculosis can be spread only from individuals who develop active disease.

Children younger than 5 years have an increased risk of developing active tuberculosis once infected, and the disease is more likely to produce disseminated and life-threatening disease. Those individuals with evidence of inactive tuberculosis on a chest roentgenogram are at equally high risk of developing active tuberculosis. A variety of other factors are believed to increase the risk of developing active tuberculosis once infection occurs.

According to a National Consensus Conference on Tuberculosis [2], chemoprophylaxis should be considered in individuals of any age who have a positive PPD along with any of the following conditions:

Hematologic reticuloendothelial malignant neoplasm

Systemic corticosteroid use in dosages greater than 15 mg of prednisone per day or other significant immunosuppressive therapy for a prolonged time

Silicosis

Chronic renal insufficiency

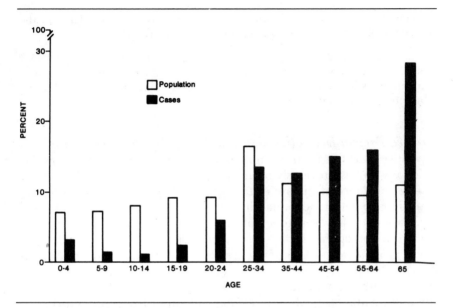

Fig. 15-2. Percent distribution of tuberculosis cases and population by age in the United States, 1980. (From Tuberculosis in the United States. Dept. of Health and Human Services/PHS, Centers for Disease Control, Center for Prevention Control, Division of Tuberculosis Control, Atlanta, Ga, 1983.)

Diabetes mellitus, particularly if the condition is poorly regulated

Conditions associated with nutritional deficiency and substantial loss of weight, including gastrectomy and intestinal bypass

Heroin addiction, regardless of the user's age

Since the mid-1960s, the number of cases of tuberculosis per 100,000 people in the United States has been generally falling for all age groups except those 65 years and older. Approximately 30 percent of all cases of active tuberculosis now occur among those 65 and older, despite the fact that they make up less than 15 percent of the population (Fig. 15-2).

─── STUDY QUESTION 15-2

Given what we know about the natural history of the disease and the measures implemented to control it, how can you explain why the peak incidence of the disease actually occurs in the 65 years and older age group?

_____ STUDY QUESTION 15-3
If all current conditions remain unchanged, what will happen to the incidence of tuberculosis in the population older than 65 as individuals born during the baby boom advance into older age?

Purified Protein Derivative Tests and Screening for Tuberculosis
A positive PPD test is an example of cell-mediated immunity in an individual who has previously been exposed to *M. tuberculosis*. Because of the low incidence of disease in the general population, mass screening campaigns to detect individuals infected with tuberculosis are no longer necessary [2]. However, tuberculosis remains an important infectious disease in susceptible groups of individuals in the United States [2]. These groups include: (1) newly arrived immigrants, refugees, foreign students, temporary foreign workers, and migrant workers; (2) new residents of nursing homes; (3) employees of nursing homes and community and mental hospitals; and (4) new inmates of prisons. Individuals within these groups are the most likely to be infected with tuberculosis and, therefore, to develop active disease. Crowding (measured as persons per room) along with intimacy of exposure to an infected case are second only to the extent of disease of the active index case in determining the probability that a contact will become infected.

Like any other screening test, PPD will have a sensitivity and specificity and will be plagued with false positive and false negative results. The occurrence of reactions to PPD when given to individuals with no history of tuberculosis or known contact with tuberculosis raised questions about false positive tests. Consequently, a standardized dosage and method of administration of PPD was developed. It was decided that Mantoux's method of intradermal inoculation was the best way of administering the PPD test. A dosage of 5 tuberculin units (TU) was chosen.

It is known from the testing of thousands of individuals all over the world who had active tuberculosis that response to PPD approximates fairly closely a normal bell-shaped distribution, with a mean of 15 to 16 mm of induration and the vast majority of reactions in the range of 8 to 24 mm. Less than 5 percent of those with known infection have skin test reactions of less than 10 mm (Fig. 15-3).

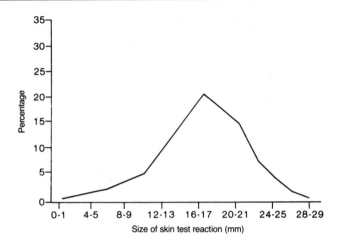

Fig. 15-3. Frequency curves of sizes of reactions to 5 tuberculin units of purified protein derivative in tuberculosis hospitals in all countries. (Adapted from Comstock GW. Epidemiology of tuberculosis. Am Rev Respir Dis 1982;125(S):8–15.)

_____ STUDY QUESTION 15-4

If 10 mm is chosen as the cutoff point and 5 percent of infected tuberculosis patients have a PPD reaction of less than 10 mm, what is the sensitivity of the test?

A reaction of 10 mm of induration that occurs after 48 to 72 hours is considered, in the United States, to be diagnostic of infection with tuberculosis. The 10-mm cutoff is not a magic number, however, since one also needs to consider the size of the reaction among those without evidence of tuberculosis in a patient population.

In the southeastern United States, interpretation of the PPD is complicated by reactions to nontuberculous mycobacteria known as atypical mycobacteria [3]. These atypicals are capable of causing human disease but are not generally spread from person to person and do not cause active tuberculosislike disease in most exposed individuals. Cross-reactivity to these organisms generally results in smaller reactions than those of *M. tuberculosis.* The situation is illustrated in Figure 15-4.

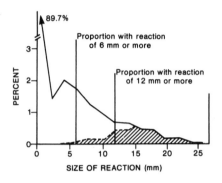

Fig. 15-4. Distribution of reactors to 5 tuberculin units of purified protein derivative among white Navy recruits from the state of Georgia, 17 to 21 years of age, who are lifetime United States residents, with estimate of the proportion infected with *Mycobacterium tuberculosis. Hatched area* = individuals infected with *M. tuberculosis; open area under curve* = those infected with atypical mycobacteria. (From Reichman [3].)

_____ STUDY QUESTION 15-5
(a) If, in Figure 15-4, 10 mm of induration is used as a cutoff between a negative and a positive test, is an individual with a PPD reaction of 10 mm more likely to be infected with *M. tuberculosis* or an atypical mycobacterium? (b) What about those with a PPD reaction of 12 mm? (c) What about those with a PPD reaction of 20 mm?

The other end of the spectrum is depicted in Figure 15-5, which shows the size of the reactions among Alaskans who, in the 1960s, had an extraordinarily high rate of tuberculosis [3]. There are no known cross-reacting atypical mycobacteria in Alaska.

_____ STUDY QUESTION 15-6
In the Alaskan population reported on in Figure 15-5, with a high incidence of active tuberculosis, what is the likely meaning of a PPD reaction of 10 mm? What about a PPD reaction of 5 mm?

False negative reactions to PPD can also occur. There are many reasons for a false negative reaction. The tuberculin that is used could become adulterated in some way as, for example, by improper storage. If

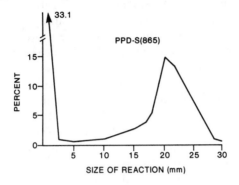

Fig. 15-5. Distribution of reactors to 5 tuberculin units of purified protein derivative among Alaskans tested in 1962. (From LB Reichman. Tuberculin skin testing. Arch Environ Health 1968;17:507. Reprinted with permission of the Helen Dwight Reid Educational Foundation. Published by Heldref Publications.)

the tuberculin is not administered properly or the test is not read and recorded properly, a false negative response may be obtained. If a patient is ill with chronic renal failure or a lymphoreticular malignancy, or if he or she is on corticosteroids or has had a recent or overwhelming infection with *M. tuberculosis,* a false negative result may also occur. In addition, up to 15 percent of individuals who are ill with disseminated tuberculosis may be PPD-negative.

Isoniazid Prophylaxis

Isoniazid is an important medication in tuberculosis prophylaxis. It meets many of the criteria for an ideal prophylactic agent. It is inexpensive and easy to take. Before considering the widespread applications of this agent, however, it is important to review the risks and benefits of isoniazid prophylaxis.

BENEFITS

Beginning in the late 1950s, the U.S. Public Health Service conducted a series of studies of isoniazid as a prophylactic agent against tuberculosis. Studies were conducted among entire populations of patients in mental institutions, communities with extremely high rates of active tuberculosis, recent household contacts of tuberculosis, and patients with evidence of old disease. In all cases, patients who were randomized to receive a year of isoniazid experienced a reduced incidence of active tuberculosis during the period of the study [4, 5].

The Public Health Service study of household contacts illustrates many of the findings of these studies [5]. This trial was conducted among approximately 25,000 household contacts of recently diagnosed tuberculosis patients. The contacts, who were free of active disease, were randomized to receive isoniazid or placebo at a dose of 5 mg per kilogram of body weight per day for a year. The overall results during the medication year can be summarized as follows:

	Placebo Group	Isoniazid Group
Active tuberculosis	62	14
No active tuberculosis	11,977	12,439

_____ STUDY QUESTION 15-7
What are the relative and attributable risks of not receiving isoniazid prophylaxis?

The reduction in active tuberculosis occurred exclusively among the approximately 50 percent of the population who were PPD-negative at the beginning of the study. What does this mean with regard to those who were PPD-positive? In addition to the effects observed during the period of medication use, the benefits of isoniazid appeared to continue beyond the duration of the medication. Follow-up data showed 17 cases of active tuberculosis occurred in the placebo group and 10 cases occurred in the isoniazid patients during the follow-up period.

A recent study of nursing home patients was conducted by Stead and colleagues [6]. This was not a controlled clinical trial, since once the efficacy of isoniazid was established in the 1960s, it was not considered ethical or feasible to conduct a controlled clinical trial. Those who did not take isoniazid in the study were primarily those patients whose physicians did not prescribe such preventive intervention. Table 15-1 displays the data for those whose skin tests recently converted.

_____ STUDY QUESTION 15-8
What are the relative and attributable risks of tuberculosis among those with recently converted skin tests who were not treated with isoniazid?

Table 15-1. Recently converted skin tests among
treated and untreated nursing home patients

	Isoniazid	Tuberculosis	No treatment	Tuberculosis
Positive test of unknown duration	534	1	3370	79
Recent converts	605	1	757	45

Source: Data from Stead and colleagues [6].

RISKS

Obviously, if isoniazid were completely without side effects, it would be beneficial to give it to large numbers of individuals to prevent the development of active tuberculosis. During the large-scale trials of isoniazid prophylaxis conducted by the U.S. Public Health Service between 1955 and 1968, the incidence of clinically overt hepatitis, according to Kopanoff and co-workers [7], was "so low and so similar in the randomly selected groups receiving isoniazid and placebo that it was assumed to be concurrent viral hepatitis." These investigators further state that "although isoniazid had been implicated as a possible hepatotoxin in a small number of case reports from 1953 to 1961, the patients who developed hepatitis were also taking other drugs" [7].

The detection of isoniazid as a cause of hepatitis was complicated by the fact that a substantial percentage of those who receive isoniazid experience an increase in their aspartate aminotransferase (AST) and alanine aminotransferase (ALT) levels, which subsequently return to normal despite continued isoniazid therapy. The difficulties of detecting and assessing any side effect came to light in a traumatic and public way when, in 1970, the U.S. Public Health Service began widely prescribing isoniazid to persons employed on Capitol Hill after seven cases of tuberculosis were identified [8]. Among 2321 individuals who received isoniazid as preventive therapy, 19 manifested clinical signs of liver disease. The data on isoniazid recipients and a matched comparison group of untreated Capitol Hill employees are as follows:

	Isoniazid Group	*Control Group*
Clinical hepatitis	19	1
No clinical hepatitis	2302	2153

Person-to-person contact between the cases did not seem likely [8].

—————————————————————————— STUDY QUESTION 15-9
In this study, what were the relative and attributable risks of hepatitis if isoniazid is taken?

As a result of the Capitol Hill experience, the Centers for Disease Control organized a national cooperative surveillance study of isoniazid [7]. A total of 13,838 persons on isoniazid were followed to assess the risk of hepatitis. Hepatitis was defined as an AST level of 250 Karmen units or more *or* an AST level of less than 250 Karmen units but an ALT level equivalent to or greater than the AST level, *and* an absence of hepatitis B surface antigen and no other apparent cause of hepatitis. Possible isoniazid-related cases of hepatitis were defined as an AST level of less than 250 Karmen units, *or* more than 250 Karmen units in the presence of other causes of liver disease, *or* 250 Karmen units or more without other biologic tests. It was found that a substantial percentage of individuals taking isoniazid had elevated liver function tests at less than 4 times their baseline levels. Liver function generally reverted to more normal levels even if isoniazid therapy was continued.

A total of 92 probable cases and 82 possible cases of isoniazid-related hepatitis occurred among assessed participants, for a rate of probable cases of 10.4 per 1000 and a rate of possible cases of 10.3 per 1000. These rates, and all rates in the study, were adjusted for the length of time participants were in the study. The study also found that nearly 60 percent of the probable cases occurred in the first 3 months of isoniazid use and only 5 percent occurred after the eighth month.

Two characteristics of patients at risk for the development of isoniazid-related hepatitis were identified: age and alcohol use. Figure 15-6 displays the risk of possible cases by age. The data for risk of isoniazid-related hepatitis in alcohol users are as follows:

Alcohol Use Status	Probable Cases (rate/1000)
Nondrinkers	6.4
Daily drinkers	26.5
Occasional drinkers	10.8

The symptoms of isoniazid-related hepatitis are typical of other hepatitis cases, including fatigue, weakness, anorexia, malaise, and nonspe-

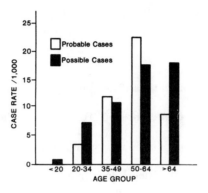

Fig. 15-6. Comparison of probable and possible isoniazid-related hepatitis case rates per 1000 participants by age group. Case rates have been adjusted for length of study and are maximal rates, since only persons known actually to have taken the isoniazid are included in the denominator. (From Kopanoff et al. [7].)

cific gastrointestinal symptoms. Continued use of isoniazid during this symptomatic interval has been shown to be associated with the development of more severe and less reversible liver disease.

—————————————————————— STUDY QUESTION 15-10
From what you know about the risk of developing tuberculosis and isoniazid-related hepatitis, what factors would you consider when comparing the risks and benefits of isoniazid prophylaxis?

—————————————————————— STUDY QUESTION 15-11
How would you weigh your knowledge of an individual patient in recommending or not recommending isoniazid prophylaxis? Specifically, what effect would a history of noncompliance or a history of alcohol abuse have on your decision?

—————————————————————— STUDY QUESTION 15-12
From what you have learned, what would you do in case A (see page 255)? Justify your answer.

—————————————————————— STUDY QUESTION 15-13
From what you have learned, what would you do in case B (see page 255)? Justify your answer.

_____ STUDY QUESTION 15-14

From what you have learned, what would you do in case C (see page 255)? Justify
your answer.

References

1. Myers JA. Tapering off of tuberculosis among the elderly. Am J Public Health
   1976;66:1101–1106.
2. National Consensus Conference on Tuberculosis. Chest 1985;87(S):1155–
   1375.
3. Reichman LB. Tuberculin skin testing: the state of the art. Chest
   1979;76(S):764–770.
4. Ferebee SH, Mount FW. Tuberculosis morbidity in a controlled trial of the
   prophylactic use of isoniazid among household contacts. Am Rev Respir Dis
   1962;85:490–509.
5. Mount FW, Ferebee SH. The effect of isoniazid prophylaxis on tuberculosis
   morbidity among household contacts of previously known cases of tuberculosis. Am Rev Respir Dis 1962;85:821–827.
6. Stead WW, Lofgren JP, Warren BA, et al. Tuberculosis as an endemic and
   nosocomial infection among the elderly in nursing homes. N Engl J Med
   1985;312:1483–1487.
7. Kopanoff DE, Snider DE, Caras GJ. Isoniazid-related hepatitis. A U.S.
   Public Health Service cooperative surveillance study. Am Rev Respir Dis
   1978;117:991–1001.
8. Garibaldi RA, Drusin RE, Ferebee SH, et al. Isoniazid-associated hepatitis:
   report of an outbreak. Am Rev Respir Dis 1972;106:357–365.

Rabies

LAWRENCE J. D'ANGELO

CHAPTER SIXTEEN

When Elisa found the raccoon cub on the wooded border of her parent's property, it seemed almost too wonderful to believe. Twelve-year-old girls are on the verge of being too big for stuffed toys, but this little fellow, who appeared quite scared, was a nice intermediate step between a real pet and that special world of store-bought soft and cuddly things. She brought it into the family garage, cleaned it up, found some fruit and cheese, and proceeded to commit herself to caring for the animal. Every day after school she would come home and play with the raccoon. No one supervised this play, and in 3 days' time Elisa had numerous cuts and scratches on her exposed skin, particularly on her arms and hands.

On the fourth day after she had adopted the raccoon, Elisa came home to find the cub listless and lying on its side. A call to the veterinarian stimulated her parents' concern. They drove the raccoon in for examination and treatment, but by early evening the cub had died. The veterinarian told Elisa's parents that the cub most likely died of rabies. This would have to be confirmed by the state laboratory, of course, but the veterinarian's suggestion to the family was to contact their physician for further advice.

The inquiry you receive from this family is different from the host of minor ailments you hear about each night on call. How will you respond?

STUDY QUESTION 16-1

What resources could you call on to assist you in providing accurate information and appropriate therapy?

Natural History of Rabies

Rabies is an ancient disease, described first in the Code of Hammurabi and noted in humans as early as 2300 B.C. It is caused by a bullet-shaped ribonucleic acid (RNA) virus that belongs to the rhabdovirus family [1]. This virus has few relatives in human virology.

After inoculation into a bite wound or onto a mucous membrane surface, the virus infects local cells. A slow replicative process then begins, usually in muscle cells. The virus spreads locally to axons and then to peripheral nerves via migration up the axoplasm. It then invades the spinal cord and, eventually, the brain [2]. The incubation period in humans is usually from 20 to 60 days, after which a nonspecific assortment of malaise, fatigue, anorexia, fever, and headache appears. The immediate prodrome of these first symptoms may be even less specific, initially presenting as apprehension, anxiety, and agitation. An acute neurologic phase follows that frequently is marked by hyperactivity, disorientation, hallucinations, seizures, bizarre behavior, nuchal rigidity, and paralysis. Abrupt changes in orientation make accurate history taking difficult. During this phase, the patient may experience the characteristic painful pharyngeal spasms when attempting to drink (hydrophobia) or when air is blown across the patient's face (aerophobia).

The second phase involving the central nervous system results in seizures, partial to complete paralysis, and ultimately, death. This usually occurs 4 to 14 days after the appearance of some clinical sign or symptoms. Many of these symptoms may follow a waxing and waning course, but death is a fairly constant feature.

Any warm-blooded animal can be infected with the rabies virus. Certain species, however, are far more likely to be infected on the basis of food preferences or because of susceptibility. In the United States, these include wild carnivores, especially skunks, raccoons, foxes, coyotes, and bobcats. The risk for domestic animals, such as dogs and cats, appears to be intermediate between the risk for carnivores and that for unlikely hosts such as rodents or rabbits. In the mid-Atlantic states, a recent widespread outbreak of rabies has occurred in raccoons. The partial domestication of these animals and their frequent choice of a suburban environment as home increases the chances that an animal infected with the rabies virus will expose others [3].

Rabies Prevention

POSTEXPOSURE VACCINATION

It was not until 1887 that Pasteur was able to make the first vaccine against rabies. This crude inoculum had a number of side effects that made the decision to initiate or undergo therapy a difficult one for both physician and patient. The live attenuated virus was replaced by an inactivated one in 1919. The resultant vaccine, as well as those that followed, were prepared from virus grown in adult animal neural tissue. Despite continued advances in the purity of these products, contamination with animal myelin led to a rate of acute neurologic complications in 1 of every 1600 persons vaccinated. This was reduced to 1 in 8000 by the use of suckling mouse brain as a system of cultivating virus, and was further reduced to 1 in 32,000 when vaccine developed from virus grown in duck embryos was introduced in the mid-1950s [4]. The final development in reducing the risk of vaccination occurred in the mid-1970s when a vaccine from virus grown in human diploid cell culture was produced. Administered as five shots on days 0, 3, 7, 14, and 28, it took almost 10 years for this product to be approved in the United States. It is now administered to approximately 25,000 persons yearly [5].

Any time that vaccine is administered, human rabies immune globulin (HRIG) is simultaneously administered with the day 0, or first, vaccination. This high-titered, specific, passive form of immunization allows for immediate protection. One-half of the product is given intramuscularly, whereas the other half is infiltrated around the bite site.

_____ STUDY QUESTION 16-2
If you decide to provide postexposure vaccination for Elisa (the girl discussed on page 269), what sort of preventive intervention does this represent?

Given the natural history of rabies infection, when the decision to initiate therapy is made, it is assumed that transfer of virus from the salivary glands of an infected animal has taken place. Since the virus may well be infecting cells locally, the key to preventing a clinical case of rabies is neutralization of infection. This can be accomplished by providing combined passive and active immunization with HRIG and human diploid strain rabies vaccine (HDSRV), respectively. It appears that only this combination is sufficient to abort an incubating infection. The use of either of these immunizing agents alone is unacceptable. One of the few recorded failures using HDSRV was in a patient who had not received HRIG [6]. When administered correctly, the combination is virtually infallible.* The original vaccine trials using HDSRV successfully protected a young boy in whom saliva from a proved rabid wolf had been inoculated in the meninges by a severe bite wound to the head and neck [8].

_____ STUDY QUESTION 16-3
Given that postexposure prophylaxis is a form of successful secondary prevention, what problems might such a successful preventive health measure create?

Tertiary prevention for rabies is futile. Once the infection is established, it usually pursues a relentless course to a fatal outcome. Intensive

---

*Recently a case of rabies was reported in a man who received both HDSRV and HRIG [7]. Although given in a timely fashion, the vaccine and the accompanying immunoglubulin were improperly administered.

supportive therapy, with carefully controlled respiratory and cardiac monitoring, offer some hope. There have been 3 reported human survivors of rabies, but only one of these appears to be well documented [9]. Attempts to treat established infection with high doses of immune globulin, interferon, and antiviral agents have been disappointing.

PRIMARY PREVENTION
Significant public health efforts have been focused on primary prevention. Since the early 1950s, the number of cases of rabies in domestic animals has dropped from more than 8000 to fewer than 300 yearly. It was this decrease, secondary to successful and legally mandated vaccination of domestic animals, that heralded a decrease in the number of human cases. One of the most successful forms of primary prevention, the vaccination of domestic dogs and cats, produces the rapid appearance of protective antibody. Unfortunately, this has not made a major impact on wild animals. Not only is vaccination in the wild contraindicated since vaccine virus can be reactivated in certain hosts, but there is no practical way to administer it to wild animals.

The destruction of infected animals is a definitive form of primary prevention. It is now well established that prior to the appearance of overt clinical symptoms of illness, dogs and cats can shed rabies virus in saliva for 10 days [10]. Therefore, dogs and cats who are potential sources of infection for humans or other animals can be quarantined for 10 days and observed. If they exhibit no sign of illness in this time, they need not be sacrificed. This is not true for wild animals, however. These animal hosts can shed virus for up to 6 months before showing signs of illness. One example is a skunk that was kept in captivity and died of rabies after having licked or bitten 26 persons in the months preceding its death [11].

Another form of primary prevention is preexposure immunization, which is similar to that provided for most other vaccine-preventable diseases. It is offered to high-risk persons such as veterinarians, animal handlers, certain laboratory workers, and persons spending more than 1 month in a foreign country where rabies is endemic in domestic as well as wild animals. Such therapy protects these individuals in the case of inadvertent exposure or when definitive therapy after exposure will be delayed. Once a high-risk individual is successfully vaccinated and the individual's titer is established, the vaccinee should receive boosters and revaccination when exposure has taken place.

Several problems do exist, however, with this sort of preventive therapy. Attempts to provide the vaccine by some route other than intramuscular injection (intradermally or subcutaneously, as cost-saving devices) have resulted in variable antibody responses [12]. In addition, patients who have received preexposure prophylaxis are also more susceptible to experiencing an adverse reaction to the vaccine when given booster injections [13]. The cumbersome details of ensuring appropriate immunization and the increased rate of side effects in those needing boosters make this approach to primary prevention less attractive than other methods. In the case of rabies, not all primary preventive strategies are equally effective; some are or will be more important than others.

In determining whether to use an immunizing agent, you need to ask certain questions. These are:

1. Is the potential vaccinee likely to have prior immunity to the illness in question?
2. Once vaccinated, can we expect an individual to be protected against infection or illness (vaccine efficacy)?
3. If protected, how long will this protection last?
4. How serious is the clinical illness we are seeking to prevent?
5. How likely is it that unvaccinated persons will acquire the illness if exposed?
6. What are the side effects of the vaccine?
7. Does the clinical value of giving the vaccine outweigh the risks and the cost?

For rabies, these questions can be easily answered.

1. Unless preexposure prophylaxis has been provided at some time previously, no one is expected to have a protective titer to rabies virus.
2. The vaccine is highly efficacious. As mentioned in the text, when human diploid strain rabies vaccine (HDSRV) is administered correctly with human rabies immune globulin, protection is virtually a certainty. However, recent evidence has questioned the success of HDSRV as a sole agent for preexposure immunization. It currently appears that of individuals receiving preexposure vaccination, only 66 percent will develop adequate protective titers. Problems with transport or interference by other concomitantly administered vaccines or medications may account for this [12].
3. Even if the vaccine is appropriately administered, it is difficult to

know exactly how long a protective titer will last. The recommendation that individuals at high risk who have been vaccinated according to preexposure protocol receive a booster every 2 years has recently been changed, owing to an increasing number and increasing severity of reaction to the booster [13].

4. Because rabies is virtually always fatal, the question about severity is moot.

5. The actual risk of acquiring rabies once exposure has occurred has been debated since Pasteur's time, but the best guess is 15 to 20 percent if the individual is not treated [2]. This number may be influenced by the location and size of the wound. Deep wounds or macerated ones or those on the head, face, or neck appear to be most capable of resulting in a clinical infection [14]. This could also be influenced by the type of local wound care received in the immediate postbite period. The current recommendation is for vigorous cleansing with soap and water. This is an effective preventive step to take and replaces previous recommendations which insisted that quartenary ammonia compounds were necessary to inactivate the virus locally [15].

6. With HDSRV, side effects after postexposure prophylaxis are rare and are confined mainly to local redness and swelling. Isolated cases of neurologic difficulties have been reported.

7. The cost of administering rabies vaccine is considerable. Let us look at risks and costs first, and then turn to considerations of how they are to be weighed against each other.

--- STUDY QUESTION 16-4

Given the following assumptions, calculate the cost of rabies vaccinations given in the United States each year.

1. Human rabies immune globulin (HRIG) costs $65 per vial (300 IU per vial)
2. Human diploid strain rabies vaccine (HDSRV) costs $63 per 1-ml dose
3. Each individual treated will receive HRIG, 20 IU per kilogram of body weight (assume 70-kg weight for each individual treated), and 5 doses of HDSRV.
4. Once a vial of HRIG is partially used, the remainder is usually discarded.
5. Twenty-five thousand individuals receive postexposure therapy yearly.

--- STUDY QUESTION 16-5

Given the assumptions in study question 16-4 as well as the following, what is the cost of preventing a case of rabies by secondary preventive intervention in the United States?

1. Approximately 20 percent of animals involved in exposures for which therapy is recommended are actually rabid.
2. Unvaccinated individuals have approximately a 20-percent chance of acquiring rabies if exposed.

Guidelines for Instituting Preventive Measures

The frightening severity of clinical rabies makes our cost analysis rather simple. We are able to see what it costs to save lives. Because of the relentless intrusion of economics into medicine, it remains an unsavory, if necessary, task to calculate the cost of saving a life, which sets up a conflict and leads to potentially volatile arguments about the worth of a human life. Considering the best form of prevention has led us to an ethical threshold. For the present, we are spared long deliberations when rabies is the disease in question. However, ethical issues may need to be considered in the future.

When confronted with a patient in whom postexposure therapy may be indicated, each practitioner must ask himself or herself the following questions: (1) Is rabies known or suspected to be present in the species of animal involved; and (2) has a bona fide exposure capable of transmitting rabies virus occurred (i.e., has potentially infected saliva or bodily secretions come in contact with an open wound)?

As mentioned earlier, wild carnivorous animals (especially skunks, raccoons, foxes, coyotes, and bobcats) are the species most likely to be infected with the rabies virus. After an individual has received a bite from or salivary exposure to such an animal, ideally the animal will be tested by immunofluorescent examination of brain tissue. Then, if indicated, postexposure therapy should be provided. If examination is not possible, exposure to a high-risk animal is reason enough to initiate therapy. Certain other wild species, such as rodents and rabbits, are unlikely hosts for the virus, and so exposure to these species does not necessitate therapy unless the animal's behavior was highly atypical or brain tissue examination of the offending animal documents rabies. Domestic animals, particularly dogs and cats, are at lower risk of being infected with rabies virus if local vaccine programs are fairly complete.

Although the preceding generalizations provide a rough guide to determining whether treatment is necessary, the risk of rabies is best ascertained by examination of the involved animal. Because we known the natural history of the disease in dogs and cats, it is appropriate to quarantine these animals for 10 days to observe them before deciding

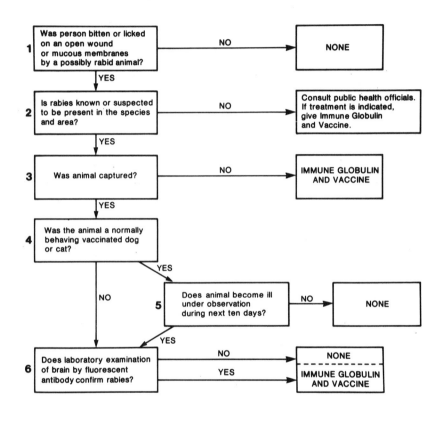

Fig. 16-1. Prophylaxis algorithm for rabies.

whether they need to be sacrificed for immunofluorescent testing of neural tissue. In contrast, it is necessary to sacrifice all suspected rabid wild animals, even those that have been domesticated, to examine brain tissue via immunofluorescent staining. This policy is the result of the unpredictable incubation period and variable clinical presentation of rabies in such animals. Regardless of the species, if there is doubt about the need for therapy, destruction of the animal and examination of its brain tissue is almost always appropriate.

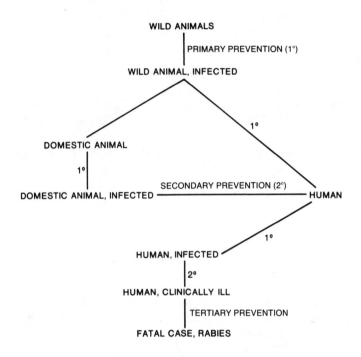

Fig. 16-2. Areas and nature of possible preventive interventions to control rabies.

If the species of animal is prone to rabies the next step is to determine whether exposure actually has taken place. To be considered a legitimate exposure, virus-contaminated saliva or other potentially infectious material, such as brain tissue, must come in contact with an open wound (including scratches or abrasions) or mucous membrane surfaces. If such contact is unlikely to have occurred, then it is probable that true exposure has not taken place and no prophylaxis is necessary. A summary of the algorithm for reaching a vaccination decision is shown in Figure 16-1.

_____ STUDY QUESTION 16-6
Given all the data presented thus far, what would you do in the case of Elisa, presented on page 269?

Future Trends

The advances in providing prevention on multiple levels for combatting rabies have been considerable. Public health professionals at the local, state, and national levels have contributed mightily to this effort. To keep rabies under control, adherence to domestic animal immunization, the outlawing of keeping otherwise wild animals as pets, and continued efforts to control the disease in wild animals will be necessary. Practicing physicians must acquaint themselves with the concepts of the preventive interventions that have been outlined (Fig. 16-2). By doing so, they will be able to participate in the effort to prevent rabies.

References

1. Murphy FA, Harrison AK. Electron microscopy of the rhabdoviruses of animals. In: Bishop DHL, ed. Rhabdoviruses. Boca Raton, Fla.: CRC Press, 1979:65–106.
2. Hattwick MAW. Human rabies. Public Health Rev 1974;3:229–274.
3. Winkler WC. Current status of rabies in the United States. In: Winkler WC, ed. Rabies: concepts for medical professionals. Miami: Merieux Institute, 1985:17–28.
4. Rubin RH, Hattwick MAW, Jones S, et al. Adverse reaction to duck embryo vaccine: range and incidence. Ann Intern Med 1973;74:643–649.
5. Anderson LJ, Winkler WC, Hafkin B, et al. Clinical experience with a human diploid cell rabies vaccine. JAMA 1980;244:781–784.
6. Devriendt J, Staroukine M, Costy F, Vanderhaeghen JJ. Fatal encephalitis apparently due to rabies: occurrence after treatment with human diploid cell vaccine but not rabies immune globulin. JAMA 1982;248:2304–2306.
7. Shill M, Baynes RD, Miller SD. Fatal rabies encephalitis despite appropriate post-exposure prophylaxis: a case report. N Engl J Med 1987;316:1257–1258.
8. Bahmanyar M, Fayaz A, Nour-Salehi S, et al. Successful protection of humans exposed to rabies infection: postexposure treatment with the new human diploid cell rabies vaccine and antirabies serum. JAMA 1976;236:2751–2754.
9. Hattwick MAW, Weiss TT, Stechschulte CJ, et al. Recovery from rabies: a case report. Ann Intern Med 1972;76:931–942.
10. Vaughn JB, Gerhardt P, Paterson JCS. Excretion of street rabies virus in saliva of cats. JAMA 1963;184:705–708.

11. Centers for Disease Control. Rabies in pet skunks. MMWR 1978;27:399–401.
12. Centers for Disease Control. Field evaluations of pre-exposure use of human diploid cell rabies vaccine. MMWR 1983;32:601–603.
13. Centers for Disease Control. Systemic allergic reactions following immunization with human diploid cell rabies vaccine. MMWR 1984;33:185–188.
14. Shah U, Jaswal CS. Victims of a rabid wolf in India: effect of severity and location of bites on development of rabies. J Infect Dis 1976;134:25–29.
15. Anderson LJ, Winkler WC. Aqueous quaternary ammonium compounds and rabies treatment. J Infect Dis 1979;139:494–495.

Down's Syndrome: Making Difficult Decisions

CHAPTER SEVENTEEN

BENJAMIN C. BLATT

The Sager Case

Approximately a month ago, I had the opportunity to speak with Jonathan Sager again, and I asked him to think about the two occasions in the recent past when he and his wife Mary had to make decisions about amniocentesis. Jonathan is a big burly man of 40, with a full reddish beard, whose approach to things in general is vigorously intellectual with occasional nervous undertones. He looks more like a logger than what he is—a violinist for a small urban symphony orchestra. His wife, Mary O'Reilly Sager, tall and pensive, can be tough and determined when necessary. She works as a lawyer for an environmental organization. I have known them both for a long time as patients and as friends.*

Mary first became pregnant in 1979, when she was 36 years old, and that is when the issue of amniocentesis first arose for the Sagers. Jonathan did not remember how he first heard about amniocentesis, but he told me:

Everyone was a little more hesitant about amniocentesis in those days. It was a little more up in the air about whether or not it was a choice for us . . . We were told by our doctor that it was up to us—that it was a decision that could go either way—we were not being urged to do amnio. I remember it as being quite an agonizing choice and what I remember was . . . that there was some chance of spontaneous abortion after the procedure, but at her age at that time it was felt that there was an equal chance of a Down's syndrome child . . . I kept saying to Mary that when you figured it out, the odds were something like 49 to 1 against having a Down's syndrome child.† You know, if someone offered a bet like that, you'd take it in a second . . .

---

*This section of the chapter is based on an interview that Jonathan Sager agreed to do with me. Names and some details have been altered to protect his and Mary's privacy. The quotations are Jonathan's words, with an occasional modification for clarity.

†Jonathan's *memory* of the odds that were presented to him nearly 3 years ago is "49 to 1." As we shall see, the actual odds of having a Down's syndrome child at age 36 are much lower (1 : 287). It is curious that Jonathan remembered them so differently. Perhaps the figures presented to the Sagers by their genetics counselor represented the odds of having a child with *any* sort of genetic abnormality, including Down's syndrome. Those odds, since they take into account genetic abnormalities in addition to Down's syndrome, would be expected to be worse: In fact, they are 1 : 161 [1], still quite far

The risk of abortion as a consequence of the procedure and Mary's age as a risk factor for Down's syndrome thus entered into the Sagers' thinking. Jonathan then elaborated the other factors that were important to them.

What I remember worrying about at the time were these several things: It seemed to me that there were so many medical technologic inventions that were quite stunning in themselves . . . but they were rushed onto line and everyone was extremely enthusiastic about them and yet, as with x-rays, it was discovered years later that there were problems with them. It wasn't clear to me what putting a needle into that environment and disturbing that environment [would do]—who knew what results that would have, what might show up from that disturbance when a child was 16, say?—beyond the obvious thing of sticking a needle into the fetus, which seemed like a minimal possibility. And it did not seem to me at that time that there had been a lot of long-term studies of kids who had come out of amnio . . .

In addition to revealing his intellectual appreciation of the possible future dangers of new technology, Jonathan made some interesting comments about his emotional reaction to the situation:

I think I also had some feeling—I don't know if it is the equivalent of the feeling of immortality or what—but I felt very strongly that nothing could happen to us . . . at a gut level, I felt that having a Down's syndrome child just wasn't going to happen to us.

Jonathan and Mary elected not to have amniocentesis during this first pregnancy. Interestingly, this decision had unexpected consequences, as Jonathan noted:

Inventions like amniocentesis create their own problems . . . you just can't will them to cease to exist because you don't want to use them. It was a more difficult pregnancy than I think it otherwise would have been, because Mary worried constantly about the fact that she might in fact have a Down's syndrome child and she hadn't taken the chance to find out about it. There were periods when she was very disturbed and upset and in tears about the choice we had made.

---

from what Jonathan recalls. When I presented him with the actual figures, Jonathan replied, "They gave us the real figures then; but even after you told me just now the true figures, I still have a memory of 1 : 49 odds."

The factors then that seemed most important in this couple's decision not to have amniocentesis during their first pregnancy were (1) their physician's neutral stand, (2) their view of the odds of having a Down's syndrome child, (3) their fear of the long-term consequences of a new technology, and (4) Jonathan's strong feeling that a Down's syndrome child would not be born to the Sagers. Now let us look at their decision-making process during Mary's second pregnancy, nearly 3 years later, when she was 39.

The second time around, there was no question about amniocentesis. Mary was at the age where they weren't really saying it was a choice. Secondly, I think, she was convinced that she didn't want to go through the horror of not knowing again . . . to a large extent, I don't think we had a lot of discussion about it . . . I felt it was just agreed; yes, she was going to do it . . . She was past the cusp. We knew the odds had gone up significantly.

When I asked Jonathan if he remembered what the odds of having a Down's syndrome child were, he told me that he couldn't remember exactly, "something like 1 : 12 or 1 : 16." Thinking about his previous comment regarding his willingness to take a bet with 1 : 49 odds without a second thought, I remarked that, assuming his estimation was correct this time, the odds were still strongly against the Sagers' having a Down's syndrome child. During the second pregnancy, however, Jonathan seemed much less frightened of the technology and much more willing to think about a Down's syndrome child as something that *could* happen to them. He replied to my remark:

The odds of 1 : 12, or whatever it was, didn't sound so great . . . not when you're talking about having a child that might actually rip your life apart and rip your family apart . . . It's not like a roulette table . . . It's not like you're just losing some money.

He went on to say: "I still had a gut-level feeling that everything would be okay, but I felt that just for our peace of mind we should go ahead with the amniocentesis."

This second time around, the Sagers did elect amniocentesis. The factors that seemed to play a part in this decision were (1) perception that the odds of a Down's syndrome child had greatly increased; (2) a strong physician recommendation in favor of amniocentesis; (3) the desire to avoid the agony of not knowing that had especially plagued Mary during the first pregnancy; and perhaps on a more emotional level, (4) Jonathan's greater comfort with the safety of the test and his doubts about his initial statement of denial: "A Down's syndrome child just [couldn't] happen to us."

In conversations with the Sagers, many key issues have surfaced about the decision to have or not to have amniocentesis. This chapter's principal mission will be to focus on the decision-making process in which patient and physician must share in wrestling with issues of secondary prevention. How can a physician help a couple such as the Sagers make the best decision? The principles of obtaining informed consent delineate the ground that must be covered by a counseling physician. These principles constitute the organizational framework of this chapter. To provide informed consent, the physician must offer adequate data, ensure sufficient understanding, and avoid coercion.

How Data Presentation Can Influence Medical Decision Making

As we have read, Mary Sager's age and its relation to the risk of having a Down's syndrome child is something that Jonathan mentioned again and again. Another of Jonathan's prominent concerns was safety of amniocentesis. Still another vital issue that he did not much mention is the accuracy of the test. We will review the data* on each of these issues as well as the challenges faced by a counseling physician in attempting to help patients such as the Sagers understand them.

CLINICAL FEATURES OF DOWN'S SYNDROME

Down's syndrome was not a medical obscurity to the Sagers, nor is it to many people. It is familiar because of its dramatic phenotypic features and because of its relative commonness.

People with Down's syndrome are short and have a characteristic facial appearance—oblique orbital fissures, flat nasal bridge, small ears, nystagmus, and mouth hung open. In addition, they are mentally deficient. The genetic defect most often associated with this condition is trisomy 21, the presence of three instead of the normal two chromosomes 21. Chromosomal translocation may also be responsible. In addition, mosa-

---

*Though a couple being counseled will undoubtedly be interested in the risk data on *any* genetic abnormality, we will discuss only the data relevant to Down's syndrome. Since this is by far the most common genetic abnormality, Down's syndrome can be used with reasonable accuracy to illustrate the issues of cytogenetic decision making. It is also the syndrome that most people know best.

icism of trisomy 21 with normal cells (46/47, +21) can occur and produce modified features of Down's syndrome. Women with trisomy 21 can become pregnant, and half of their children will have the syndrome. People with trisomy 21 mosaicism also have a higher incidence of Down's syndrome children, and unfortunately, many of these people—because their condition is undiagnosed—only discover their genetic problem after they have had their first Down's syndrome child.

Down's syndrome leads to many tragic consequences beyond mental retardation. Cardiac malformations may cause death in infancy in one-third of individuals. In addition, Down's syndrome children are at higher risk for many other congenital anomalies and for leukemia.

Mental retardation, however, is the feature of the syndrome most prominent in many people's minds. How severe is the mental retardation seen in Down's syndrome, and what is its resultant monetary (as well as emotional) cost? One set of experts notes that the average intelligence quotient (IQ) scores of adults with Down's syndrome range between 25 and 50 (an IQ greater than 50 is considered the educable range) [2]. They emphasize, however, that IQ scores can be misleading; Down's syndrome adults can be taught tasks (e.g., running a tractor) that normal children might have difficulty performing [2]. Another group of experts estimates that 20 percent of Down's children are educable [3]. The latter group paints a grim picture, assuming only those with IQs in excess of 50 could work, and then only at half the productivity of an average person. Based on a survey done in Scotland, these investigators estimate that 25 percent of those afflicted with Down's syndrome will need permanent care by age 15, 50 percent by age 25, 75 percent by age 35, and 100 percent by age 45. If these estimates are correct, caring for Down's syndrome children could result in a huge financial outlay for society.

As mentioned above, the commonness of Down's syndrome, as well as its distinctive appearance, makes it familiar to large numbers of people. How common is Down's syndrome? What is the risk for a couple of having a baby afflicted with Down's syndrome? The incidence rate is one measure of risk and approximates the probability of developing a disease. In the case of Down's syndrome, the incidence is approximately 1 in 800 live births. This information might be useful to a couple such as the Sagers. However, even more useful would be information that might pinpoint factors which would place them at special risk. One such factor might be a history of a previous Down's syndrome child (evidence for subclinical trisomy 21 mosaicism). Jonathan Sager recognized maternal age as a factor. In fact, there appears to be a strong relationship between

Table 17-1. Risk of having a live child with Down's syndrome
related to maternal age (1-year intervals from age 20 to 49)

Maternal age (yr)	Risk	Maternal age (yr)	Risk	Maternal age (yr)	Risk
20	1 : 1923	30	1 : 885	40	1 : 109
21	1 : 1695	31	1 : 826	41	1 : 85
22	1 : 1538	32	1 : 725	42	1 : 67
23	1 : 1408	33	1 : 592	43	1 : 53
24	1 : 1299	34	1 : 465	44	1 : 41
25	1 : 1205	35	1 : 365	45	1 : 32
26	1 : 1124	36	1 : 287	46	1 : 25
27	1 : 1053	37	1 : 225	47	1 : 20
28	1 : 990	38	1 : 177	48	1 : 16
29	1 : 935	39	1 : 139	49	1 : 12

advanced maternal age and risk (Table 17-1). Compared to a 20-year-old woman, a woman of 35 years has an approximately 5 times greater chance of having a Down's syndrome child, and a woman 45 years old has an approximately 60 times greater chance.

_____ STUDY QUESTION 17-1
Using Table 17-1, it is now possible to answer the Sagers' questions about their personal risk more precisely. What was the risk of bearing a Down's syndrome baby for Mary at age 39 as compared to her risk at 36?

PREVENTION OF DOWN'S SYNDROME
At this time, the only way to prevent the birth of a Down's syndrome child once conception has occurred is detection of the abnormality before birth and interruption of the pregnancy. Amniocentesis is the most commonly used method for early detection. Approximately 20 years ago, Steel and colleagues [4] first cultured and karyotyped amniotic fluid cells. Once cell culture and karyotyping became possible, amniocentesis—removal of fetal cell–containing amniotic fluid from the amniotic sac—was used more and more for early detection of genetic and biochemical abnormalities. The technique is performed with local anesthesia under ultrasonic guidance using a small-bore (often 20-gauge) needle, and it is done during the second trimester when enough fluid has accumulated to minimize fetal risk. In medical circles, amniocentesis

has a good reputation. Nonetheless, patients (as well as their physicians) have many concerns about any invasive procedure, especially one involving a mother and her unborn child.

In one sampling of women considering amniocentesis [5], the women interviewed listed their concerns as follows:

Concerns	No. of women (%)
Risk of spontaneous abortion	29 (39%)
Risk of fetal injury	27 (36%)
Not knowing what to expect	19 (24%)
Diagnosis	10 (14%)
Pain	12 (16%)
Other	1 (0.1%)
No concerns	16 (22%)

Physicians can be of great assistance with the issues of not knowing what to expect and fear of pain. However, what can a physician tell a couple such as the Sagers about the risk of injuring the fetus with the needle, or of causing bleeding or infection in the mother, or of involuntarily precipitating an abortion? How accurate is the test in detecting Down's syndrome? Might the couple decide to have an abortion on the basis of a positive test only to find at autopsy that the fetus was normal and healthy? Let us look at data that will help answer some of these questions.

Safety of Amniocentesis
In 1976, the National Institutes of Child and Health Development (NICHD) conducted a prospective study in nine different medical centers involving 1040 subjects who decided to have amniocentesis [6]. Once a subject entered the study, the investigators searched for a control patient who was not a candidate for, or who elected not to have, amniocentesis. Randomization, the hallmark of a controlled clinical trial, was not used in this study.

_____ STUDY QUESTION 17-2
Can you explain why randomization was not used?

Because of the nature of the selection process, the subject group turned out to be substantially older (p $<$.001) than the control group (older women tended to elect amniocentesis), introducing a potential bias to the study. In addition, it should be mentioned that a stated goal of the study was to have 1000 subjects and 1000 controls, so that a doubling in frequency of selected important adverse occurrences in the amniocentesis group would be statistically significant at the 5-percent level of probability. The number of subjects and controls chosen determine the study's statistical power (how small a true difference between subjects and controls can be demonstrated to be statistically significant).

According to the study, the adverse consequences affecting the mother within 1 week of the procedure were:

Amniotic fluid leakage	12
Vaginal bleeding	11
Premature labor pains	2
Spontaneous abortion	1
Amnionitis	1

Comparison of study subjects with controls showed no difference in the incidence of toxemia, vaginal bleeding, placenta abruptio or previa, or infection. Similarly, the two groups showed no substantial difference in the incidence of complications of labor or delivery, except that cesarean section was performed more often in subjects (17.9 percent) than in controls (12.4 percent). Hence, there were only two serious maternal complications in the amniocentesis group: one case of amnionitis and one of presumably induced abortion. Overall, this is very reassuring information.

The overall rate of fetal loss for the amniocentesis patients was 3.5 percent (36 cases) compared to 3.2 percent (32 cases) for the controls, not a statistically significant difference.

_____ STUDY QUESTION 17-3
Would you tell the Sagers (or any couple asking your advice) that their fears that amniocentesis might induce abortion are groundless?

_____ STUDY QUESTION 17-4
In the NICHD study [6], the risk difference for fetal loss between subjects (3.5 percent) and controls (3.2 percent) is 0.3 percent. Could the study be somehow exaggerating this difference, and if so, how? (In considering this question, note that the spontaneous rate of fetal loss varies with age: The older the person, the higher the rate. Also note, as was previously mentioned, that in the NICHD study, the study group was substantially older than the control group.)

_____ STUDY QUESTION 17-5
Could there actually be a substantially increased risk for subjects over controls
that this study is not reflecting? How might you explain this? (Remember the
limitations of the statistical power of the study.)

An observed difference that does not reach statistical significance may
have several interpretations. The effect of age as a selection bias and the
relatively small number of study participants, with its propensity to lead
to type II errors, can greatly modify the way one thinks about these
numbers and how one ultimately advises one's patients. In light of the
abortion risk data from the NICHD study [6], it would probably be most
prudent to suggest to a couple considering amniocentesis that the risk
of induced abortion is extremely small but nonetheless there.

_____ STUDY QUESTION 17-6
Assume that you routinely make the prudent suggestion to your patients that
there probably is a slight risk of induced abortion with amniocentesis. How
might your interpretation of the data influence a 38-year-old woman (risk of
bearing a Down's syndrome child is 1 : 175) who has finally conceived after 10
years of trying?

Other potential untoward fetal consequences were considered in the
NICHD study. The following were found not to differ substantially between the infants of subjects and controls:

Birth weight

Prematurity

Apgar scores

Congenital anomalies (other than chromosomal)

Neonatal jaundice, seizures, or respiratory distress syndrome

Neonatal deaths

Status after 1 year (deaths, infection, growth, physical examination,
intelligence)

In addition, no evidence of needle injury was found in the subject
group. Nevertheless, a further qualification must be made. One disad-
vantage of many clinical trials is that they are short-term. The NICHD
trial did have 1-year follow-up, but infant intelligence cannot be ade-

quately assessed at 1 year. It is possible that the study failed to discover mental deficits that might manifest themselves later.

_____ STUDY QUESTION 17-7
(a) Based on the data provided, what do you conclude about the overall safety of amniocentesis for mother and fetus? (b) Are there any limitations in generalizing these results to the population at large?

Diagnostic Accuracy of Amniocentesis
Of the 1040 women undergoing amniocentesis in the NICHD study [6], 950 had the procedure performed for cytogenetic indications, and in 90 the procedure was done to check for possible inherited metabolic disorders. The number of positive tests were as follows:

Cytogenetic abnormalities	19
Metabolic abnormalities	15
Sex determinations (male) for X-linked disorders	11

The NICHD investigators state that six diagnostic errors were made, one in metabolic diagnosis and five in cytogenetic diagnosis. Three of the latter were incorrect sex determinations, and two concerned women in whom amniocentesis was negative for Down's syndrome but who bore children with trisomy 21 (false negatives). No false positive results occurred for Down's syndrome (i.e., no case tested positively for trisomy 21 in normal babies). The investigators thus calculated a diagnostic accuracy* of 99.4 percent, a very impressive figure. However, no test is perfect. Pretest probability has to be taken into account, and the higher the pretest probability for disease, the lower the risk of a false positive result.

THE SAGERS' DECISIONS AND THEIR CONSEQUENCES
Having reviewed the principles of data presentation, let us reiterate the bases on which Jonathan and Mary Sager made their decisions and see what the results were. During the first pregnancy, the Sagers took into account their particular risk based on Mary's age. However, the strong odds in their favor (1 : 294), their distrust of the safety of this relatively

_____
*Diagnostic accuracy of a test is defined as the number of correct diagnoses minus the erroneous diagnoses (false positives and false negatives) resulting from the test, divided by the total number of tests.

new technique (though the NICHD study was out by that time), and Jonathan's strong belief that "it won't happen to us" convinced them not to undergo amniocentesis. It is interesting to note that concern about diagnostic accuracy did not surface much in the Sagers' deliberations, and equally interesting is the emotional element in their (and in our) reasoning. Mary gave birth to a normal healthy girl, whom the Sagers named Meg.

During the second pregnancy, new factors came into play. Mary had worried profusely about the possibility of a genetic problem during the first pregnancy, and she did not want to go through that again. In addition, Jonathan's perception of the risk (though it only changed from 1 : 294 to 1 : 137 was that it had greatly increased. Mary had midsemester amniocentesis, and trisomy 21 was diagnosed. Mary and Jonathan painfully decided to proceed with a saline abortion.

Ensuring Understanding and Minimizing Bias

DECISION ANALYSIS

Data on age as a risk factor and on test safety and accuracy had a lot to offer the Sagers in their struggle to decide whether amniocentesis was necessary. However, major decisions seldom are made by objective criteria alone.

During the first pregnancy, Jonathan had a gut-level feeling that their child would not have Down's syndrome and believed that the odds were so good that "if someone offered a bet like that, you'd take it in a second." During the second pregnancy, though, the odds had only advanced from 1 : 294 to 1 : 137. Nonetheless, Jonathan felt the odds had "gone up significantly," especially "when you're talking about having a child that might actually rip your life apart." Thus, during the first pregnancy, Jonathan focused on one side of the coin—the 294 : 1 odds *against* having a Down's syndrome baby—whereas during the second pregnancy, he focused on the opposite side of the coin—the 1 chance in 137 that *favored* a Down's syndrome baby. Undoubtedly, Jonathan's fear of technology played a major role in the first decision-making process. The greater familiarity with technology lessened his fear of the procedure the second time around, and the anguish of not knowing and the fear of having a child that might "rip your life apart" took over and shaped his thinking. Strong emotional factors (perhaps magnified in their impact by the importance of a major medical decision) can thus lead a person to interpret similar data in diametrically opposite ways.

The physician, when counseling, must do more than merely summarize the data. He or she has the even more formidable task of helping a patient sort through his or her emotions to discover which are promoting his or her best interests and which are impeding them. Furthermore, during all this, the physician is obliged to monitor his or her own biases to ensure that they do not adversely interfere with the decision-making process of a patient.

Recently, a number of new approaches have been developed to help the counseling physician collaborate with patients faced with major medical decisions. One such approach is called decision analysis. We will look at this approach as it applies to the amniocentesis decision.

The Nondirective Model Versus Decision Analysis

The genetic counselor, in the traditional *nondirective model,* supplies the couple with information about risks and probabilities, and then encourages them to sort through the information and make a decision. However, because the couple may not be used to dealing with the mathematic complexities of numerous different probabilities in a complicated decision, this nondirective approach may seem overwhelming.

Pauker and Pauker [7], in a 1979 report on amniocentesis, proposed an alternative to traditional nondirective counseling: decision analysis. In an adaptation of their amniocentesis model, seven possible outcomes are summarized:

Amniocentesis Not Performed
1. Spontaneous abortion
2. Unaffected child
3. Affected child

Amniocentesis Performed
4. Spontaneous abortion
5. Elective abortion after a positive result
6. Unaffected child after a negative result
7. Affected child after a negative result

These outcomes are then arranged in a decision tree (Fig. 17-1).

The patient is asked to consider each possible outcome and assign it a utility score on a scale from 0 to 100. A score of 100 represents the most desirable outcome, the one with the greatest utility or lowest burden. A score of 0 represents the least desirable outcome, the one with the lowest

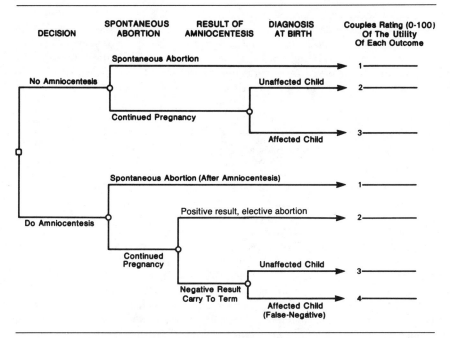

| DECISION | SPONTANEOUS ABORTION | RESULT OF AMNIOCENTESIS | DIAGNOSIS AT BIRTH | Couples Rating (0-100) Of The Utility Of Each Outcome |

Fig. 17-1. Options and alternative outcomes of amniocentesis as a decision tree. The square node denotes the decision, whereas each circular node denotes a chance event. (Adapted from Pauker and Pauker [7].)

utility or greatest burden. The patient then fills in these utilities on the decision tree. Once this has been done, each of the patient's utilities is multiplied by the probability of the event occurring. For example, if a patient feels the burden of spontaneous abortion induced by amniocentesis is high, she might give it a utility score of 30. The probability of such spontaneous abortion occurring, as we know from the NICHD study [6], is 3.5 percent. (One can calculate a weighted utility for this possible outcome by multiplying 30 by 3.5.) The weighted utilities (probability × utility) are added for the three possible outcomes if amniocentesis is not performed and separately for the four possible outcomes if amniocentesis is performed. The counselor then recommends the alternative with the highest overall weighted utility, i.e., the highest probability of producing a favorable outcome given the decision maker's values.

_____ STUDY QUESTION 17-8

A 38-year-old woman (odds of bearing a Down's syndrome baby, 1 : 175) who had been trying unsuccessfully to get pregnant for the past 10 years has finally become pregnant. Although she does not like the idea of voluntary abortion, she believes that bringing a Down's syndrome child into the world is worse. How do you think she would rate the following two possible outcomes on the decision tree?

Spontaneous abortion as a result of amniocentesis

Bearing a Down's syndrome baby after not having amniocentesis

_____ STUDY QUESTION 17-9

Assume that a 36-year-old woman believes that voluntary abortion is always morally wrong. In addition, she and her husband feel that they would be wrong to abort a Down's syndrome baby because "any human life is precious and besides, some Down's syndrome children can learn enough to work and be relatively independent." However, this couple has told you that they are considering amniocentesis because if they have a Down's syndrome baby, they want to know in advance so they can prepare psychologically and financially. As you can see by looking at the decision tree in Figure 17-1, there is no place for the choice "amniocentesis for prognosis." One advantage of decision analysis is that it is flexible enough to incorporate such new options. How might you alter the decision tree in Figure 17-1 to allow for amniocentesis for prognosis?

Advantages of Decision Analysis

One of the major advantages of decision analysis as a counseling technique is that it allows patients to integrate the probability data and their value judgments about each potential outcome in a logical way under the guidance of a professional well-versed in handling the data. At the end of the process, the couple (or individual) is directed to a decision consistent with the data and consistent with their beliefs. Decision analysis should thus minimize the chances of a patient with strong beliefs becoming so confused by the data that he or she does not know what to choose. Decision analysis is quantitative and allows the physician and patient to weigh alternatives mathematically and precisely. Also it allows the physician and patient to break down decisions into components, thus allowing them to isolate and further explore areas of confusion. For all these reasons, decision analysis can help the patients clarify complex situations and reach a decision consistent with their beliefs.

Finally, decision analysis does help with some of the more emotional aspects of decision making. To a degree, it allows the individual or couple to incorporate feelings and beliefs into the decision-making process. For example, Jonathan and Mary Sager, during the second pregnancy, did not want to go through the agony of not knowing again. This in part reflects their fear of the consequences of having a Down's syndrome baby. Referring to the decision tree in Figure 17-1, they could take this into consideration by assigning a very high utility to doing an amniocentesis and discovering a genetic abnormality. Also, decision analysis might have persuaded Jonathan to be more logical about the change in the age-related risk of Down's syndrome. However, a number of Jonathan and Mary's emotional responses, which powerfully affected their decision-making process, do not easily fit into the decision analysis model. How would you figure in Jonathan's "gut reaction" that everything would be okay, or Jonathan's and Mary's fear of new invasive technology (how can one incorporate fears of outcomes not yet known or knowable)? Also, what influence did physician biases have on Mary's and Jonathan's decision making? (During the first pregnancy, their doctor was neutral, but during the second, he strongly favored amniocentesis.) How can one account for physician bias in decision analysis?

BEHAVIORAL DECISION THEORY: A CRITIQUE
OF THE DECISION ANALYSIS MODEL
Decision analysis is an elegant and powerful technique that can go far in helping ordinary people integrate complex probabilities with their personal beliefs. However, as we have seen, it also has some disadvantages. In an article critiquing decision analysis, Eraker and Politser [8] point out that people often do not make the choices that decision analysis would advise them to make. To explain this phenomenon, the researchers cite a body of psychologic research known as behavioral decision theory. Behavioral decision theory notes that persons asked to make decisions in grossly unfamiliar areas have difficulty quantifying their utilities. Perhaps amniocentesis was just such a novel situation for Jonathan and Mary Sager during the first pregnancy. Behavioral decision theory also notes that decision analysis assumes that people's values are defined well enough to quantitate; however, many people are not sure of what they want. Finally, behavioral decision theory points out that people often make substantial errors in making judgments. These errors are attributable in part to biases that are already established in the patient's thinking or that are introduced by the way the physician presents information.

Presentation Bias

To gain a better appreciation of how presentation can bias decisions, let us consider a scenario taken from a study by McNeil and colleagues [9]. Put yourself in the place of a patient with lung cancer. Lung cancer treatment sometimes involves an operation on the lungs. Most patients are in the hospital for 2 or 3 weeks and have some pain around their incision. They spend a month or so recuperating at home, after which they generally feel fine.

Radiation therapy for lung cancer involves the use of radiation to kill the tumor. It requires coming to the hospital approximately 4 times a week for 6 weeks. Each treatment takes a few minutes, and during the treatment, patients lie on a table as though they were having a chest roentgenogram. During the course of the treatment, some patients develop nausea and vomiting, but at the end of the 6 weeks, they also generally feel fine. Thus, after the initial 6 or so weeks, patients treated with either surgery or radiation therapy feel about the same. Now consider the following and decide which treatment you would prefer:

FRAME 1.   Of every 100 people having surgery, *10* will die during treatment, *32* will have died by 1 year, and *66* will die by 5 years. Of every 100 people having radiation therapy, *none* will die during treatment, *23* will die by 1 year, and *78* will have died by 5 years.

The data in this frame summarizes the experience of many hospitals. How would you choose to be treated? Now consider new information pertaining to a specific hospital and make a new choice on the basis of these data.

FRAME 2.   At this single hospital, 10 percent of the patients who have surgery die during the perioperative period. The patients who survive treatment have a life expectancy (i.e., average number of remaining years) of *6.8* years. Life expectancy of all patients who undergo surgery (including those who die in the postoperative period) is *6.1* years. With radiation therapy, nobody dies during treatment, and life expectancy of the patients who undergo radiation therapy is *4.7* years.

At this hospital, which treatment would you prefer? After considering both frames, was your decision for both the same? The basic information was! The study population in McNeil's article [9] preferred radiation to surgery 42 percent of the time in the first frame and 25 percent of the time in the second.

_____ STUDY QUESTION 17-10
How did the presentation of the data differ in the first and second frames?

Availability Bias

Another type of bias is termed *availability*. This bias, however, is not introduced by the physician but preexists in the mind of the patient. Consider the following example. A 42-year-old man develops polyuria and polydipsia and is found to have a random blood glucose level of 640 mg per deciliter. His physician advises insulin therapy, but the patient refuses, explaining that his brother died last year of an insulin overdose. This man's distortion in judgment is the result of his tendency to assess the likelihood of an event by the ease with which relevant instances can be recalled. As Eraker and Politser [8] point out, "Availability suggests that judgments will be influenced by both direct experience with death of friends and relatives as well by indirect exposure through movies, books, television and newspapers."

JUDGMENT ANALYSIS

Clearly, many factors can bias and distort a person's judgment. Decision analysis can be very useful in helping people understand and grapple with the elements of complex medical decisions, but to work well, decision analysis requires intact judgment. Persons in the highly emotional throes of life and death decisions (such as whether or not to have amniocentesis) may be medically and legally competent to make medical decisions but, very understandably, have judgment distortions. Even if they are able to face such major medical decisions calmly, their own preexisting biases or physician-introduced biases may impair their judgment.

In summary, the decision analysis model implies that merely supplying data (the nondirective model) to patients making decisions is insufficient. Rather, decision analysis suggests that the patients must be assisted in integrating their values with the data in a logical way to arrive at the best decision. As we have seen, however, behavioral decision theory emphasizes that formal decision analysis often is inadequate because people in stressful situations make faulty judgments. A faulty judgment plugged into a decision analysis formula results in a faulty decision.

Behavioral decision theory thus raises a critical issue. How can a counseling physician help his patient avoid judgment distortion? A possible solution employs a method we shall call *judgment analysis*.

First, the counseling physician must be aware of "red flags" that suggest such a problem in judgment is occurring. These can be sought in two areas: (1) the patient's emotional status, and (2) the patient's behavioral consistency. With regard to emotional status, patients whose responses suggest depression, extreme anxiety, bewilderment, or ambivalence will probably be more likely to have impaired judgment. Also, patients who suggest actions that are inconsistent with previous expressions of fact or belief are equally suspect.

If impaired judgment is suspected, two techniques are especially useful to the counseling physician: (1) exploring the patients thinking process, and (2) emotion management. In the first, the physician asks the patient to share with him or her the thinking behind his or her judgments. The physician can then, in a supportive way, point out biases and inconsistencies between beliefs and decisions. In the second, the physician helps the patient control emotions such as severe anxiety that may be impeding the patient's ability to make clear judgments.

APPLICATIONS OF VARIOUS COUNSELING METHODS

Now that we have seen ways in which people apply logic, judgment, values, emotion, and bias to decision making, let us return to the question posed early on: How can the physician best help a patient arrive at a major medical decision consistent with his or her needs and beliefs? In this chapter, we have discussed three major counseling methods that can help the physician in his or her quest toward this ideal. The first, the *nondirective model,* involves presenting data accurately and understandably and then encouraging the patient to make an independent decision.

The second counseling method, *decision analysis,* also relies on accurate data presentation but, unlike the nondirective model, does not leave the patient to decide alone. It provides a technique by which the physician takes an active role in helping the patient integrate the data with his or her beliefs and values.

The third counseling method, *judgment analysis,* is a method to minimize interference from factors that undermine the soundness of a person's judgment. It relies on exploring the patient's thinking process behind the judgments he or she makes and on emotion management. Judgment analysis can be integrated into the decision analysis and the nondirective models.

To provide better understanding of these three major counseling approaches, let us look at some specific examples and see which of these methods you might apply.

(a) How might you help a mathematically naive woman integrate the various probabilities in the amniocentesis decision into her decision-making process? (Probabilities to be considered include the risk of the procedure to the fetus, the risk of the procedure to the mother, the risk of inducing abortion, the risk of a false positive chromosome test, and the risk of a false negative chromosome test.) (b) How might you counsel a 36-year-old woman who has religious reservations about abortion but who requests referral for amniocentesis "because of the high risk of a Down's syndrome baby once you get to be older than 35"?

In the words of Jonathan Sager, this is an age of "so many medical technological inventions that are stunning in themselves." Certainly amniocentesis fits this description. But as Jonathan and Mary Sager discovered, this stunning technology brought with it agonizing choices that people never previously had to confront. Nevertheless, the counseling physician, with skillful use of the techniques we have discussed, can aid his patients to make as fully informed and reasonable a decision as possible among the choices they face.

References

1. Hook EB, Chambers GC. Estimated rates of Down syndrome in live births by one year maternal age intervals for mothers age 20 to 49 in a New York State study: implications of the risk figures for genetic counseling and cost-benefit analysis of prenatal diagnosis programs. In: Bergman D, Lowry RB, Trimble BK, et al., eds. Numerical taxonomy of birth defects and polygenic disorders—birth defects 5 Vol. 13, part 3A. New York: Liss, 1977, pp. 124–141.
2. Smith DW, Wilson AA. The child with Down's syndrome. Philadelphia: Saunders, 1973.
3. Hagard S, Carter FA. Preventing the birth of infants with Down's syndrome: a cost-benefit analysis. Br Med J 1976;1:753–756.
4. Steel MV, Breg WR Jr. Chromosome analysis of human amniotic fluid cells. Lancet 1966;1:383.
5. Davies BL, Terence DA. Factors in a woman's decision to undergo genetic amniocentesis for advanced maternal age. Nursing Res 1982;31(1):56–59.
6. NICHD National Registry for Amniocentesis Study Group. Midtrimester amniocentesis for prenatal diagnosis. JAMA 1976;236(13):1471–1476.

7. Pauker SP, Pauker SG. The amniocentesis decision: an explicit guide for parents. Birth defects: original article series, 1979 (The National Foundation);15(5c):289–324.
8. Eraker SA, Politser P. How decisions are reached: physician and patient. Ann Intern Med 1982;97:262–268.
9. McNeil BJ, Pauker SG, Sox HC, Tversky A. On the elicitation of preferences for alternative therapies. N Engl J Med 1982;306:1259–1262.

Tertiary Prevention

PART SIX

Use of Oral Acyclovir
for Genital Herpes

CHAPTER EIGHTEEN

WALTER A. STEIN

CASE A. In your primary care practice, the physician's assistant confers with you regarding the treatment plan for a 35-year-old divorced woman complaining of symptoms of recurrent genital herpes. She was diagnosed in your office 2 years ago as having a painful initial episode of genital herpes. The history obtained today reveals a typical picture of recurrent genital herpes. She has episodes of vesicular eruptions on the external left labia every 4 to 12 weeks. This patient complains of prodromal symptoms of moderately severe shooting pains in the left buttock within the 24 hours before the development of papular genital lesions. She also admits to localized pain and itching approximately 12 hours before the skin lesions appear. The lesions themselves begin as small 2- to 3-mm erythematous macular lesions and progress to vesicles. The vesicles crust over after several days and completely heal within 2 weeks. Your patient is status–post tubal ligation. She would like to be placed on some form of therapy to minimize the impact genital herpes has had on her life. She is particularly interested in relief of symptoms over the next 4 months.

Natural History of Genital Herpes

Genital herpes is a sexually transmitted disease. There may be as many as 500,000 or more new cases per year in the United States [1]. Prevention of recurrent infection is an emotionally important and clinically difficult problem. Once a patient has contracted herpes, the clinician's efforts are directed at prevention of spread of recurrent attacks.

In 1962, the two serologic types of herpes simplex virus (HSV) were recognized [2]. Most infants have been exposed to herpes simplex virus type 1 (HSV-1) by 18 months of age, as demonstrated by antibody formation [3]. Many patients with HSV-1 are asymptomatic whereas others have an illness of gingivostomatitis with vesicles that may be accompanied by fever. HSV-1 seems to have a predilection to enter cells of the trigeminal ganglion and remain latent after the primary infection.

Herpes simplex virus type 2 (HSV-2) initial infections usually occur after puberty and the initiation of sexual activity. As with HSV-1, many HSV-2–infected individuals do not experience clinical manifestations. After primary infection, HSV-2 appears to reside in the sacral dorsal root ganglia in its latent state.

The most unusual aspect of herpes infection is that recurrences occur in the presence of circulating antibody and sensitized lymphocytes. Although HSV-2 has been considered venereal and HSV-1 nonvenereal, a change in the epidemiology seems to be an increase in the number of patients with type 1 virus in genital lesions and type 2 virus in oral lesions [4]. Initial episodes of HSV-2 may cause urinary retention and encephalitis (2500 cases per year) [4]. They may also predispose to spontaneous abortions and prematurity [5].

The symptoms and signs of recurrent genital herpes usually are localized to the genital area. The duration of an episode ranges from 8 to 12 days. Prodromal symptoms occur in approximately half of the cases, and range in onset and severity from a mild tingling sensation ½ to 48 hours before the eruption to shooting pains of a sacral neuralgia perceived in the legs, buttocks, or hips 1 to 5 days before frank skin lesions appear. Symptoms are more frequent and severe in women.

The affected area in recurrent genital herpes appears to be smaller than in primary infections. Viral shedding takes place for approximately 4 days after the onset of lesions, with crusting of lesions taking nearly 4 to 5 days. The average time from onset of lesions to complete healing is approximately 10 days. Viral shedding can take place even without lesions but is more likely to start with the formation of lesions, especially early in the clinical course. The herpes simplex virus can be transmitted to others during periods of asymptomatic shedding.

Approximately 80 percent of patients with a primary HSV-2 genital infection will develop a recurrence within 12 months. The mean interval between primary episode genital herpes infection and a recurrence is 120 days, compared to the mean of 42 days between episodes in recurrent disease. The frequency and severity of recurrent episodes varies in the same individual as well as among different individuals. Although it has not been clearly established, emotional stress, heat, moisture, pregnancy, oral contraceptive use, climate change, and trauma may trigger recurrent genital herpes infections.

Herpes simplex virus infection is of great clinical importance and concern to pregnant women. It has been transmitted to newborns through congenital and intrapartum routes. During the first trimester, higher rates of spontaneous abortion have been reported in women with herpetic cervicitis than in those pregnant women without evidence of herpetic cervicitis. Premature delivery has been associated with herpetic cervicitis during the last trimester of pregnancy [6].

To review the salient points, typical recurrent genital herpes infections are unilateral and mild in comparison to primary infections; an individual's expression of the disease varies widely over time; and in pregnant women, both primary and recurrent genital herpes infections present challenging clinical management problems.

Potential Goals of Therapy

There are a number of potential goals of therapy for genital herpes infection. These include: (1) preventing initial infection in those who come in sexual contact with the disease; (2) preventing initial infection in children born of infected mothers; (3) shortening the pain and local manifestations in the clinical course of the initial disease; (4) reducing the acute systemic complications of the initial disease; (5) preventing the development of latency; (6) preventing subsequent clinical recurrence among those with established latent infections; (7) reducing transmission from those with established latent disease; and (8) eradicating established latent infection.

_____ STUDY QUESTION 18-1

Which of these goals could potentially be accomplished by a safe and effective vaccination given to sexually active individuals prior to exposure?

_____ STUDY QUESTION 18-2

Which of these goals could potentially be accomplished by a safe and effective drug that is able to prevent additional lesions and stop viral shedding during the initial episode only? (Note: This drug does not eradicate the virus.)

_____ STUDY QUESTION 18-3

Which of these goals might be accomplished by a drug that successfully prevents clinical disease and viral shedding in patients with recurrent genital herpes? (Note: This drug does not eradicate the virus.)

Acyclovir

Although no treatment has been shown to satisfy all the goals of therapy for genital herpes, acyclovir is an approved form of treatment that comes closest to accomplishing those goals for a safe and effective drug for initial and recurrent disease. Let us look at the data supporting the efficacy of acyclovir as well as the reservations concerning its use. It is clear that the advent of acyclovir represents a breakthrough in the treatment of human viral infections. It is the only antiherpes virus medication in current use that depends on a virus-mediated metabolite to be effective. After intracellular uptake requiring phosphorylation, acyclovir becomes effective in antiviral action. Acyclovir triphosphate inhibits herpes simplex virus deoxyribonucleic acid and is chain terminating [7]. The phosphorylating enzyme thymidine kinase (TK) is only present in virus-infected cells, and acyclovir becomes effective only in those cells. Since acyclovir is activated by TK herpes simplex virus intracellularly, those strains that produce little or no TK would be essentially resistant to the drug.

Once a patient has contracted a herpes infection, the clinician can provide only tertiary prevention for that individual. This means that although no therapy will cure the patient of the disease, there is still a disease state to treat that is recurrent in nature and has implications for spread. The options for use of oral acyclovir in treating genital herpes are: (1) chronic suppression therapy; (2) patient-initiated therapy; (3) physician-initiated therapy; and (4) no therapy at all. How does one choose an option? One must consider issues of safety and effectiveness as well as the relative utility and indication for each of these four options.

EFFICACY

It may be especially difficult to assess the efficacy of a drug for genital herpes through uncontrolled clinical trials. There is a great deal of variation in the frequency of attacks even within the same individual. Patients are most likely to be enrolled in a study at a time of frequent attacks. Consequently, even without treatment, they are likely to have less frequent attacks during the subsequent treatment phase of the study. This phenomenon is known as regression to the mean or return to the average. Regression to the mean can deceive clinicians into believing that an ineffective therapy is effective. Let's look at some of the available data from controlled clinical trials on the use of oral acyclovir.

Suppression Therapy

Douglas and colleagues [8] reported a doubleblind study of acyclovir to suppress recurrences of genital herpes infection. Patients eligible to enter the study had had six or more episodes of HSV-2 genital herpes in the preceding year, were in general good health, were not pregnant if female, were not receiving immunosuppressive therapy, and were not experiencing a clinical recurrence at the time of enrollment.

Patients were randomized in a doubleblind fashion in blocks of six, so that one-third of the patients took 200 mg of acyclovir 5 times daily (acyclovir-5), one-third took acyclovir twice daily (acyclovir-2), one-sixth took placebo 5 times daily (placebo-5), and one-sixth took placebo twice daily (placebo-2). The medication was taken for a period of 4 months. Patients were followed for adverse effects through telephone surveys and were examined in clinic once monthly and at any time of a suspected recurrence of genital herpes. After the 4 months of therapy, patients were similarly followed for an additional 4 months without treatment.

This permitted the investigators to compare pretreatment, treatment, and posttreatment data. The demographic and clinical characteristics of patients in each pretreatment group were very similar.

In all groups combined, 143 patients completed the 4 months of therapy. Ninety-four percent of the placebo patients had a recurrence during this 120-day period, whereas 29 percent of the acyclovir-5 and 35 percent of the acyclovir-2 patients experienced a recurrent genital herpes outbreak. Analysis of survival data indicates that acyclovir recipients had a statistically significant ($p<.001$, Mantel-Cox test) and substantial reduction in the number of clinical recurrences beginning 5 days after therapy was initiated. The average interval from initiation of therapy to the first clinical recurrence was 18 days in one placebo group compared to more than 120 days in both acyclovir-treated groups. The frequency of recurrences for the acyclovir groups returned to their pretreatment levels during the 4 months following discontinuation of therapy. The data from this study can be summarized as follows:

	Acyclovir-5 Group	Acyclovir-2 Group	Combined Placebo Groups
Total no. of patients	45	51	47
No. of patients with recurrence	13	18	44

_____ STUDY QUESTION 18-4
Calculate the relative risk of a recurrence and attributable risk for placebo versus acyclovir 5 and acyclovir 2.

_____ STUDY QUESTION 18-5
If acyclovir were widely used in clinical practice, what secondary or dynamic changes may occur that were not observed in the controlled clinical trial?

Episodic Recurrence Therapy
In a controlled study of the treatment of recurrent herpes with oral acyclovir, Reichman and co-workers [9] studied 212 patients in a two-part method. In part A of the study, 212 patients received physician-initiated treatment for a recurrence of genital herpes after a clinic visit within 48 hours of symptoms. Some received acyclovir and others placebo. In part B of the study, 165 of the same patients from part A self-initiated therapy. They were told to begin treatment as soon as possible after the onset of a recurrent episode of genital herpes and then return for monitoring as part of the study.

Table 18-1. Results of physician-initiated therapy for genital herpes

Observed characteristic	Acyclovir (mean ± S.E.)	Placebo (mean ± S.E.)	Statistical significance
Duration of viral shedding (days)	2.1 ± 0.1	3.1 ± 0.3	p < .001
Time to crusting (days)	2.2 ± 0.2	2.2 ± 0.2	p < .05
Time to healing (days)	6.3 ± 0.3	7.4 ± 0.3	p < .01
Duration of pain (days)	2.8 ± 2	3.1 ± 0.3	NS
Development of new lesions during therapy (%)	16	24.5	

S.E. = standard error; NS = not significant.
Source: Adapted from Reichman and colleagues [9].

Each patient received the same drug in both parts of the study. The patients in this study had frequent recurrences of genital herpes, averaging from 10 to 13 per year. All were 18 years of age or older, the average being older than 30 years. There were no statistically significant differences between the patients in the two groups in terms of age, sex, or duration of disease.

Each patient was treated with 200 mg of acyclovir or placebo-5 times per day for 5 days. Among the characteristics that were observed and compared were: the duration of viral shedding; the time of lesion crusting; the time of healing; the duration of pain; and the development of new lesions. Table 18.1 summarizes the results of part A for all lesions, including the new ones that developed.

———————————————————————— STUDY QUESTION 18-6
Are you impressed with these results? Is this a clinically important or impressive decrease in pain and other measured characteristics?

The data from part B, patient-initiated treatment, are summarized in Table 18-2.

———————————————————————— STUDY QUESTION 18-7
Are you more impressed by these results than those for physician-initiated therapy?

Table 18-2. Results of self-initiated therapy for genital herpes

Observed characteristic	Acyclovir (mean ± S.E.)	Placebo (mean ± S.E.)	Statistical significance
Duration of viral shedding (days)	2.1 ± 0.2	3.9 ± 0.3	p < .001
Time to crusting (days)	2.4 ± 0.2	3.9 ± 0.3	p < .001
Time to healing (days)	5.7 ± 0.3	7.2 ± 0.5	p < .001
Duration of pain (days)	3.0 ± 0.3	3.4 ± 0.3	NS
Development of new lesions during therapy (%)	7.3	21.7	

S.E. = standard error; NS = not significant.
Source: Adapted from Reichman and colleagues [9].

_____ STUDY QUESTION 18-8
Let us assume that subsequent studies confirm that patient-initiated therapy is
an effective method for reducing the symptoms and spread of recurrent genital
herpes. What factors need to be considered in individual patient selection?

SAFETY
There are several dilemmas associated with long-term acyclovir therapy.
Long-term effects on all organ systems have not been well studied or
documented. There is even less information available regarding teratogenic effects of this drug on humans. All studies have required that
women not be pregnant and also that they be using acceptable birth
control methods.

In reviewing the package insert provided for acyclovir, you are re-
minded that this drug is in category C for teratogenic effects. The insert
states that acyclovir ". . . should not be used during pregnancy unless
the potential benefit justifies the potential risk to the fetus." There are
no clinical trials of acyclovir with pregnant women.

_____ STUDY QUESTION 18-9
(a) Based on what you know about acyclovir's efficacy and safety, which treatment option would you use for the patient in case A? (b) Would you decide
differently if she had not had a tubal ligation and was not using dependable
birth control?

The *Physicians Desk Reference* also states, "The safety and efficacy of orally administered acyclovir in the suppression of frequent episodes of genital herpes have been established only for up to 6 months. Thus, this regime should be considered only for appropriate patients and only for 6 months until the results of ongoing studies allow a more precise evaluation of the benefit/risk assessment of prolonged therapy."

Once a drug is approved, physicians are permitted to prescribe for indications beyond those approved. Let us look at one situation you might encounter, and see how you would decide.

CASE B.   A 29 year-old, single male patient has just finished a course of 6 months of suppression therapy with acyclovir for recurrent genital herpes. He appears to have responded well, having had one recurrence with vesicles and one other episode in which he experienced sacral pain but had no skin lesions. He has been off acyclovir for 8 weeks and is back in your office asking for another 6-month supply. Prior to his suppression therapy, he averaged one episode of genital herpes every 2 months. Since being off acyclovir, he has had two episodes. He feels that you have liberated him and would like to continue using the drug. He has been buying it for $59 per 100 tablets and feels this is a small price to pay for such a good amount of relief.

_____ STUDY QUESTION 18-10

What issues are raised by prescribing more long-term therapy for this patient? What would you do?

References

1. Becker TM, Blount JH, Guinan ME. Genital herpes infestations in private practice in the United States, 1966 to 1981. JAMA 1985;253(11):1601–1603.
2. Schneweis KE. Zum Antigenen aufhau des Herpes simplex Virus. Z Immunitatsforsch 1962;124:173–196.
3. Plummer G. Serological comparison of the herpes viruses. Br J Exp Pathol 1964;45:135.
4. Holmes K, Per Anders M, Sparlins PF, et al. Sexually transmitted diseases. New York: McGraw-Hill, 1984.
5. Naib ZM, Nahmias AJ, Josey WE, et al. Association of maternal genital herpetic infection with spontaneous abortion. Obstet Gynecol 1970;35:360.
6. Nahmias AJ. Perinatal risk associated with maternal genital herpes simplex infection. Am J Obstet Gynecol 1971;10:6.
7. Lerner AM. Editorial. Ann Intern Med 1982;96(3):370–371.

8. Douglas JM, Critchlow C, Benedetti J, et al. A double-blind study of oral acyclovir for suppression of recurrences of genital herpes.
9. Reichman RC, Badger GJ, Mertz GJ, et al. Treatment of recurrent genital
herpes simplex infections with oral acyclovir. JAMA 1984;251(16):2103–
2107.

Atrial Fibrillation, Stroke, and Anticoagulation

CHAPTER NINETEEN

L. GREGORY PAWLSON

CASE A.   Mrs. E. L. is an 85-year-old woman who moved into a retirement home following the death of her husband. She has mild glaucoma and cataracts, with accompanying visual impairment, and a 3-year history of mild, congestive heart failure for which she takes hydrochlorothiazide, 25 mg each day. You are called to see her for dyspnea. The patient states that she experienced increasing shortness of breath over the past 48 hours without chest pain or other symptoms. Physical examination reveals that her pulse is rapid and irregular, with an apical rate of 120 and a radial pulse of 76. She also has a few inspiratory rales and 3 + pitting edema. An electrocardiogram confirms the presence of atrial fibrillation that was not apparent on an electrocardiogram done 4 months ago. You decide to admit her to the hospital. In the hospital, you are successful in controlling her ventricular rate, but the patient remains in atrial fibrillation.

Should Mrs. E. L. be encouraged to accept anticoagulation to reduce her risk of stroke?

CASE B.   Mr. R. B. is a 95-year-old man who comes into your office with a complaint of chronic constipation. On physical examination, you find, among other things, that he has an irregular pulse, with an apical rate of 80. The electrocardiogram reveals atrial fibrillation, with a ventricular rate of 80. A previous medical record obtained indicates that the atrial fibrillation was present on an electrocardiogram done 6 years ago.

Do you recommend to Mr. R. B. that he be anticoagulated to reduce his risk of stroke?

Uncertainty in Decision Making

The preceding cases illustrate a form of prevention often called tertiary prevention. In tertiary prevention, we seek to prevent a complication (in this case, stroke) of an established condition (atrial fibrillation) rather than to prevent the condition (primary prevention) or to detect it at an early stage so that clinical expression of the disease can be prevented (secondary prevention). Tertiary prevention is common in clinical medicine, but many clinicians do not fully recognize that the intervention is preventive. For example, the treatment with penicillin of a mild pharyngitis that proves, on culture, to be positive for beta-hemolytic streptococci is more justified as a means of preventing peritonsillar abscess or rheumatic fever than as a direct measure to alleviate the discomfort of sore throat. If considered this way, many clinical decisions may be classified as tertiary prevention.

As we have seen in previous chapters, the answers to questions about whether to screen for a risk factor or whether to intervene with a preventive measure may not be obvious. In this chapter, we focus on atrial fibrillation and stroke to demonstrate the use of formal decision analysis to assist in deliberations concerning the use of prevention in situations of relative uncertainty. In addition, we will illustrate decision making about prevention for a small group or even an individual and explore the effect of advanced age with high baseline mortality on decisions to use preventive measures.

Atrial Fibrillation

Atrial fibrillation can occur in the absence of rheumatic heart disease and does so with a probability that increases with age. In atrial fibrillation, the orderly effective contraction of the atria are lost, and a very rapid (280 or greater) atrial rate is present. In the elderly without a history of rheumatic heart disease, fibrosis of the sinoatrial node and conducting system often is the immediate cause of atrial fibrillation and, in most patients, is associated with ischemic heart disease. However, it is not clear whether fibrosis is always secondary to ischemia or whether it also occurs with aging alone. Attempts at chemical or electric cardioversion often are only temporarily effective. The ventricular rate, however, is usually controllable.

INCIDENCE AND PREVALENCE

A number of studies have documented an increase in the incidence and prevalence of atrial fibrillation with age. Svanborg and colleagues [1] reported a prevalence of 4 percent in men and 2 percent in women in a random sample of 70-year-olds in Gotheborg, Sweden. The Framingham study in the United States revealed an increasing incidence with age, with a cumulative 22-year incidence of 39.7 per 1000 men and 29.9 per 1000 women, or an incidence of 1.72 per 1000 persons per year in men and 1.35 in women [2]. A number of studies using ambulatory monitoring have noted a much higher prevalence, reporting atrial fibrillation, especially in paroxysmal bursts, in up to 20 percent of persons older than 70 years [3].

EMBOLIC STROKE AND ATRIAL FIBRILLATION

The term *stroke* applies to a prolonged (greater than 48 hours) or permanent loss of neurologic function owing to an alteration in blood supply to the brain. There are, by clinical and pathologic criteria, three basic kinds of stroke—hemorrhagic, embolic, and thrombotic—although any single stroke may have characteristics of more than one of these types. In most populations, thrombotic strokes are much more prevalent, with hemorrhagic and embolic strokes together accounting for fewer than 35 percent of all strokes. In terms of overall occurrence among all strokes, based on clinical studies, approximately 15 to 25 percent of strokes are believed to be embolic in origin. This general range is supported by autopsy [4] and, more recently, by computed tomographic studies [5]. However, as we shall see, the incidence of embolic stroke is substantially increased in patients with atrial fibrillation.

Older studies of stroke generally relied on the clinical picture to classify a stroke by type. The clinical data were supplemented first by autopsy studies or arteriograms and more recently by computed tomographic scanning. Embolic strokes generally have a very sudden onset, giving little or no warning. They tend to be fairly massive, and most studies document between 20 and 35 percent immediate mortality, with severe permanent disability occurring in more than 50 percent of survivors [6–8]. It is unclear whether recurrent strokes cause the same morbidity and mortality. One study indicates a lower mortality with a second stroke (12 percent versus 38 percent for a first stroke), whereas other studies of recurrent stroke report mortality of 22 to 30 percent.

Strokes have long been recognized as a complication of atrial fibrillation in patients with rheumatic heart disease. However, it was not until Wolff and colleagues [9] reported on the Framingham study that the full extent of the risk was known in patients without rheumatic heart disease. In a cohort study of more than 5000 people followed for 24 years, the Framingham investigators were able to assess the relative risk of stroke in the presence of atrial fibrillation.

_____ STUDY QUESTION 19-1

Using the Framingham study data in Table 19-1, determine the relative risk and the attributable risk of stroke in the presence of atrial fibrillation.

Examination of the Framingham study data shows that the risk of stroke from atrial fibrillation is greatest at the onset of the atrial fibrillation (Table 19-2).

Table 19-1. Rate of stroke per 1000 person-years
adjusted for age, sex, and presence of hypertension

	Person-years	Strokes	Observed rate	Expected rate*	Observed/expected rate
No atrial fibrillation or rheumatic heart disease (RHD)	109,051	311	2.87	3.11	0.92
Atrial fibrillation only (no RHD)	481	20	41.48	7.43	5.60
Total	109,532	331			

*Based on data adjusted for age, sex, and hypertension.
Source: Data adapted from Wolff and colleagues [9].

Table 19-2. Relationship of time of onset of atrial fibrillation to risk of stroke

	% of All strokes with atrial fibrillation	Estimated relative risk
Time of onset of atrial fibrillation at time of stroke	25	—
1 year before stroke	14	15.5
1–3 years before stroke	8/year	9.0
>3 years before stroke	4/year	4.4
Total	100	5.6

Source: Adapted from Wolff and colleagues [9].

_____ STUDY QUESTION 19-2
What factors related to the way the initial Framingham data analysis was done
(Table 19-1) might indicate that the relative risk may be an underestimate? (Hint:
Remember that the atrial fibrillation had to be present on an examination prior
to the stroke to be included in Table 19-1.)

_____ STUDY QUESTION 19-3
Calculate the percentage of *total* strokes that could be eliminated if we could
prevent all strokes owing to known atrial fibrillation. (Hint: Use 5.1 as the relative risk and 0.0044 as the percentage of all persons at risk of stroke who had
atrial fibrillation.)

After an initial embolization, it appears that an individual is at high risk of a recurrent event. Recurrence in the Framingham study was approximately 25 percent, with nearly half of the recurrences in the first 6 months after the initial stroke [9]. Most studies have supported this high rate of recurrence after an initial embolus, given the presence of atrial fibrillation [7, 10, 11].

EFFICACY OF ANTICOAGULATION

Surprisingly, there are no controlled clinical studies of the efficacy of oral anticoagulants in preventing stroke in nonrheumatic atrial fibrillation. Such a study, which would have to compare treated to untreated patients with atrial fibrillation, has not been done for logistic reasons, among others. To conduct a study with (1) the usual limit of type-I errors of 5 percent; (2) a rather liberal type-II error margin of 30 percent; and (3) an assumption of a 50-percent reduction in stroke by the use of anticoagulants would require a minimum sample size of 1367 persons with atrial fibrillation in each of the two experimental groups, for a total of 2734 people [12].

_____ STUDY QUESTION 19-4

What is the minimum size of the population of persons aged 70 that would have to be screened to obtain 2734, assuming that 30 percent of the persons screened would volunteer for the study (an optimistic assumption) and that all patients with atrial fibrillation, regardless of duration or prior treatment, may be included? (Hint: Use the data of Svanborg and co-workers noted earlier) [1].

The problems of conducting a controlled clinical trial force us to rely on a number of retrospective studies, most with unmatched controls, or studies of related but not identical conditions. In addition, the standard anticoagulation therapy has changed substantially over the past 10 years, making the results of some earlier studies less useful. One major change involves better standardization of the prothrombin time test used to control oral anticoagulant dosage. Extrapolation from older studies is further complicated by the recent realization that the dose of heparin or oral anticoagulants required for optimal management varies widely and is particularly problematic in the elderly.

A study by the Cerebral Embolism Study Group [6] indicated that the incidence of recurrent stroke in the presence of atrial fibrillation in the immediate (2-week) post–cerebral infarction period can be reduced with anticoagulant therapy from approximately 10 percent to nearly 4 percent. Other less-well-controlled studies tend to confirm these findings [10, 11]. Thus, immediate anticoagulation with heparin in persons with atrial fibrillation who have had a stroke usually is preferable. Whether patients with no prior stroke benefit from long-term anticoagulation is less obvious.

_____ STUDY QUESTION 19-5
Why is it inappropriate to extrapolate from short-term to long-term anticoagulation?

   The most useful data on long-term anticoagulation and stroke occurrence are shown in Table 19-3 [13, 14]. The best evidence for the efficacy of anticoagulation comes from a study done in a population entirely different from persons with nonrheumatic atrial fibrillation [13]. In this randomized study, patients were given oral anticoagulants to prevent recurrent myocardial infarction. As a secondary finding of the study, it was noted that the incidence of stroke was 31.3 per 1000 patient-years of observation in the placebo group versus 19.0 per 1000 patient-years in the treated group. Although this result was not statistically significant, (p = .18), the authors believed that it suggested the efficacy of long-term anticoagulation.
   It is important to note that this study did not set out to examine atrial fibrillation or stroke. Therefore, we must be cautious in drawing any conclusions from this data. Nevertheless, it is of interest that the placebo group had 21 strokes, only 1 of which was hemorrhagic, whereas in the anticoagulated group, 9 of 13 strokes that occurred were hemorrhagic. Thus, anticoagulation appeared to reduce the rate of embolic and thrombotic stroke by more than 80 percent, at the cost of a smaller increase in the incidence of hemorrhagic stroke. These hemorrhagic strokes were important. They tended to be massive and often were fatal in this group of patients who had survived a myocardial infarction, most of whom *did not* have atrial fibrillation. The distribution of thrombotic, embolic, and hemorrhagic strokes in the control group was similar to that of the general population in that thrombotic stroke made up 75 percent of the total.
   Other useful data are derived from a retrospective study of a mixed population of patients with atrial fibrillation who were treated with oral anticoagulants [14]. The percent reduction in stroke or percent efficacy achieved by anticoagulation was 45 percent.

319

Table 19-3. Efficacy of anticoagulation in systemic embolization

| Study | Study type | Study population | End point | Study duration (years) | Incidence of event per 1000 patient-years | | Percent efficacy |
					No AC	AC	
Szekely [14]	Retrospective	Rheumatic heart disease and atrial fibrillation	All emboli	7.7	69.1	38.5	45
Sixty Plus Reinfarction Study Group [13]	Randomized trial	Post–myocardial infarction	All strokes	2.0	31.3	19.0	40

AC = anticoagulation.

COMPLICATIONS OF ANTICOAGULATION
Both of the common anticoagulants, heparin and warfarin, can cause severe side effects, of which hemorrhage or bleeding is the most prominent. The importance of recent changes in the administration and monitoring of heparin and warfarin use was noted earlier. Recent studies of complications that reflect these changes are lacking, so we must rely again on approximations. The investigators who studied anticoagulation use after myocardial infarction [13] reexamined their data for the incidence of complications from oral anticoagulants [15] and found there were eight intracranial bleeds in the anticoagulated group and one in the control group, yielding respective rates of 11.6 and 1.5 per 1000 patient-years of observation. However, the *total* number of strokes was reduced by 40 percent.

Since it is sometimes impossible to determine the exact type of stroke, we will consider here only extracranial complications of anticoagulation. Intracranial bleeds will simply be considered as a stroke, which will affect the number and outcome of strokes associated with anticoagulation therapy.

Major extracranial bleeds occurred at the rate of 40.8 per 1000 patient-years and resulted in 102 hospitalization days per 1000 patient-years. Older studies cite somewhat higher rates, with Pollard and associates [16] reporting 11 major episodes in 139 cases followed for an average of 18 months (or a rate of 52 per 1000 patient-years) (Table 19-4). It is of interest that in the myocardial infarction study, 40 percent of the cases of major bleeds, were associated with an underlying condition that contributed to the bleed [15]. The same study cites nonreferenced data from a registry in Holland of a rate of 1 fatal extracranial bleed per 1000 patient-years.

Earlier data suggested the elderly are at greater risk from complications of anticoagulation [17], but more careful monitoring and generally lower doses of anticoagulants are now used. Recent studies, such as the post–myocardial infarction study, have not demonstrated a substantial increase in complications of anticoagulation with age. However, few, if any, of these studies involve individuals who are older than 80 years or who have other major risk factors for bleeding such as a history of falls.

Decision Analysis: Anticoagulant Therapy for Atrial Fibrillation?
Given the data just presented, deciding whom to anticoagulate is not clear-cut. Should we recommend anticoagulation to all persons with

Table 19-4. Complications from oral anticoagulation

Study	Year	Type	Patient population	Complication probability per year		Effect of age
				Minor	Major	
Sixty Plus Reinfarction Study Group [15]	1982	Randomized trial	Post–myocardial infarction, 78 yr	0.114	0.041	None
Pollard et al. [16]	1962	Retrospective	All indications	0.221	0.052	Not mentioned
Coon and Willis [17]	1974	Retrospective	All indications	0.182	0.065	Increase with age

nonrheumatic atrial fibrillation, only those patients with recent-onset atrial fibrillation, or only patients of a certain age with certain characteristics? More specifically, what should we recommend to the two patients whose cases are presented at the beginning of this chapter? There is no randomized doubleblind study to provide an easy answer to our questions. Furthermore, even if there were a randomized study, it is very unlikely that it would include enough patients in the 85-and-older age group to make the conclusions of the study directly applicable to the clinical situations presented in cases A and B. This lack of a direct answer is typical of the uncertainty of many clinical decisions, especially those involving older patients. Often, we resort to an intuitive guess, or appeal to expert opinion (usually in the form of a consultation). The technique of formal decision analysis can also be used to assist in our efforts to advise patients about their options.

DRAFTING A DECISION TREE

In case A, the patient is an 85-year-old woman with mild congestive heart failure who has experienced the recent onset of atrial fibrillation. A first action dictated by the clinical situation is to decide whether to institute anticoagulant therapy. We will represent this choice by a decision node with two branches, anticoagulation and no anticoagulation (Fig. 19-1). To this must be added the potential outcomes that could befall our patient. The most important possible outcome is a stroke. This event can be represented by a chance node with branches for stroke or no stroke. If the patient has a stroke (again in the simplest terms), the patient may either die from the stroke or survive. To represent this, we can create another chance node on the stroke branch, which now has two more branches, namely death and survival. These two branches, death and survival, represent the outcome of the overall clinical situation for someone who is anticoagulated and has a stroke. Since they represent an end state, they are called terminal branches, with an outcome at the end of each branch.

_____ STUDY QUESTION 19-6
List some likely events that are not included in the decision tree depicted in Figure 19-1.

From the answer to study question 19-6, it should be apparent that we have neglected some issues that may be important in our decision to institute anticoagulant therapy or in the patient's decision about whether

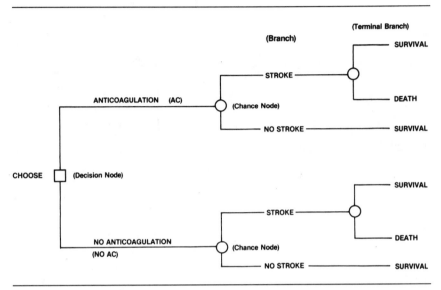

Fig. 19-1. Simple decision tree.

to accept anticoagulation. For example, we did not include the possibility that the patient could have an adverse response to anticoagulation. In this regard, we should note that the intracranial manifestations of anti-coagulant complications (e.g., hemorrhagic stroke or intracranial bleed) are accounted for within the rate of strokes of all types associated with anticoagulation. However, major extracranial bleeds are not infrequent, may be serious, and therefore, should be considered in our decision tree. In addition, the outcome of a stroke is clearly more complex than either survival or death. In some instances, a major disability resulting from the stroke may be more feared by the patient than death. Finally, if the patient survives the stroke or does not have a stroke, he or she could die from other causes. This is especially true in the case of an 85-year-old woman with congestive heart failure and atrial fibrillation due to athero-sclerotic cardiovascular disease.

STUDY QUESTION 19-7

Diagram a decision tree that incorporates the additional chance events and out-comes just noted for the 85-year-old woman with atrial fibrillation.

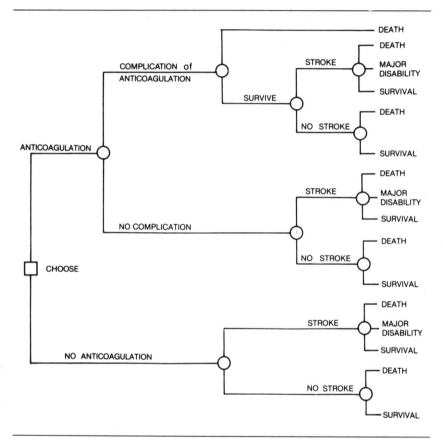

Fig. 19-2. Second-level decision tree: Is it better to anticoagulate patients with nonrheumatic atrial fibrillation?

One way of representing the tree required to answer study question 19-7 is shown in Figure 19-2, yet even this representation is somewhat simplified. For example, the outcome of stroke could be graded to include mild, moderate, or major disability, or the complications of anticoagulation could be graded on a similar scale. As is apparent from comparing Figures 19-1 and 19-2, the complexity of the tree rapidly increases as chance nodes and outcomes are added. A major problem confronting the decision analyst is how complex to make any given decision tree. One method often used is to start with a relatively complex tree and "prune" those branches that, after initial analysis or review, are shown to be highly improbable or clinically absurd. In the present situation, we will assume that the tree in Figure 19-2, while not totally complete, is adequate for purposes of analysis. Note that we could, if desired, add other branches at our initial point (such as "do an echocardiogram") or additional decision nodes or branches anywhere in the tree.

_____ STUDY QUESTION 19-8

Using the tree in Figure 19-2 as a guide, what data appears to be needed or relevant to our decision making?

It should be apparent that one important use of a decision tree is to help organize our thoughts about clinical situations, especially in determining what information we will need to arrive at a rational decision. In particular, a decision tree can help by making explicit the possible outcomes and important variables to consider.

The process of decision analysis need not focus on an absolute decision. Rather, it provides a way to measure and compare the relative probabilities and utilities of the likely outcomes of alternative choices being considered. As we shall see, decision makers must consider, *before* arriving at a formal decision, whether they agree with the numerical expressions of the probabilities and utilities assigned to such outcomes as stroke, major disability, and death.

RISK ANALYSIS

Risk analysis aims to determine the probability of each potential outcome of the two possible decisions, to anticoagulate or not to anticoagulate. First, we must estimate the probability of each chance event along every branch of our decision tree. For example, we must calculate the probability of death given a complication from anticoagulation in a patient with atrial fibrillation and congestive heart failure. The probabilities can be taken directly from the literature, if available, or can be estimated based on expert opinion or inferences from appropriate study data. Although the use of subjective probabilities does introduce additional imprecision, such estimates form part of almost every clinical decision process. Furthermore, in formal decision analysis, we are able to test the range of our estimates over which our eventual decision remains the preferred option.

Figure 19-3 shows the probabilities and utilities that we will apply to our decision concerning the 85-year-old woman with recent-onset atrial

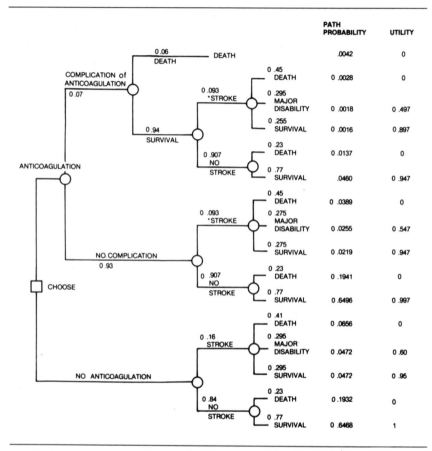

Fig. 19-3. Decision tree with probabilities and utilities for an 85-year-old woman with recent onset of atrial fibrillation. The probabilities and utilities shown represent our baseline or best-guess probabilities and utilities. (*The probability of stroke given anticoagulation is equal to the probability of stroke without anticoagulation × [1 − the efficacy of anticoagulation].)

fibrillation. Our best estimates of the probabilities are drawn from the literature discussed previously. Information from controlled clinical trials was given additional weight if it applied directly to the situation at hand. The probabilities used in developing our decision analysis are summarized in Tables 19-5 through 19-7.

Once we have specified each of the probabilities for intervening chance events, we can calculate the probability of every final outcome simply by successively multiplying the probabilities on each pathway leading to that outcome (see Fig. 19-3).* It should be noted that the probabilities of all the terminal positions for the entire tree will add up to more than one. However, since we begin with a decision node, the probabilities of the terminal branches (pathways) for each of our possible choices at the decision node *should* equal 1. For instance, for the decision not to anticoagulate, the probabilities are: $0.0656 + 0.0472 + 0.0472 + 0.1932 + 0.6468 = 1$.

Probabilistic Dominance
In special situations, the risk analysis alone may allow us to choose one option over another. This will happen when one of our choices yields a lower probability than the other choices for each and every adverse outcome that can occur in the decision tree. This phenomenon is termed probabilistic dominance. When there are only two potential outcomes, such as death and survival, one merely determines which choice produces the greater probability of survival. This is the case when we use

---

*The probability of surviving or dying given atrial fibrillation, stroke, and patient aged 85 (or 95) years is a *compound* probability derived using the method of Beck and colleagues (18). Age adjustment is done by adjusting the survival at age 65 to age 85; then:

$$\text{Mortality rate} = \frac{1}{\text{LE baseline}} + \frac{1}{\text{LE with disease}} + \frac{1}{\text{LE without disease}}$$

where LE = life expectancy

It assumes that cerebrovascular disease accounts for 15.9 percent of all deaths at age 85 and cardiovascular disease for 50 percent, and that 1-year survival for a woman of 65 with a stroke is 75 percent and with congestive heart failure is 85 percent (see Table 19-6). The interaction factor in the compound probability results from the fact that death from a stroke and atrial fibrillation secondary to cardiovascular disease is embedded in the probability of dying from all causes. In a younger population, this interaction factor would be trivial. However, stroke and other cardiovascular deaths are so common in older persons that part of the death from all causes is "contaminated" by death from cardiovascular disease.

Table 19-5. Probability estimates

Variable	Baseline rate	Range
No anticoagulation: stroke outcome		
None	0.45	0.30–0.60
Major disability	0.30	0.25–0.50
Death	0.25	0.15–0.35
Anticoagulation		
Efficacy	0.42	0.20–0.60
Risk of complication		
Major	0.07	0.04–0.10
Death*	0.06	0.015–0.10
Stroke outcome		
None or minor	0.39	0.25–0.50
Major disability	0.33	0.25–0.55
Death	0.28	0.15–0.40

*Risk of death given complication.

Table 19-6. Probability of dying in 1 year (using declining exponential method)

Woman, 85 years old	
Baseline	0.15
CHF + AF	0.23
CHF + AF + stroke	0.41
CHF + AF + stroke − AC	0.45
Man, 95 years old	
Baseline	0.34
AF	0.49
AF + stroke	0.62
AF + stroke − AC	0.66

CHF = congestive heart failure; AF = atrial fibrillation; AC = anticoagulation.

Table 19-7. Risk of stroke

Patient parameter	Baseline rate	Range
85-year-old woman		
Baseline	0.013	
Recent-onset atrial fibrillation	0.16	0.08–0.24
95-year-old man		
Baseline	0.022	
Chronic atrial fibrillation	0.07	0.05–0.09

Table 19-8. Risk profile for an 85-year-old woman using baseline assumptions

Outcome	Treatment options		Gain[a] (loss)
	No anticoagulation (N = 10,000)	Anticoagulation (N = 10,000)	
Survival			
No stroke			
No complication	6468	6496	28
Complication[b]	—	460	(460)
Stroke			
No disability	472	235 (16)[c]	237
Disability	472	273 (18)[c]	199
Total survive	7412	7464	52
Death			
Stroke	656	417 (28)[a]	239
Complication[b]	—	42	(42)
All other	1932	2078 (137)[c]	(9)
Total dead	2588	2537	51

[a]Gain indicates less adverse outcome among anticoagulated patients.
[b]Total complications (survived and dead) = 700.
[c]Number included who also had complications.

the simplified decision tree in Figure 19-1. When we use our more complex tree in Figure 19-2, there can be no probabilistic dominance because we have one event—that is, complications from anticoagulation that appear only in the outcome related to anticoagulation. Thus, when more than two potential outcomes exist or if all outcomes do not occur as a result of all the alternatives being considered, we need to decide the relative utility of the potential outcomes.

Risk Profile
Let us take a look at how a risk profile might be done for an 85-year-old woman with recent-onset atrial fibrillation. Figure 19-3 illustrates how we might assign probabilities to the different outcomes (ignore the utilities for now). Table 19-8 illustrates how we can combine the probabilities into a risk profile. This risk profile demonstrates the outcomes we would expect if 10,000 similar 85-year-old women with new-onset atrial fibrillation were assigned to anticoagulation and 10,000 to no anticoagulation therapy. Our table shows that for the 10,000 people treated with anticoagulation, there are 237 fewer persons who have a stroke with no disability, 199 fewer with a stroke and a major disability, and 51 fewer

deaths, although 700 people will suffer major complications from anti-coagulation (the 42 persons who will die from the complication are included in the overall deaths). We might, at this point, be willing to say that 700 major complications from anticoagulation is a reasonable loss for fewer strokes, fewer disabilities, and fewer overall deaths.

A risk profile for a 95-year-old man presents a picture that is much less clear (Fig. 19-4, Table 19-9). We see that of 10,000 similar 95-year-old men that would be treated, there would be 82 fewer strokes with no disability and 56 fewer strokes with a major disability. However, 700 additional people would suffer major complications from anticoagulation with a net increase of 8 deaths overall.

UTILITY ANALYSIS

We can, in decision analysis, incorporate into the decision process numerical expressions that quantify the relative value or utility of various outcomes. The process of applying utilities to our decision tree and then evaluating the tree is known as utility analysis. To perform a utility analysis, we will need to assign a utility to each potential outcome of the tree. These utilities can be assigned by the physician, the patient, or some other decision maker. Utilities can be expressed in multiple ways as, for example, quality-adjusted years of survival, costs and benefits in terms of dollars, or as relative preference for different outcome states. There are a variety of ways to assign utilities to outcomes, and there is a large and growing body of literature on the subject [19].

Assigning Utilities to Outcomes

The simplest method of assigning utilities is to ask the decision maker to apply his or her personal values to different outcomes based on an equal-interval scale with arbitrary end points (Fig. 19-5). The usual convention is to allow survival with no therapy and no adverse effects to be equal to 1 and death to be equal to 0. The assumption is usually made that death from whatever cause has the same value and that death is the worst possible outcome. However, there is nothing to prevent us from deciding that some types of deaths are less desirable than others or that some outcomes are worse than death.

Whereas life and death are relatively easy to assign to opposite ends of the scales, intermediate states—such as stroke with a major disability—are harder to compare with one another and with death or survival without stroke. Therefore, the method of simply placing utilities on an interval scale may not adequately reflect actual values. One commonly

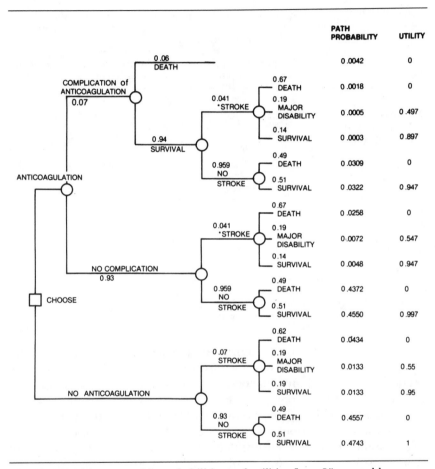

		PATH PROBABILITY	UTILITY

Fig. 19-4. Decision tree with probabilities and utilities for a 95-year-old man. The probabilities and utilities shown represent our baseline or best-guess probabilities and utilities. (*The probability of stroke given anticoagulation is equal to the probability of stroke without anticoagulation × [1 − the efficacy of anticoagulation].)

Table 19-9. Risk profile for a 95-year-old man using baseline assumptions

| Outcome | Treatment options | | Gain[a] (loss) |
	No anticoagulation (N = 10,000)	Anticoagulation (N = 10,000)	
Survival			
No stroke			
No complication	4743	4550	263
Complication[b]	—	322	(322)
Stroke			
No disability	133	51 (3)[c]	82
Disability	133	77 (5)[c]	56
Total survive	5009	5000	(9)
Death			
Stroke	434	276 (18)[c]	158
Complication[b]	—	42	(42)
All other	4557	4681 (309)[c]	(124)
Total dead	4991	4999	(8)

[a]Gain indicates less adverse outcome among anticoagulated patients.
[b]Total complications (survived and dead) = 700.
[c]Number included who also had complications.

used method to improve on our ability to specify utilities is termed the *reference gamble.* Another is known as the *trade-off technique.* In the reference gamble, the individual or group of individuals is asked to answer a series of questions regarding their willingness to take the risk of a shortened life with no adverse outcome compared to the risk of some adverse outcome. In our example, we might ask: What probability of death would you risk to ensure that you will not have a major disability from a stroke, such as paralysis of one side of your body but with retention of some speaking ability? Alternatively, we can phrase the question as a trade-off: How much of a year of life in your present state of health would be equivalent to a year of life with a major disability from a stroke, such as paralysis of one side of your body but with retention of some speaking ability? Obviously, the way the information is presented or framed is extremely important. If such a process is followed, the intermediate outcomes can then be assigned utilities in relation to the best or worst outcome.

We interviewed a number of elderly patients in clinical situations similar to those of cases A and B and posed the question: What part of a

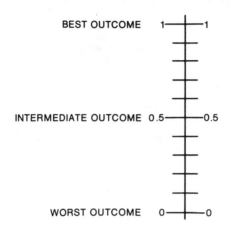

Fig. 19-5. Equal-interval scale for utility. This type of scale generally goes from 0 to 1 or 0 to 100, where 0 equals the worst outcome.

year of life in your present state do you feel is of equivalent utility to a year of life with a major disability from a stroke, including paralysis of one side of your body but with retention of some speaking ability? The results are summarized in Table 19-10. The average for the group was that a year of life with major disability was equal to only 30 weeks of life in their present state. That is, the disability "cost" 22 weeks of life. Thus, the utility of a year of life with a major disability is equal to 30/52 or approximately 60 percent of a year of life with no major change in their physical status. The utilities assigned to suffering a complication of anticoagulation or stroke with disability or of having to take anticoagulation were derived in a similar fashion.

Many people who are learning decision analysis are dismayed by the need to derive explicit utilities for various outcomes such as life or death or life with a major disability. Yet every clinical decision that we make involves implicitly assigning relative importance to various outcomes. There is little evidence that our intuitive guesses will be better in the aggregate than using a more formal decision analysis process. At times, the formal process of assigning utilities may help us realize that our utilities are very different from those held by the patient. Thus, decision analysis may help clarify our patients' preferences.

Table 19-10. Patient assignment of utility for various outcomes

Outcome	Equivalent loss in longevity (weeks)	Utility*
Stroke, no disability	3	0.95
Stroke with disability	22	0.60
Complication of anticoagulation	3	0.95
Taking anticoagulation	15	0.997
Death	—	0

*Utility = 1 − (equivalent loss/52).

Calculating Weighted Utilities

Figures 19-3 and 19-4 display our decision trees for cases A and B, with one set of probabilities and utilities assigned to each case. To take into account these probabilities and utilities, we calculate a weighted utility for each potential outcome by multiplying the utility by the probability of each outcome. Adding together the weighted utilities for each potential outcome of the choices (anticoagulation and no anticoagulation) produces an overall weighted utility for each option. Let us review these steps:

First, we multiply the utility of each outcome of our decision to anticoagulate (such as a stroke with major disabilities) by the probability that it will occur. This produces our weighted utilities. Next, we add up the weighted utilities for all outcomes emanating from a decision to anticoagulate. This will provide us with a single overall measure of the consequences of our decision and equals the overall weighted utility. Now, we repeat this process for a decision not to anticoagulate. Finally, we compare the overall weighted utility of a decision to anticoagulate to the overall weighted utility of a decision not to anticoagulate. In decision analysis terms this process is known as folding back decision trees.

Applying the fold-back methodology to our two cases brings us the results shown in Table 19-11. We can see that under the assumptions we have made, the overall weighted utility of anticoagulation is higher in the case of the 85-year-old woman. In contrast, for the 95-year-old man, the option favored by the overall weighted utility is *not* to anticoagulate. The choice not to anticoagulate, however, seems to be preferable by a very narrow margin. (Remember that the numbers have no absolute meaning; only their relationship to one another is meaningful.)

One of the most powerful aspects of decision analysis is that we can

Table 19-11. Overall weighted utilities using baseline assumptions

Woman, 85 years old	
Anticoagulation	0.7282
No anticoagulation	0.7176
Man, 95 years old	
Anticoagulation	0.4932
No anticoagulation	0.4943

now go back and test how "robust" or solid our decision is by doing a sensitivity analysis.*

SENSITIVITY ANALYSIS

A sensitivity analysis is a reevaluation of our tree substituting a series of alternative probabilities or utilities for our baseline or best-guess estimates. Through the use of a computer, a relatively large number of alternative probabilities or alternative utilities can be tested. In addition, a multiway analysis can be done by varying two or more values at the same time. Although essentially any probability or utility can be chosen for analysis, it is most useful to choose those that are most uncertain and have the most clinical relevance for the decision.

Using the technique of sensitivity analysis, we can determine how robust our decision is in the face of varying clinical situations. We can also see whether our final choice is affected by changes in some of our estimates. Figures 19-6 and 19-7 illustrate a three-way sensitivity analysis for our two cases. We have chosen to vary the efficacy of anticoagulation,† the probability of having a stroke, and the rate of complications from anticoagulation. In the figures, the area above the curved lines contains the values of the three variables for which the decision to anticoagulate has the higher overall weighted utility. The line itself traces the threshold or toss-up values for the variables of efficacy and probability of stroke. The area below the line contains the variable values for which the decision not to anticoagulate has a higher overall weighted utility.

One variant of a sensitivity analysis is termed a *threshold analysis.* In a

---

*There are also a growing number of methods to measure the statistical certainty of the difference between two overall weighted utilities resulting from a decision node.
†*Efficacy of anticoagulation* means the percentage of the strokes that could be eliminated among those with atrial fibrillation. It is the same as attributable risk of no anticoagulation.

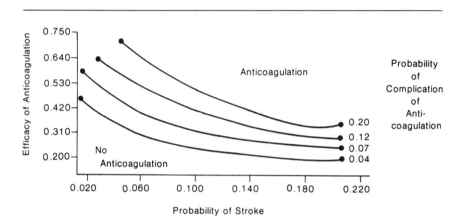

Fig. 19-6. Sensitivity analysis for an 85-year-old woman. The region above and to the right of each curved line contains the values of the variables on the horizontal and vertical axes for which the decision to anticoagulate has a higher overall utility. (*Baseline assumptions.)

threshold analysis, we calculate the numerical value for a particular variable at which the weighted utility of the branches of our decision node would become equal. In other words, we determine the numerical measure of a particular variable at which the overall weighted utility of the two decisions are equal. For example, in the case of our 85-year-old woman, we can calculate the overall weighted utility for the efficacy of anticoagulation at which the overall weighted utility of two branches of the decision node (i.e., to anticoagulate and not to anticoagulate) are equal. In essence, the threshold value for any variable is the value at which the decision "turns" from one choice to another. If our clinical data suggest that it is very unlikely that such a threshold or toss-up value will occur in our usual practice, our initial decision can be said to be robust (i.e., unlikely to be altered by changes in the variable under consideration).

The decision to anticoagulate the 85-year-old woman is very robust. Given our baseline 7 percent rate of complications of anticoagulation and 18 percent probability of stroke, the efficacy of anticoagulation

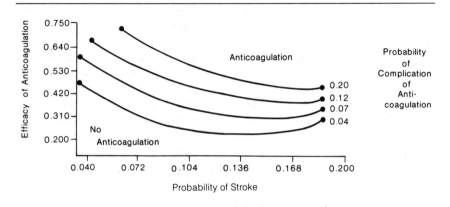

Fig. 19-7. Sensitivity analysis for a 95-year-old man. The region above and to the right of each curved line contains the values of the variables on the vertical and horizontal axes for which the decision to anticoagulate has a higher utility. Baseline assumptions: efficacy of anticoagulation = 0.42; probability of stroke = 0.072; probability of complication = 0.07.

would have to be less than 20 percent instead of our baseline estimate of 42 percent before the overall weighted utilities would favor no anticoagulation. This low efficacy appears to be outside what the literature would suggest in our patient (see Beck and Parker [20]). They could, however, occur in a patient who was expected to be very noncompliant with medication.

In the case of chronic atrial fibrillation in the 95-year-old man, very small changes, well within our range of uncertainty, do affect our choice. This situation, referred to as a toss up, occurs more frequently than we generally care to acknowledge. We have a toss-up when the value of the outcomes resulting from either decision is approximately the same.

——————————————————————————————— STUDY QUESTION 19-9
Faced with a toss-up for our 95-year-old man, how would you proceed?

Finally, let us review the effect of age and, more specifically, initial life expectancy. Initial life expectancy in our example is the life expectancy of the patient if he or she does not have a stroke. Age manifests itself primarily through increasing both the incidence of stroke and the death rate (i.e., shorter life expectancy). The major effect of increasing mortality from all causes is to limit the magnitude of the benefit that can occur from successful anticoagulation relative to a younger population with a lower overall death rate. When initial life expectancy is very short, the overall weighted utility of both choices becomes small because nearly everyone dies regardless of treatment. The choice with the highest overall weighted utility can easily change based on small changes in the probabilities or utilities of specific outcomes. Thus, it is not surprising that as the age of our patients increases, the decision becomes more difficult.

_____ STUDY QUESTION 19-10
Why is life expectancy, rather than age, the more important consideration?

ASSESSING THE RESULTS OF DECISION ANALYSIS
At times, the results of decision analysis may not seem intuitively reasonable to you. For instance, you might believe that anticoagulation is not the best decision for our 85-year-old woman or you may be strongly opposed to anticoagulating the 95-year-old man. One way to test your intuition is to apply the decision analysis technique using the probabilities and utilities that you believe are most appropriate in this situation or modifying the tree. If the calculation supports your intuition, then the case can be discussed from the standpoint of whose tree, probabilities, or utilities are more valid.

If you still believe anticoagulation is not the best decision despite a decision analysis that suggests anticoagulation, the following factors may be contributory:

1.   The decision analysis here and in most applications does not distinguish between bad outcomes that occur in the immediate versus the more distant future. In other words, the utility of death is not discounted for time. Thus, you or the patient may have a strong preference for delaying the poor outcomes even if this increases their probability of occurring.*

2.   You may be risk aversive. You may prefer the assurance of accepting current risk to taking on a new, difficult-to-assess risk such as

_____

*There are a variety of techniques to overcome this objection (see Beck and Pauker [20]).

anticoagulation. Risk aversion or risk-taking tendencies can be partially incorporated into the utilities. The degree of overall risk aversion, however, may not be fully reflected in the utilities of specific outcomes. Thus, a patient may still be uncomfortable with a decision that incorporates his or her utilities for specific outcomes. This should prompt a search for the barrier to communication or action that underlies the discrepancies. Not only risk aversion but many other psychologic factors can affect the degree to which decision analysis can truly mirror our own or our patients' feelings [21].

In summary, using the techniques of decision analysis to advise us, it would appear that the decision to use anticoagulation to prevent a stroke in an individual similar to the woman in case A would be favored, whereas the decision to anticoagulate the 95-year-old man in case B would be a toss-up. The results from this analysis can be generalized to other patients using the sensitivity and threshold analyses that were done here. If the set of probabilities and utilities of a patient with chronic atrial fibrillation falls within the anticoagulate area of our sensitivity analysis, we can conclude that prophylaxis should be used.

Decision analysis can be applied in a wide variety of situations concerned with prevention in which no compelling answer from the literature is available. Thus, even though we may lack a decisive study showing the unequivocal value of a preventive measure in every possible individual at risk, we can still apply prevention in a defined group or even on a case-by-case basis using decision analysis. Decision analysis can assist us in determining which individuals would benefit, from both our perspective and theirs, from the intervention.

_____ STUDY QUESTION 19-11

Using Figure 19-6, determine the appropriate course of action for an 85-year-old woman for whom you estimate the probability of complications of anticoagulation as approximately 0.12 (or 1 chance in 8), a probability of a stroke of 0.06 (or just over 1 chance in 17), and an efficacy if anticoagulation of 0.42.

_____ STUDY QUESTION 19-12

Using Figure 19-7, determine the appropriate course of action for a 95-year-old man with a probability of complications of approximately 0.07, a probability of stroke of 0.16, and an anticoagulation efficacy of 0.42.

_____ STUDY QUESTION 19-13

Using Figure 19-6, determine the appropriate course of action for an 85-year-old woman with a probability of complications of 0.20, a probability of stroke of 0.14, and an anticoagulation efficacy of 0.42.

References

1. Svanborg A, et al. Seventy year old people in Goteborg, Sweden: a population study in an industrialized Swedish city. Acta Med Scand (Suppl) 177;61:5–37.
2. Kannel WB, Abbott RD, Savage DN, et al. Epidemiologic features of chronic atrial fibrillation. N Engl J Med 1982;306:1018–1022.
3. Abdon NJ, Zettervall O, Carlsson J, et al. Is occult atrial disorder a frequent cause of nonhemorrhagic stroke? Stroke 1982;13:832.
4. Hinton RC, Kistler NP, Fallon TT, et al. Influence of etiology of atrial fibrillation on systemic embolization. Am J Cardiol 1977;40:509–514.
5. Dainj KR, Ackerman RH, Kistler JP, et al. Computed tomography of cerebral infarction. Comput Tomogr 1977;1:71–86.
6. Cerebral Embolism Study Group. Embolic stroke: a random trial. Stroke 1983;14:668–676.
7. Sage JI, Van Uitert RL. Risk of recurrent stroke in patient with atrial fibrillation and non-valvular heart disease. Stroke 1983;14:537–540.
8. Sherman, DG, Goldman L, Whiting RB, et al. Thromboembolism in patients with atrial fibrillation. Arch Neuro 1984;41:708.
9. Wolff PA, Dawber TR, Thomas HE, et al. Epidemiologic assessment of chronic atrial fibrillation and risk of stroke: The Framingham Study. Neurology 1978;28:973–77.
10. Kelley RE, Berger JR, Alter M, et al. Cerebral ischemia and atrial fibrillation. Neurology (NY) 1984;34:1285–1291.
11. Hart RG, Coull BM, Hart D. Early recurrent embolism associated with non-valvular atrial fibrillation. Stroke 1983;14:688–693.
12. Wilson DG. Chronic atrial fibrillation in the elderly. J Am Geriatr Soc 1985;33:298–302.
13. Sixty Plus Reinfarction Study Group. a double blind trial to assess long-term oral anticoagulant therapy in elderly patients after myocardial infarction. Lancet 1980;1:989–993.
14. Szekely P. Systemic embolism and anticoagulant prophylaxis in rheumatic heart disease. Br Med J 1964;1:1209–1212.
15. Sixty Plus Reinfarction Study Group. Risks of long-term oral anticoagulant therapy in elderly patients after myocardial infarction. Lancet 1982;1:64–68.
16. Pollard JW, Hamilton MJ, Christensen NA, et al. Problems associated with long-term anticoagulant therapy. Circulation 1962;25:311–317.
17. Coon WW, Willis PW. Hemorrhagic complications of anticoagulation. Arch Intern Med 1974;133:386–391.

18. Beck JR, Pauker SG, Gottlieb JE, et al. An approximation of life expectancy (the DEALE). Am J Med 1982;73:889–897.
19. Weinstein MC, Feinberg HV. Clinical decision analysis. Philadelphia: Saunders, 1980.
20. Beck JR, Pauker SG. Anticoagulant and atrial fibrillation in the bradycardia-tachycardia syndrome. Med Decision Making, 1981;1:285–301.
21. Eraker S, Politser P. How decisions are reached: physician and patient. Ann Intern Med 1982;97:262–268.

Conclusion

PART SEVEN

CHAPTER TWENTY

Putting Prevention into Practice

RICHARD K. RIEGELMAN
KATHLEEN K. DAVIS
GAIL J. POVAR

Let us return to our original case of aspirin and Reye's syndrome and see if you're ready to read between the lines of the official recommendations.

Reye's syndrome is a rare, life-threatening disease of children, characterized by vomiting, hepatic abnormalities, and mental changes that may progress to coma and death. Reye's syndrome usually follows viral infections, especially influenza and chickenpox. The treatment of Reye's syndrome, once diagnosed, is largely supportive, with no known cure available. Recently, the use of aspirin but not acetaminophen has been suggested as a contributory cause of Reye's syndrome.

One of your patients brings in a bottle of children's aspirin and reads you the official recommendations, which state: Children and teenagers should not use this medicine for chickenpox or flu symptoms before a doctor is consulted about Reye's syndrome, a rare but serious disease

Based on what you've learned, you should be prepared to characterize the problem and evaluate the solutions. List the questions you would want to answer in order to understand and interpret the recommendation.

You might have asked the following:

1. What data are needed to establish aspirin as a contributory cause of Reye's syndrome?
2. What are the risks and benefits of using aspirin compared to the alternatives?
3. When, in the natural history of the disease, is the intervention occurring?
4. Who is the target of the intervention?
5. How is the recommendation being implemented?
6. What intervention options are being rejected and why?

Characterizing the Problem

Controlled clinical trials are often used to establish all three criteria of contributory cause. Knowing that Reye's syndrome is a rare disease, you appreciate that a controlled clinical trial will not be feasible. Alterna-

345

tively, you would ask about the retrospective or case-control studies that might establish the existence of a strong association with a large relative risk and attributable risk.* In the case of a retrospective study, you would expect a carefully designed research effort to ensure that the children with Reye's syndrome took the aspirin before the syndrome developed. This is important since you know that aspirin could be taken to treat the symptoms of Reye's syndrome, thus confusing which came first. You would also want to be sure that the study avoided the potential for recall error. Parents of Reye's syndrome children could easily search their memory and recall more aspirin use than control group parents without Reye's syndrome children.

Even if well-designed retrospective studies of aspirin and Reye's syndrome are available, you would realize that some doubt would remain. A natural experiment might help reduce that doubt by establishing that altering aspirin use alters the incidence of Reye's syndrome. A natural experiment, however, would require successful intervention to reduce the use of aspirin among children.

Risks and benefits may be hard to weigh when risk of the disease is low but serious and the benefits are frequent but small. The risks and benefits of aspirin use may be sidestepped to some extent because there is an acceptable alternative, acetaminophen, which is not known to be associated with risk of Reye's syndrome.

Evaluating the Solutions
We are now able to address the when, who, and how of intervention. We currently know that tertiary prevention after the development of Reye's syndrome is largely ineffective, as is secondary prevention once early Reye's syndrome appears. Thus, primary prevention before the development of Reye's syndrome is the focus of our intervention. Not surprisingly, *whom* to target and *how* to intervene have become the most controversial issues. Remembering that we may intervene at the level of the individual, the group at risk, or the population level, we could choose between the following types of interventions:

---

*Knowing that until recently aspirin was widely used among children, you would also know that if the attributable risk were large, the population attributable risk would also be large.

On the individual level, clinicians might stop prescribing aspirin for children with acute febrile illness, especially potential chickenpox or influenza, or clinicians might attempt to educate individual parents not to use aspirin for childhood fevers.

Intervention directed at the risk group level might include placing a warning on children's aspirin bottles that advises against the use of aspirin for acute febrile illness, or working through the schools or parent-teacher associations to warn parents to avoid use of aspirin for their children.

Intervention directed at the population level might include mass media warnings or removal of children's aspirin from the nonprescription market.

The choice among implementation strategies—namely, information, motivation, and obligation—depends on our evaluation of the effectiveness of each method and our willingness to restrict individual freedom of choice to protect individuals against health risks.

Reading Between the Lines

Having thought through the problems and potential solutions, we are now much better prepared to read between the lines of the official recommendations. Current policy is directed at primary prevention, at the group at risk, and through information directed to patients and doctors. Among the policy options being rejected are the option to rely solely on individual permissive efforts at the doctor-patient level and the option legally to remove children's aspirin from the nonprescription market, thereby restricting its availability in children's form. Underlying these recommendations is the assumption that doctors and patients to whom the facts are available will take the necessary protective actions and that groups at risk are being effectively reached, so more obligatory methods are not necessary. What do you think?

Testing Your Mastery of Important Concepts

At times, you may want to do more than read between the lines of the official recommendations. You may want to analyze the original data and draw your own options and conclusions. To do this, you need to have mastered the tools, contained in the introductory chapters and illustrated in the cases, for characterizing the problem and evaluating the solutions.

To test your mastery of some of these concepts, see if you can answer the following questions, again using aspirin and Reye's syndrome as an example (see the Appendix for answers).

1. Imagine that a case-control or retrospective study found an approximate relative risk of 10 for the relationship between aspirin and Reye's syndrome. A relative risk of 10 implies that:
   a. a strong association exists between aspirin use and Reye's syndrome.
   b. aspirin is a contributory cause of Reye's syndrome.
   c. aspirin use is necessary for the development of Reye's syndrome.
   d. aspirin use is sufficient for the development of Reye's syndrome.
2. If the relative risk is 10, the attributable risk associated with aspirin use is:
   a. 10 percent.
   b. 50 percent.
   c. 75 percent.
   d. 90 percent.
   e. 95 percent.
3. The attributable risk implies:
   a. the maximum percentage reduction in Reye's syndrome that can be expected in a community.
   b. the maximum percentage reduction in Reye's syndrome that can be expected among those who use aspirin.
   c. the risk of Reye's syndrome if aspirin is used compared to the risk of Reye's syndrome if aspirin is not used.
   d. the odds of Reye's syndrome if aspirin is used compared to the odds of Reye's syndrome if aspirin is not used.
4. To establish aspirin definitively as a contributory cause of Reye's syndrome, one needs to establish that:
   a. aspirin is associated with Reye's syndrome.
   b. aspirin use is associated with subsequent development of Reye's syndrome.
   c. aspirin use is associated with subsequent development of Reye's syndrome and reduced use of aspirin reduces the incidence of Reye's syndrome.

    d. Reye's syndrome occurs only after aspirin use.
5. If parents of children with Reye's syndrome make an extra effort to search their memory for use of aspirin before the onset of Reye's syndrome, this may produce a study design problem called:
    a. recall bias.
    b. reporting bias.
    c. selection bias.
    d. confounding variable.
6. If aspirin use is associated with Reye's syndrome 1 time in 1 million uses in children, how many times must aspirin be used to be 95 percent confident of observing at least 1 case of Reye's syndrome?
    a. 100,000.
    b. 1,000,000.
    c. 3,000,000.
    d. 10,000,000.
7. The official warning label implies that which of the following types of analysis has been performed?
    a. cost-benefit analysis.
    b. cost-effectiveness analysis.
    c. decision analysis.
    d. risk-benefit analysis.
8. The decision to intervene by preventing exposure to aspirin among children is an example of which of the following types of prevention?
    a. primary prevention.
    b. secondary prevention.
    c. tertiary prevention.
    d. none of the above.
9. The decision to label aspirin with warnings against use for children and teenagers with symptoms of chickenpox or influenza represents a decision to direct a preventive intervention at:
    a. the individual level.
    b. the group at risk.
    c. the population level, including those who are not at risk.
    d. none of the above.
10. From the patient's point of view, requiring warning levels on aspirin represents the following form of preventive intervention:
    a. an information approach aimed at allowing a voluntary or permissive choice.
    b. a motivation approach aimed at persuading individuals to change their behavior by providing incentives.

    c. an obligation approach aimed at requiring behavior change by re-
       quiring individual action.
    d. none of the above.

Checklist of Questions to Ask

As you attempt to characterize the problem and evaluate the solutions,
the following checklist of questions to ask should be used as a guide.

ESTABLISHING CONTRIBUTORY CAUSE AND MEASURING IMPACT
1. Is there an association between the cause and the effect?
    a. Do differences in rates of disease between populations or over time
       support the existence of a group association between the cause and
       the effect?
    b. Are there well-designed retrospective (case-control) studies that es-
       tablish an individual association between the cause and the effect?
2. Has the cause been shown to precede the effect?
    a. Are there prospective (cohort) studies which establish that the
       cause precedes the effect?
    b. If prospective studies are not available, are there well-designed ret-
       rospective studies that allow you to imply that cause precedes the
       effect?
3. Is there evidence that altering the cause alters the effect?
    a. Are there well-designed controlled clinical trials establishing the
       third criteria of contributory cause?
    b. If controlled clinical trials are not available, are there well-observed
       natural experiments which establish that altering the cause alters
       the effect?
4. If the evidence for contributory cause is equivocal, have the ancillary
    criteria of contributory cause been fulfilled?
    a. Is there a strong association between the cause and the effect?
    b. Is there a consistent association in different populations studied?
    c. Has a dose-response relationship been established between the
       cause and the effect?
    d. Is there evidence of biologic plausibility supporting a cause and
       effect relationship?
5. What is the strength of the relationship between the cause and the
    effect? What is the impact on individuals, groups at risk, the
    community?
    a. What is the relative risk (or odds ratio)?

b. What is the attributable risk?

c. What is the population attributable risk?

SCREENING FOR DISEASE CONTROL

1. Does the disease cause a substantial morbidity or mortality leading to a substantial impact on society or a substantial impact on an identifiable subgroup?

2. Are there risk factors which can be identified before the development of clinical disease that can be modified to prevent the appearance of clinical disease or can serve to identify high-risk groups to facilitate the early detection of disease?

3. Does treatment begun during the asymptomatic preclinical phase result in a better outcome than treatment that awaits the appearance of symptoms?

   a. Could lead-time bias explain an apparent improvement in outcome among those screened?

   b. Could length bias explain an apparent improvement among those screened?

   c. Could patient self-selection explain the apparent improvement in outcome among those screened?

4. Is there a testing approach that makes it feasible to detect or rule out disease effectively at the asymptomatic preclinical phase and is acceptable in terms of patient safety, acceptance, and cost?

EVALUATING POTENTIAL INTERVENTIONS

1. What are the potential benefits of the intervention?

   a. Has the efficacy of the intervention been demonstrated in well-designed studies?

   b. Has the effectiveness of the intervention been demonstrated in clinical settings similar to your own?

   c. Are changes in effectiveness, such as the occurrence of resistance, likely if large-scale application occurs?

2. What are the potential risks of the intervention?

   a. How does the timing of occurrence and severity of the known risks compare to the known benefits?

   b. Has the intervention been applied to enough individuals to make rare but serious risks unlikely?

   c. Has the intervention been studied long enough to make new long-term risks unlikely?

3. Have the benefits and risks been compared?
   a. Has a risk-benefit analysis been done, allowing the conclusion that for selected individuals the benefit outweighs the risk?
   b. Has a decision analysis been performed, weighing the risks and benefits of alternative interventions?
4. Have costs been considered in evaluating the intervention?
   a. From whose perspective have the costs been calculated—the individual, a third-party payer, or society?
   b. What costs were included?
   c. Was the intervention shown to be cost saving, cost effective, or most cost effective?

SELECTING A STRATEGY FOR IMPLEMENTATION

1. When, in the natural history of the disease, should intervention occur: primary prevention, before the disease has occurred; secondary prevention, in the asymptomatic disease state before symptoms of clinical disease have occurred; or tertiary prevention, after manifestations of clinical disease but prior to the occurrence of preventable complications?
2. Who should be the target for the intervention: the individual patient, those with risk factor(s) for the disease, or a general population including individuals not at risk?
3. How should the intervention occur: through information designed to provide voluntary choice, through motivation designed to persuade using incentives, or through legal obligation requiring change?
4. In deciding on a strategy for intervention, have the following been taken into account: the effectiveness of the strategy chosen, the effect of the intervention on freedom of choice, the financial cost of the strategy chosen, and the social consequences of implementing the strategy chosen?

Appendix

2–1. When case-fatality rates are very high as in the case with lung cancer, mortality rates approximate incidence rates. However, if there was improvement in the treatment of lung cancer or better methods for early detection, the mortality rates might decline despite a constant or even increasing incidence rate.

2–2. (a) To assess whether changes are artifactual or real, we first consider whether artifactual changes are likely. These increases in this situation are not likely to be owing to artifactual differences. Over this period of time, lung cancer mortality is unlikely to be affected by changes in the definition of the disease, efforts to search for the disease, or the technology available for detecting the disease. The ability to diagnose lung cancer at least at the time of death has been present throughout this time period. Thus, these changes probably represent real changes in the mortality rate and the incidence rate of lung cancer. The rates have been standardized for age, so changes in the age distribution of the population are not the cause of the increased mortality.

(b) The existence of real changes leads us to think about possible risk factors that may explain the changes. Cigarette smoking is known to have increased in frequency among men during the decades before 1930. In women, the increase began several decades later. Thus, the pattern of increasing lung cancer among men before the increase among women is compatible with a hypothesis that the changes are related to cigarette exposure.

(c) These trends do not necessarily imply that the mortality from lung cancer will continue to increase. Early detection or better treatment may affect future mortality. In addition, in recent years the frequency of smoking has declined, especially among men. Thus, the high current rate among men may represent a cohort effect, reflecting the high degree of exposure in previous years. In future years, as cohorts of men who have smoked less reach older ages, the incidence and death rates from lung cancer may decline.

2–3.

$$\tfrac{1}{2} - 1 \text{ pack} = \frac{59.3}{3.4} = 17.4$$

$$1 - 2 \text{ packs} = \frac{143.9}{3.4} = 42.3$$

$$2 + \text{ packs} = \frac{217.3}{3.4} = 63.9$$

2–4.

$$2 + 2 + 3 = 7$$

2–5.

$5 \times 10 = 50$

2–6.

$$AR = \frac{RR - 1}{RR} = \frac{20 - 1}{20} = \frac{19}{20} = 95\%$$

2–7. Using Figure 2-3, if the relative risk is 20 and the prevalence of the risk factor is 50 percent, the population attributable risk equals 90 percent.

2–8. A large attributable risk implies that for individuals who smoke cigarettes, most of the lung cancer that occurs is associated with cigarette smoking. When both are high and the disease is a common cause of mortality, it implies that cigarette smoking is an important risk factor for individuals who smoke and for society as a whole. Remember, however, that a risk factor does not necessarily imply a cause and effect relationship.

2–9. The prospective studies establish that cigarette smoking is associated with lung cancer (criterion 1) and that cigarette smoking precedes the development of lung cancer (criterion 2). They do not establish criterion 3 (i.e., altering the cause alters the effect).

2–10. The size of the relative risks and the large number of individuals involved establish the strength of the association. The existence of three different studies with very similar results establish the consistency of the association. The increasing mortality ratios (estimates of relative risk) with increasing exposure to cigarettes establish the existence of a dose-response relationship.

2–11. Randomization of individuals to smoke cigarettes and not smoke cigarettes would be required for a controlled clinical trial. When the evidence of risk as established by retrospective and prospective studies is large and there are no medical dangers of avoiding exposure, it is generally considered unethical to randomize patients. Even if it were ethical, it is hard to imagine that such a study would be feasible.

2–12. These data suggest that altering the cause alters the effect. This is the third and final criteria for contributory cause. The evidence, however, is not as strong as can usually be obtained from a controlled clinical trial. It is possible that those who stopped smoking were less prone to lung cancer for some other reason. However, when a controlled clinical trial is not possible, this type of evidence is usually considered adequate to establish this final criteria of contributory cause.

2–13. In general, this is the type of data used to establish biologic plausibility.

2–14. A contributory cause does not require that every smoker develop lung cancer or that only cigarette smokers develop lung cancer. Despite the strong evidence that cigarette smoking is a contributory cause of lung cancer, cigarette smoking is neither a necessary nor sufficient cause of lung cancer.

3–1. The Framingham Study* clearly demonstrated that hypertension may be regarded as a disease or a risk factor associated with subsequent development of such cardiovascular diseases as stroke, congestive heart failure, myocardial infarction, and intermittent claudication. Hypertension has a high prevalence in the adult population. Approximately 15 percent of adults in the United States have a diastolic blood pressure above 95 mm Hg on at least one home reading, as documented in more than 150,000 persons in the Hypertension Detection and Follow-up Program. Thus, criterion 1 is satisfied since hypertension is a common disease (as shown by the Hypertension Detection and Follow-up Program) and results in a high proportion of adverse outcomes (as shown by the Framingham Study).

3–2. Criterion 2 is satisfied in the case of hypertension, as illustrated by substantially decreased mortality among individuals whose disease was identified on screening and treated early. Controversy exists on the ideal lower level for defining hypertension, but general agreement exists that screening for high blood pressure identifies a modifiable risk for vascular disease.

3–3. Lead-time bias and length bias could not have explained these results. Thus, hypertension satisfies criterion 3.

3–4. Hypertension is a unique situation in which the screening test itself (i.e., blood pressure recording) is the gold standard for diagnosis of

*Kannel WB. Hypertension, blood lipids and cigarette smoking as co-risk factors in coronary heart disease. Ann NY Acad Sci 1978;304:128–139.

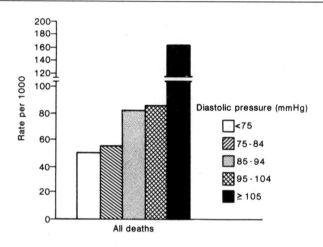

Mortality among white U.S. men, aged 30 to 59, from all causes in 10 years according to diastolic blood pressure at entry. (Adapted from IS Wright and DT Fredrickson. Cardiovascular diseases: guidelines for prevention and care. Washington, DC: US Department of Health, Education and Welfare, 1973. DHEW publication no. [HSM] 73-7022.)

the condition. The test is very safe, acceptable to the patient, and affordable. In addition, a wide variety of effective treatments exist that can reduce the mortality and morbidity which result from hypertension. Problems with sensitivity and specificity do occur because of the volatile nature of blood pressure and the resultant difficulty in defining a level for any one individual.

A more difficult problem is determining the best blood pressure level to use to define hypertension. As the figure illustrates, on the average, the lower the blood pressure, the lower the risk. This holds true well below a diastolic blood pressure of 95 mm Hg. Thus, if treating hypertension were risk-free, it would be reasonable to define hypertension as diastolic blood pressure well below 90 mm Hg. However, as one lowers the limits for diagnosing hypertension, it is important to recognize that

The benefits to be gained per individual treated are less.

The number of individuals who require treatment is increased enormously.

The potential for side effects is increased by virtue of the large number of individuals requiring treatment.

General agreement exists that early detection and treatment of cases of elevated blood pressure above 140/95 is safe, acceptable, and affordable. Controversy still exists as to whether detection of lower blood pressure levels and their classification and treatment as hypertension is safe, acceptable, and affordable.

4–1.   This type of controlled clinical trial enables one to assess the efficacy of alcoholex. The double-blind randomization to experimental and control groups and subsequent follow-up establish all three criteria of contributory cause or efficacy at least for this population.

Efficacy in a controlled clinical trial, however, must be distinguished from effectiveness in clinical practice. If the study group were especially motivated to take the medication, especially prone to alcohol-induced liver disease, or in some other important way different from a particular physician's clinical population, the results might not be as impressive when used in that clinical practice.

4–2.   The rule of three states that one needs to observe 3 times the number of individuals in the denominator of the incidence rate to be 95 percent sure of observing at least 1 case of the side effects. Thus, if the incidence of bladder cancer is 1 case per 3000 persons, each using it for 5 years, then one would need to observe 3×3000, or 9000, individuals to be 95 percent sure of finding 1 case of bladder cancer.

4–3.   The diagram on p. 358 illustrates one type of decision tree that could be used to approach this problem.

4–4.

Death from complications of alcoholex	$0.01 \times 0 = 0$
Survival of complication of alcoholex with no subsequent disease	$0.02 \times 90 = 1.8$
Survival of complication of alcoholex but disease develops	$0.03 \times 50 = 1.5$
No complications of alcoholex and no subsequent disease	$0.85 \times 100 = 85.0$
No complication of alcoholex but disease develops	$0.09 \times 60 = 5.4$
	93.7

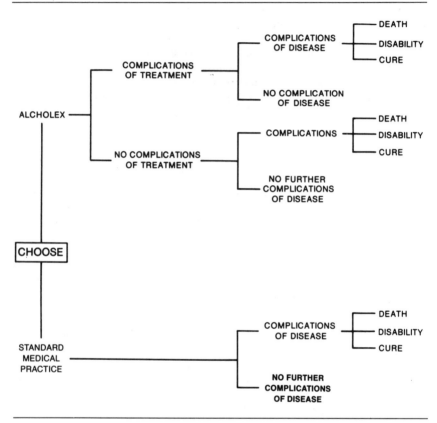

Decision tree comparing the option to use alcoholex in patients with medical complications of alcoholism and the option to use standard medical treatment of the complications of alcoholism.

4–5.

No disease	$100 \times 0.7 = 70$
Disease with subsequent death	$0 \times 0.05 = 0$
Disease with subsequent disability	$50 \times 0.1 = 5$
Disease with subsequent cure	$80 \times 0.15 = \underline{12}$
	87

What can you conclude from this sensitivity analysis? This sensitivity analysis is useful when we compare these numbers to the previous ones for the curative approach. We previously found a weighted utility of 74 for the curative approach. Now, being more optimistic, we obtain an 87 for the curative approach. From study question 4-4, we found that for alcoholex we obtained a 93.7. Thus, if we are accurate in our other assessments of probability and utility, alcoholex is the preferred approach even if the curative approach does considerably better than we originally estimated.

4–6. (a) 3. (b) 1, 2, 3. (c) 2, 3.

4–7.

$$\text{Cost effectiveness} = \frac{(Cp + Cse) - Ct}{(Eli + Em) - Ese}$$

$$= \frac{(\$3,700,000 + \$100,000) - \$800,000}{(250 + 150) - 100} = \frac{\$3,000,000}{300} = \$10,000$$

A cost-effectiveness ratio of $10,000 tells us the cost of obtaining 1 year of life at full health for one individual. This may consist of extending one individual's life for 1 year or several individuals' lives for parts of a year, or it may reflect the change of disability to full health for one or more individuals.

4–8. This question will have different answers depending on the justifications you consider most important and relevant.

5–1.

1. Primary, individual	6. Secondary, risk group
2. Primary, population	7. Secondary, population
3. Primary, risk group	8. Primary, population
4. Tertiary, individual	9. Tertiary, individual
5. Secondary, individual	

5-2.

Intervention implementation strategies for the problem of cigarette smoking

Target group	Information	Motivation	Obligation
Individual	Educational pamphlets handed out by doctor.	Doctor-patient contact. Reward system: patient purchases a frill with money saved from not smoking.	Doctor threatens not to continue relationship. Doctor refuses to prescribe birth control pills.
Risk group	Warning on cigarette packs.	Increase insurance rates for cigarette smokers: tax on cigarettes.	Banning cigarettes from worksite.
Population	Public service announcements on television.	Corporate antismoking campaign: Reward department in which largest decrease in the number of smokers occurs (creates peer pressure).	Make cigarettes illegal (hypothetically), and screen urine randomly for nicotine.

5–3.   The informational strategies should look familiar; they are in common use. Similarly, the individual risk group and total population motivational strategies are apparently generally acceptable to our society, given their broad use. However, the idea of engaging an entire office in the effort to get the smokers within it to quit may to some appear coercive (how much peer pressure is too much?) or invasive (what does such a program do to interoffice dynamics?). How likely is victim blaming in such a situation? In addition, a tax on cigarettes may be argued to be socially discriminatory, as the wealthy may be better able to ignore such a disincentive than the poor? Is such a trade-off acceptable? How would one justify it politically or ethically?

The obligatory strategies also generate problems. Whose values should take precedence in the doctor-patient relationship? Should a physician have the option of threatening to discontinue a relationship with a patient, presumably for the patient's benefit? We already have smoke-free work places. Here the argument of damage to the passive smoker supersedes the rights of the smoker to behave as he or she wishes, but a great deal of research had to prove that such "passive smoking" posed a risk before this argument could prevail. Finally, the notion of random screening of urine for drugs raises such major issues as privacy rights and risks of incorrect labeling of individuals owing to false positive or false negative tests. Cigarettes are a drug, and similar concerns therefore apply. Consider the advantages (in terms of the cost to the health care system, prevalence of disease, risk to others, and the effect of cigarette smoking on job effectiveness, for instance) that would be vital to advocating such a program.

6–1.   The correlation between cholesterol level and CHD establishes group associations. Remember that group associations do not establish that the individuals with high cholesterol are themselves the ones who develop CHD.

6–2.   To fulfill the criteria for contributory cause, it is necessary to show that altering the cause alters the disease. Individuals in the diet plus cholestyramine group had a substantial subsequent decrease in their total plasma cholesterol level and a substantial reduction in their risk of having a fatal or nonfatal CHD event. Thus, the LRC-CPPT has been accepted as evidence that cholesterol is a contributory cause of CHD, at least among men with a cholesterol level exceeding 265 mg per deciliter.

6–3.   Relative risks compared to group 1 are, for group 3, 1.08; for group 4, 1.79; and for group 5, 2.19.

6–4.   The relative risk for groups 3 and 4 are 1.18 and 1.90, respectively.

6–5.   For group 3, attributable risk $= \dfrac{78 - [(61 + 72)/2]}{78} \times 100 = 14.7\%$

6–6.

$$PAR = \frac{0.10\,(2 - 1)}{0.10\,(2-1) + 1} = 9\%$$

6–7.   This PAR implies that large reductions in the incidence of CHD in the population requires more than reductions of cholesterol levels of this magnitude. It may require, among other things, very low levels of cholesterol, protracted periods of reduced cholesterol, or simultaneous reductions in multiple risk factors. A combined approach is more likely to have a substantial impact on the age-adjusted incidence of CHD.

6–8.   Data collected during the LRC-CPPT study show various gastrointestinal tract cancers have a slightly higher incidence rate in the cholestyramine group. Thus far, only a small number of extra cancers from multiple sites have been found. Long-term follow-up is currently under way to assess the full impact of any cancer risk.

6–9.   This question will have different answers depending on the justifications you consider most important and relevant.

6–10.   The effect of lowering cholesterol for those with cholesterol levels below 265 mg per deciliter is a critical issue since there are so many individuals with these mildly elevated levels. In fact, most CHD occurs among the large group with mildly elevated levels. Unfortunately, data on this issue cannot be obtained directly from the LRC-CPPT study. In formulating their recommendations, the NIH panel assumed that the constant percentage risk reduction exhibited by the LRC-CPPT would continue for initial cholesterol levels lower than 265.

6–11 through 6–14.   These questions will have different answers depending on the justification you consider most important and relevant.

7–1.   These data demonstrate only that estrogen deficiency is *associated* with osteoporosis and that it *precedes* the disease, the first two criteria for contributory cause. It does not demonstrate that altering the cause will alter the effect.

7–2.   (a) Data does not have to be statistically significant to have meaning or provide valuable information. (b) Possible explanations for the lack of statistical significance in this study include the possibility that the numbers were too small or the study was not carried out for a long enough period of time.

7–3.   Although ideal, the controlled clinical trial described is not feasible owing to the long lag time between the menopause and the acceleration in hip fractures, as illustrated in Figure 7-2. Because of this lag time, a follow-up period of at least 20 to 30 years would be required, a task that is severely limited by logistic and economic difficulties.

7–4.   Based on the numbers in Table 7-3, the relative risk (RR) for ERT equals 0.42. The relative risk for estrogen deficiency is the inverse of this (1/0.42), which equals 2.4. This value can be inserted into the formula for attributable risk (AR) as follows:

$$AR = \frac{RR - 1}{RR} = \frac{2.4 - 1}{2.4} = 0.58 \text{ or } 58\%$$

The same can be done for calcium deficiency:

$$RR = \frac{1}{0.62} = 1.6$$

$$AR = \frac{RR - 1}{RR} = \frac{1.6 - 1}{1.6} = 0.38 \text{ or } 38\%$$

7–5.   Because of the long lag time needed for the development of renal calculi or nephrocalcinosis and the probable low prevalence of such complications, such a study would require a large number of people and many years of follow-up.

7–6 through 7–13.   These questions are meant to be an exercise in risk-benefit analysis using the information presented in this chapter regarding osteoporosis. With the exception of the case in question 7-6, consensus with regard to therapy is not expected. The goal of the exercise is not to come up with the correct answer, but rather to demonstrate your ability to identify the issues at hand in each case and to deal with them in such a way as to enable you to come to a logical, defendable decision.

The answers should center around calcium supplementation and ERT, but exercise, although only briefly mentioned in this chapter, is a well-accepted and effective form of prevention and treatment of osteoporosis and should be emphasized as concomitant therapy in each case. The issues to be addressed in each case are itemized below.

7–6.   Any woman who experiences premature menopause, whether owing to oophorectomy or ovarian failure, is at increased risk of osteoporosis because of the increased number of postmenopausal years she will experience. It is thus standard practice to treat such women with estrogen and progesterone replacement, at least until the age of natural menopause but ideally until the end of life. Assuring an adequate calcium intake and recommending exercises are also important and should be mentioned.

7–7.   A risk-benefit analysis of ERT should be discussed for this patient and should include the following factors: First, this patient's risk of osteoporosis is increased by her racial background (white) and tobacco use. Her obesity is protective against osteoporosis. Second, her risk of endometrial cancer is increased by her obesity and nulliparity. Third, her smoking and family history of myocardial infarction increase her risk of coronary artery disease and increase the potential impact of the unfavorable changes in the ratio of high-density to low-density lipoproteins associated with exogenous progesterone use.

7–8.   The following factors should be identified in the risk-benefit analysis of ERT in this patient: First, this patient's risk of osteoporosis is increased by her racial background (white), tobacco use, inactivity, and thin body habitus. Second, her gravidity and parity are protective against endometrial cancer. Finally, her smoking history contributes to her risk of coronary artery disease, but her lack of family history is favorable as compared to the patient in the preceding question.

7–9.   The analysis of this case should include the same factors mentioned in the two previous cases, in addition to the presence of diabetes mellitus. It is apparent that this patient is at high risk for both coronary artery disease and osteoporosis.

The major issue in this case is the lack of risk for endometrial cancer owing to hysterectomy. This allows the option of ERT without progestins, eliminating the issue of their unfavorable effects on the patient's lipoprotein profile and their potential impact on the risk of coronary artery disease. However, many authorities would argue this point since

data with regard to ERT and breast cancer are inconclusive and progesterone is known to antagonize or complement estrogen effects at
the breast as well as the endometrium.*† Estrogen and progesterone
should always be given in combination, regardless of the presence or
absence of an endometrium according to some authorities.

It should be considered that the patient with diabetes mellitus is particularly prone to atherosclerotic disease and may thus be at substantial
risk to suffer the consequences of the increased thrombogenicity that
has been associated with exogenous estrogens in some studies. She
would also be at greater risk to develop severe complications of cholelithiasis should this develop as a consequence of ERT.

7–10. This patient's racial background (black) substantially reduces her risk
for developing osteoporosis. Members of the dark-skinned races do,
however, carry some risk of developing the disease and fracturing
bones in late life. A thorough history should be obtained and, if other
risk factors for osteoporosis are present, ERT should be considered.
Exercise and adequate calcium intake should also be recommended,
as they should to everyone.

7–11. In this case, there are two major issues that should be addressed. First,
the postmenopausal acceleration in bone loss owing to estrogen deficiency is believed to be temporary, lasting only 7 to 10 years. Institution of ERT after this time period is therefore controversial. The potential benefit of ERT in this patient may thus be reduced, whereas
the risks associated with it are unchanged. Data on patients with established osteoporosis are limited. In one such study, discussed in Chapter
7, patients with vertebral spine fractures were treated with ERT and
calcium.§ The results suggest continued effect several years after
menopause.

The second major consideration in this case has to do with fracture
threshold. Once fracture threshold has been reached, one might argue, prevention of further bone loss is of limited value and the risks
of therapy may outweigh the benefits. This too is very controversial.
It is important to mention that hip fractures occur later than vertebral
fractures and so may require a greater amount of bone loss before

*Gompel A, Malet C, Spritizer P, et al. Progestin effect on cell proliferation and 17-beta-hydroxy
steroid dehydrogenase activity in normal human breast cancer in postmenopausal women. J Am
Endocrinal Metabol 1986;63:1174.
†Gambrell RD, Massey FM, Castaneda MA, Boddie AW. Estrogen therapy and breast cancer in
postmenopausal women. J Am Geriatr Soc 1980;28:251–257.
§Riggs BL, Seeman EE, Hodgson SF, et al. Effect of the fluoride calcium regimen on vertebral
fracture occurrence in postmenopausal osteoporosis. N Engl J Med 1982;306:446–450.

fracture threshold is reached. Thus, in this patient, treatment may still protect against hip fracture, the more devastating consequence of osteoporosis.

7–12. Here, the patient's gender (male) is at issue as well as his established osteoporosis. ERT is not an accepted form of therapy in men, and so the discussion should focus on calcium supplementation and exercise. It is important to mention that there are as yet no available studies evaluating the effect of calcium on the prevention of bone loss in men.

7–13. The risk of renal calculi should be weighed against the risk of osteoporosis in each case. It is important to mention that accepted practice in the prevention of additional renal calculi is calcium restriction. Monitoring 24-hour urine for calcium may be important in discovering hypercalciuria in a particular patient, but whether this is necessary only for those at risk for developing calculi or for everyone on calcium supplementation has not been established.

8–1. Immunization with a live-virus vaccine derived from an agent not completely shed by the host (viral latency) requires long-term observation of individuals receiving the vaccine to ascertain not only the protective effect (the absence of the development of varicella after exposure) but also the lack of occurrence of vaccine-related complications and long-term side effects (zoster).

8–2. To determine the risk of herpes zoster development among vaccinated subjects, one could select a group in which, over a short follow-up period, the occurrence of zoster is very high (i.e., children with leukemia). By using a high-risk group, one could measure the risk of herpes zoster development with and without the vaccine. This has, in fact, been done [24].

8–3.

Risk among those receiving placebo = 38/446

Risk among those receiving vaccine = 0/468

In evaluations of vaccines, the relative risk is called the protective efficacy ratio. In this instance, the protective efficacy ratio is infinite, since none of the vaccine recipients developed the disease. This is unusual in vaccine efficacy trials but does indicate that the vaccine confers a high rate of protection in this study population.

8–4.   These data indicate that there was not a single case of varicella among household contacts of vaccine recipients and that there were four cases among contacts of placebo recipients. This suggests that the vaccine is very protective in the people who receive it, even when these people come in close contact (household exposure) with a case of varicella. Normally, 80 to 90 percent of susceptible household contacts will develop the disease.

8–5.   There are three principal criteria to be considered. First, is the patient susceptible to varicella? Second, what is the nature of exposure to varicella? Third, is the patient in a high-risk group for the development of complications from varicella?

8–6.   VZIG should be given, as the patient is in a high-risk category (age 30). The fact that he can afford to pay for it is reassuring, but not a criterion by itself for using VZIG.

8–7.   (a) This immunocompromised patient was exposed 4 days before your encounter with her, the maximum elapsed time (96 hours) for which VZIG is optimally effective. In this case, VZIG would not offer protection. (b) Possibly, postexposure administration of vaccine has been employed up to 5 days after exposure. (c) The patient probably is not susceptible, since even in persons who have a negative history of chickenpox and who have reached adulthood, 90 to 95 percent have detectable antibody to varicella.

8–8.   (a) Evidence from several field trials with the varicella vaccine suggests that the vaccine could offer protection to the patient under these circumstances. The vaccine has also been given in postexposure instances, with subsequent protection from disease. (b) On the other hand, VZIG is an available protective measure that may be a more safe alternative in an immunosuppressed patient. Should VZIG immunization fail to protect this patient, vidarabine and acyclovir are available and have been shown to be effective in the treatment of varicella in immunosuppressed subjects. The drawbacks of passive VZIG immunization are the short-lived period of protection and its expense. Active immunization with live-virus vaccine would confer longer protection and avoid possible readministration of VZIG should exposure recur.

8–9.   The major determinants would be: (1) the extent to which a vaccination program could be applied such that near-universal rates of immunization are reached; (2) the length of immunity; and (3) the possible role that booster immunity plays in maintenance of immunity. This latter concept postulates that initial immunity to varicella is strengthened by continuing exposures to infected persons over the course of one's life. The extent to which this booster effect, acquired either naturally or through immunization, confers protection is not clear.

8–10.   The Japanese data, the American trials in immunosuppressed children, and the date of Weibel and colleagues lead to the following conclusions:

Attenuated live-virus varicella vaccine is highly immunogenic and that immunogenicity confers protection against the disease.

Protection is good in immunosuppressed children and even more effective in healthy children.

The vaccine appears to be truly attenuated in that no symptoms appeared in healthy children who received it. Fever and some vesicles appear in immunosuppressed recipients, but without serious consequences.

The 5-year follow-up data from Takahashi suggest a very small risk of herpes zoster in vaccinated patients.

The Brunell data [10] further suggest that the risk of herpes zoster even among immunocompromised children is small.

Questions regarding the length of immunity and the optimal type of protective immunity remain unanswered.

8–11.   Assuming these characteristics, a case could be made for immunization of all healthy children against varicella. One would need also to assume that rates of immunization would be high enough to protect the pediatric population. Data accumulated thus far would suggest that a vaccine with these characteristics would be of benefit to immunocompromised patients as well. The danger of this approach, however, is that loss of immunity after 10 years may increase the incidence of chickenpox among adults, in whom it often results in more complications.

9–1.   The subtypes chosen for the vaccine have been selected from those most commonly cultured from the blood of patients with *Streptococcus pneumoniae* infections. This has allowed the developers to produce a vaccine directed at those cases associated with severe infection. The use of blood cultures was required since sputum samples taken from patients with pneumonia may be contaminated by nasopharyngeal flora. Transtracheal aspirations have not been a practical means of sampling the cases of pneumonia. Thus, it is still not clear how well blood culture subtypes correlate with the subtypes causing pneumonia. Nasopharyngeal cultures have not been used as the basis for a vaccine since a small percentage of the population carry *Streptococcus pneumoniae* as normal flora in the nasopharynx.

9–2. To determine the percentage effectiveness against disease caused by the 14 subtypes, one must multiply 98 percent fourteen times (0.98^{14} = 0.754 = 75.5%). This must be done because the success against each subtype is independent of the success against other subtypes. This calculation measures the efficacy against all types combined. One multiplies the efficacy against individual types to determine the degree of protection afforded against pneumococcal disease caused by any of the 14 subtypes. Thus, if the vaccine prevented 98 percent of the infection caused by each of the subtypes, its overall protective effect against subtypes included in the vaccine would be slightly more than 75 percent.

9–3. The use of a high-risk population greatly reduces the sample size required to demonstrate statistically significant results. If one is dealing with a population in which the risk of disease is less than 5 per 1000 per year, it would require well over 10,000 individuals in each group to be able to demonstrate statistical significance for a true reduction of 50 percent in the incidence of disease.

Another advantage of using a high-risk population is that those at high-risk of disease are also those most likely to benefit from the therapy. If one has performed the necessary preliminary assessments of the vaccine, it often is considered most ethical to subject first those at high risk of disease to the risks inherent in a clinical trial since they are also the ones who are most likely to benefit.

9–4.

(a) Relative risk $= \dfrac{\text{risk among those receiving placebo}}{\text{risk among those receiving the vaccine}} = \dfrac{160/3007}{17/1493} = 4.4$

(b) In vaccine trials, the relative risk is often called the protective efficacy ratio. A relative risk of 4.4 implies that, on average, those receiving the placebo had 4.4 times the risk of developing pneumococcal pneumonia as those receiving the vaccine.

9–5.   Note that pneumococci cultured from the nasopharyngeal secretion was among the criteria used to identify pneumonia as pneumococcal pneumonia. This was true for pneumonia in both the vaccine and placebo groups; thus, the effect may have balanced itself out in part. The use of nasopharyngeal secretion to detect pneumococci, however, may have affected the accuracy of the estimated relative risk.

9–6.   The calculation of absolute risk requires that one take into account the incidence of disease in a particular population. For instance, if the incidence of disease is 1 in 100 without the vaccine, and the relative risk is 4.4, then the incidence of disease may be reduced to 1 in 440 by use of the vaccine. On the other hand, if the incidence of the disease is 1 in 10,000. It may be reduced to 1 in 44,000 by the vaccine. Thus, the incidence of disease in the group using the vaccine needs to be taken into account when estimating the effect of the vaccine on the absolute risk of disease.

9–7.   This is a question of attributable risk. Attributable risk or protective efficacy rate for a vaccine trial asks the question: How much of the disease occurred in those who did not receive the vaccine?

$$\text{Attributable risk} = \frac{\text{incidence in the placebo group} - \text{incidence in the vaccine group}}{\text{incidence in the placebo group}}$$

$$= \frac{160/3007 - 17/1493}{160/3007} = 78\%$$

9–8.   It is possible to reconcile these results if one assumes that chronically ill elderly individuals, unlike young healthy individuals, do not produce an antibody response that is adequate to prevent pneumonia. Their antibody response may still be adequate to prevent bacteremic disease. The Veterans Administration study was not designed to assess the impact of the vaccine on bacteremic disease. A much larger sample size would be required to address this issue using a controlled clinical trial.

9–9.   The recommendation to immunize all adults with chronic illness that predisposes them to pneumococcal infection or its complications needs to be questioned in light of the Veterans Administration study. The recommendation was made before the results of that study were known. The Veterans Administration study suggests that at least those adults older than 55 years with these types of chronic diseases do not receive adequate protection from the vaccine to prevent pneumococcal pneumonia or pneumococcal bronchitis.

9–10.   One would at least like evidence that these groups of individuals are capable of generating an antibody response to pneumococcal vaccine. Multiple myeloma patients generally have a substantial reduction in their antibody response, whereas sickle-cell patients are capable of response to most subtypes.

9–11.   If pneumococcal vaccine were effective only against bacteremic disease, it would still have the potential for saving lives by preventing mortality from the most severe disease. However, presumably the ability to reduce mortality and morbidity among those with preexisting cardiovascular and pulmonary disease would be lower because these individuals may die owing to cardiac and pulmonary failure secondary to pneumococcal pneumonia. Even if only bacteremic disease were affected, those with immunosuppressive diseases and splenic dysfunction may still benefit from vaccination since their risk of death usually is secondary to bacteremic disease.

9–12.   This measure merely estimates the cost of obtaining 1 additional year of life for one individual. It does not imply that each individual will live 1 year longer or that the average individual will live 1 year longer. The results mean that for every $6000 spent on the vaccine program, a total of 1 year of healthy life (or its equivalent in reduced disability) will be gained.

9–13.   If pneumococcal vaccine is only effective in preventing bacteremic disease, then the incidence of disease in the cost-effectiveness analysis may be in the range of only 0.08 per 1000 rather than 1.4 to 2.3 per 1000. The greatest effect of this change would be on the cost-effectiveness ratio for healthy individuals older than 65. For these people, the net cost per healthy year gained is likely to increase dramatically, making it very expensive to obtain a healthy year of life using the pneumococcal vaccine.

9–14.   Your answers to this question reflect the ethical values, political beliefs, and social priorities that ultimately determine how a cost-effectiveness assessment is translated into policy.

10–1.

$$\text{Mortality ratio} = \frac{\text{observed no. of lung cancer deaths}}{\text{expected no. of lung cancer deaths}} = \frac{450}{81.7} = 5.5$$

10–2. The figures in Table 10-1 suggest that smoking and asbestos are *multiplicative* risks: A 5-fold risk from asbestos together with a 10-fold risk from smoking results in a 50-fold risk of lung cancer death.

10–3. This attributable risk compares smoking asbestos workers to nonsmoking unexposed men. Thus,

$$\text{Attributable risk} = \frac{601.6 - 11.3}{601.6} = 98.1\%$$

10–4. Provided "regular inhalation" means regular inhalation for a working lifetime, this risk is well above the Supreme Court's threshold for action.

10–5.

	Pros	*Cons*
1. Banning		
Practical issues	Stops all exposure	Alternatives may be less effective or more dangerous
Cost	No costly retooling	Industry closes
Ethical issues	Eliminates risk to worker	Obligates all society to protect group at risk
2. Engineering controls		
Practical issues	Reduces exposure effectively	
Cost		Costly to risk imposer and, hence, to society
Ethical issues	Protects group at risk; obligates risk imposer	
3. Protective equipment		
Practical issues	Reduces exposure somewhat	Less effective than banning or engineering controls;

	Pros	Cons
		masks may be uncomfortable, ill-fitting, must be removed to talk, and so on
Cost	Costs less than engineering controls	
Ethical issues		Major obligation is on the group at risk and not on the group imposing the risk

10–6.

	Pros	Cons
1. Individual action		
Practical issues	Easy for employer	Not effective at reducing risk; employers have no financial incentive to spend money to make work places safer; few effective ways for workers to protect themselves
Cost	Cheap for companies	Costly for workers
Ethical issues	Companies have more freedom	Workers are rarely fully informed of the risks; risk imposed on worker; no penalty for risk imposer
2. Compensation and individual litigation		
Practical issues	Easy for employer in the short run; lawsuits may (years later) force employers to clean up work places	Not very effective; no immediate incentive to clean up work places (diseases may take years to manifest); few workers actually are compensated
Cost	Cheap in the short run for companies; financial compensation to injured workers	Short-run incentive not to clean up work place; company may go bankrupt later owing to lawsuits; lawsuits very expensive for all parties

	Pros	*Cons*
Ethical issues	Some compensation for injured worker; freedom for company	Question of ability of money to compensate for dying of cancer at age 50, limited freedom of choice for worker

3. Group action and litigation

	Pros	*Cons*
Practical issues	Somewhat better chance of compelling employers to make work place safer; theoretically, workers and company can negotiate acceptable level risk	Financial cost of litigation may be prohibitive; uncertain outcome of litigation; unequal contest (e.g., sued company can declare bankruptcy and not pay)
Cost	Inexpensive in the short run for companies; greater chance of compensating workers	Costly in the long run; high cost of litigation for all parties
Ethical issues	Some financial compensation for worker; some responsibility for company; freedom for company and workers to choose	Burden of illness still on worker; worker has limited choices

4. Regulation

	Pros	*Cons*
Practical issues	Effective protection	Requires enforcement
Cost	May be less costly than illness in the long run	Costly to company; costs to enforce
Ethical issues	Does not impose risk on worker; imposes duty on risk imposer (company)	Obligatory: less freedom

10–7. Options include:

Individual action: Informing workers of the risk

Compensation: Encouraging workers who are already sick to seek compensation or legal help, and helping them with medical reports

Group action: Helping or educating community or workers' groups to identify hazards and reduce the risk

Regulation: Actively advocating societal action to reduce the risk for all workers.

The decision is yours.

11–1. (a) The old are at greater risk of death from automobile accidents than the young, according to Table 11-1 (28.2 per 100,000 for 1- to 4-year-olds versus 65.5 per 100,000 for 65- to 74-year-olds). (b) A much greater number of years of life are lost among the young since a death among the young results in a loss of many years of expected life compared to a death among those 65 to 74 years old.

11–2.

$$\text{Relative risk} = \frac{\text{probability of developing the disease if the factor is present}}{\text{probability of developing the disease if the factor is absent}}$$

$$= \frac{146/33{,}200 \text{ (not buckled)}}{2/6300 \text{ (buckled)}} = \frac{0.0043975}{0.0003174} = 13.85$$

11–3.

Attributable risk

$$= \frac{\text{incidence of disease among those with the risk factor} - \text{incidence of disease among those without the risk factor}}{\text{incidence of disease among those with the risk factor}}$$

$$= \frac{146/33{,}200 - 2/6{,}300}{146/33{,}200} = 92.8\%$$

11–4. To perform a prospective study, an enormous number of individuals would have to be assessed for seat belt use and followed over many years.

11–5. No, Dr. Scherz attempts to control for speed by his epidemiologic finding that most automobile crashes in the 0-1 to 4-year-old group occur at low speeds (< 40 mph).

11–6.   First, the sample size (35 patients) is very small. Second, there is no verification of whether the child was buckled up. Dr. Kanthor simply asked the mothers.

11–7.   The Reisinger and Williams study had a larger sample size than Kanthor's study. Also, in the former, the parents were not aware that they were in a child restraint study, there was no preselection of patients. Finally, verification of the use of a child restraint was objective.

11–8.   It is very difficult to change behavior by education alone, and even motivational efforts (such as free car seats) may fail.

11–9.   Having a control group in a neighboring state observed at the same time helps control for seasonal cycles and trends. For example, maybe it was too hot to buckle up in August 1977 but not in April 1978. Perhaps parents in both states in August 1977 were exposed to a newspaper article questioning the value of child restraints. The use of a control state helps demonstrate that the change in Tennessee represents more than a general trend toward increased use.

11–10.   Child restraint laws can increase usage of child restraints.

11–11.   Child restraints *could actually be* less effective in more severe crashes, or parents who exceed the speed limit might be less likely to buckle up their children.

11–12.   (a) Child restraint laws seem to increase usage of child restraints. (b) These studies do not guarantee that child restraint usage increases will continue at the same level, but other studies have been done that show increased usage a number of years after enactment of child restraint laws.

11–13.   This seems unlikely.

11–14.   Possible methods of decreasing automobile fatalities among adolescents include:

   1. Use of airbags: Reduce risk of noncompliance. Also, these probably are better at higher speeds[1] (Note: There have been eight reported cases of vertebral column damage in high-speed accidents where seatbelts were used.[2])

[1]Status report. The human cost of airbag delay. Vol. 14, No. 14, Sept. 7, 1979.
[2]Ibrahaim KN. Lap seat belts useful but can injure children. JAMA 1981;245(22):2281.

2. Drinking and driving laws[3]: In France, these resulted in a decrease in motor vehicle crashes but not permanently. Laws may gradually change people's attitude. (In the United States, groups such as Mothers Against Drunk Drivers [MADD] and Students Against Drunk Drivers [SADD] may have an impact.)

3. Increases in age of licensure: Of course, this would decrease teenage death, but parents may not like it.[4]

4. Nighttime curfews: In four states that currently have curfews (8 PM to 4 AM), there has been a decrease in crashes involving 16-year-olds (ranging from a 25-percent decrease in Louisiana to a 69-percent decrease in Pennsylvania).[5]

5. Raising the drinking age to 21: In states where this has been adopted, there has been a decrease in teenage fatalities. In the early 1970s, more than half of the states lowered the drinking age, then reversed these decisions between 1976 and 1981 by raising the drinking age to 21. An average decrease of 28 percent in nighttime fatalities involving younger drivers was the result. The data from 26 states between 1975 and 1984 were reanalyzed, and a 13-percent decline in fatalities was found.[4]

6. Seat belt laws: Australian studies have shown a 20- to 75-percent increase in usage but only a 20-percent decrease in mortality.[6, 7] Such studies have focused on specific groups and observational techniques rather than anecdotal end points. They seem to show a definite increase in restraint usage after new child restraint laws were passed.

12–1. Table 12-4 shows that the smaller the lesion is at the time of diagnosis, the more limited is the disease. Table 12-5 shows that survival is directly related to the degree of spread. Lesions detected at less than 1 cm frequently are curable, and even those that are larger but with no spread to lymph nodes are associated with good survival rates. Table 12-5 also shows that at a time when most lesions are 1 cm or larger and palpable on physical examination, the vast majority have local invasion and more than 20 percent are associated with diseased lymph nodes. Physical examination, therefore, is useful in detecting some breast can-

[3]Status report. Drinking-driving laws: what works? Vol. 16, No. 5, April 16, 1981, p. 6.
[4]Status report. Teens and autos: a deadly combination. Vol. 16, No. 14, Sept. 23, 1981, pp. 1–11.
[5]Preusser DF, Williams AF, Zador PL, et al. The effect of curfew laws on motor vehicle crashes. Law and Policy Quarterly, Feb. 1983.
[6]Ontario Ministry of Transportation. The human collision. 2nd ed. 1975, p. 12.
[7]Robertson LS, Williams AF. International comparison of the effects of motor vehicle seat belt use and child restraint laws. Insurance Institute for Highway Safety, May 1978.

cer in early stages, but other tests are needed to identify unpalpable small lesions.

12–2.

1. Both mammography and physical examination made separate, substantial contributions to detection of breast cancer.
2. When breast cancer is detectable by only one screening method, the probability of positive lymph nodes is considerably lower.
3. Decreased mortality in the study group, compared to the control group, may be largely attributable to the increased detection of early lesions.
4. The decreased mortality was demonstrated only in the 50- to 60-year-old age group.

12–3.   Over the decade between the two studies, the sensitivity of mammography had improved in the 40- to 50-year-old age group, remaining about the same in the 50- to 60-year-olds. Physical examination appears to have become less sensitive than mammography, possibly because of earlier presentations. Table 12-8 displays this apparent change.

12–4.   In the first year of a screening program, the cases detected reflect the disease that is present at the time. Some of these cases may have been present for an extended period of time. Once the population has been screened, and preexisting cancer has been removed, the cancers detected in subsequent screenings reflect new cancers or cancers that have developed to a stage at which they are now detectable by the screening tests. Therefore, the cancer detection rate in the first year reflects the prevalence rate, whereas the cancer detection rate in the following years represents the incidence rate of new cancers.

12–5.   The following chart can be used to calculate sensitivity and specificity. The true positives (55.8) comprise the cancer detection rate. The false negatives (8) come from the interval detection rate. The false positives (302.3) represent the difference between the biopsy rate (358.1) and the cancer detection rate (55.8). The true negatives reflect all the other women per 10,000 screened.

	Cancer present	Cancer absent	
Positive screening	55.8	302.3	358.1
Negative screening	8	9634	9642
	63.8	9936.3	

(a) Sensitivity $= \dfrac{\text{true positive tests}}{\text{all patients with cancer}} = \dfrac{55.8}{63.8} = 87\%$

(b) Specificity $= \dfrac{\text{true negatives}}{\text{all patients without cancer}} = \dfrac{9634}{9936.3} = 97\%$

12–6.

(a) Positive predictive value (that a positive screening test means cancer):

$$\dfrac{\text{True positives}}{\text{All positive screening tests}} = \dfrac{55.8}{358.1} = 15.5\%$$

(b) Negative predictive value (that a negative test means cancer detected within the year):

$$\dfrac{\text{True negatives}}{\text{All negative screening tests}} = \dfrac{8}{9642} = 0.1\%$$

12–7. Remember that the BCDDP population included women aged 35 to 74 years old, with a median age of 49.5. If one is screening a predominantly young group, the predictive values will change since the prevalence of breast cancer in a particular population strongly affects the predictive value. For a population of younger women, who have a lower prevalence of breast cancer, the positive predictive value would be lower than in the BCDDP study, and the negative predictive value slightly lower. Conversely, in an older population, or in a population in which the individuals all had positive family histories of breast cancer, the prevalence of breast cancer and the positive predictive value would be higher, and the negative predictive value slightly higher.

Although you might be discouraged by such a low positive predictive value, remember that a screening test is not intended to diagnose disease. A good screening test must be good at ruling *out* disease (low negative predictive value) and must be able to define a population that needs further evaluation by a gold standard test—in this case, breast biopsy.

12–8. (a) The data and recommendation support yearly mammography for a 50-year-old woman. (b) The answer to this question relies on *your* application of both the data and other variables (e.g., your professional values).

13–1.   This is an important general question since these data often are available. Certainly, the data provided imply that early detection may alter outcome because presumably more tumors would be in a localized stage at detection and therefore a better survival rate would apply. However, one must consider other explanations. For example, the progression of the tumor in some patients may be much slower, explaining both detection in an earlier stage and longer survival, regardless of the time of detection [see Dales et al., ref. 11].

13–2.   On initial examination, more cancers were found than expected. When one first screens a previously unscreened group, many earlier asymptomatic cancers are discovered that would ordinarily have been discovered only at a more advanced symptomatic stage. On subsequent examinations, fewer cancers were found than expected. The most likely explanation is that we are now discovering only incidence cancers, not prevalence cancers. Incidence cancers are those that appeared since the last screening examination. When we screen a new, previously unscreened group, we pick up prevalence cancers, which are all those present since they appeared, not limited in time to a screening interval. Moreover, in this particular study, all polyps discovered were removed. If polyps truly develop into cancers, we have thus prevented new cancers. By what amount were there fewer incidence cancers than expected? Gilbertsen and Nelms state that only 13 new cancers occurred and approximately 87 to 90 were expected (i.e., an 85-percent reduction). However, Morrison* has pointed out that the 27 prevalence cancers, had they not been discovered and removed, would have been incidence cancers in the follow-up period and must be added to the 13 cancers for a total of 40 cancers as compared with 87 to 90 expected (i.e., a 56-percent reduction.)

(b) Table 13-3 shows that on initial examination, tumors were more localized than expected, with an improvement in 5-year survival rate. Let us now look at subsequent examinations. Remember, all polyps found were removed. The results show a marked decrease in the number of new cancers found, all of which were localized. The 85-percent overall survival rate becomes more impressive when we know that none of the deaths were in fact from cancers discovered on the examination. In other words, this screening program with removal of polyps led to prevention of death from rectal cancer.

*Morrison AS. Screening for chronic disease. Oxford: Oxford University Press, 1985, p. 101.

13–3.   Lead-time bias is unlikely to explain the results since the effects of lead time diminish with prolonged follow-up, as occurred in the Minnesota study [see Gilbertsen and Nelms, ref. 8]. The data in this study were analyzed separately for cases detected on initial and follow-up screenings. This makes it unlikely that length bias explains the improved outcome in the screened population. Patients who have a personal or family cancer history could be expected to attend a cancer detection clinic and to be at higher risk for developing cancer, as well as to exhibit health-seeking behavior that could lead to earlier diagnosis and better outcome. Clearly, patient self-selection bias is operative in these studies but should not invalidate the data. Overdiagnosis seems unlikely in view of the less-than-expected number of interval cancers discovered. One would like more information on the sources of the epidemiologic data providing the comparison and expected cancer rates. The reader must arrive at a final conclusion and screening policy on his or her own. We are impressed that this uncontrolled follow-up study does demonstrate marked benefit from early detection.

13–4.   (a) The diet with rare red meat and high-peroxidase vegetables gives a higher, presumably false, positive rate. (b) The authors would choose rehydration and a diet of no red meat and fresh fruits and vegetables for the 3 days preceding and 2 days of the collection. (c) This diet plan should result in maximizing sensitivity and minimizing false positive findings at 0.6 percent (specificity, 99.4 percent).

13–5.

(a) Sensitivity for carcinoma

$$= \frac{\text{no. of Hemoccult-positive patients with carcinoma}}{\text{total no. of patients with carcinoma}} = \frac{14}{27} \times 100 = 51.9\%$$

(b) Sensitivity for adenomas of less than 1 cm

$$= \frac{2}{45} \times 100 = 4.4\%$$

(c) Sensitivity for adenomas of more than 1 cm

$$= \frac{10}{44} \times 100 = 22.7\%$$

(d) Specificity for negative studies

$$= \frac{\text{no. of patients without disease with negative test}}{\text{all patients without disease}} = \frac{60}{66} \times 100 = 90.9\%$$

13–6.

$$\frac{\text{Predictive value of}}{\text{positive test}} = \frac{\text{true positives for colorectal cancer}}{\text{true positives plus false positives}}$$

$$= \frac{14}{34} \times 100 = 41.2\%$$

13–7.

	Disease-positive (N = 3)	Disease-negative (N = 997)
Positive test	(true positives) $0.52 \times 3 = 1.6$	(false positives) $0.04 \times 997 = 39.9$
Negative test	(false negatives) $0.48 \times 3 = 1.4$	(true negatives) $0.96 \times 997 = 957.1$

$$\text{Predictive value positive} = \frac{\text{true positives}}{\text{true positives + false positives}}$$

$$= \frac{1.6}{1.6 + 39.9} \times 100 = 3.9\%$$

$$\text{Predictive value negative} = \frac{\text{false negatives}}{\text{false negatives + true negatives}}$$

$$= \frac{1.4}{1.4 + 957.1} \times 100 = 0.15\%$$

The predictive value positive tells us what percent of patients with a positive test actually have the disease. Because the prevalence of the disease in a general (average-risk) population is relatively low, false positives greatly outnumber true positives and lead to a low predictive value. We can improve the yield by screening a higher-risk population or by maximizing specificity without sacrificing sensitivity.

The predictive value negative tells us what proportion of patients with a negative test actually have the disease.

13–8.

Sensitivity = 52%

Specificity = 96%

Prevalence = 9 per 1000

	Disease-positive (N = 9)	Disease-negative (N = 991)
Positive test	(true positives) 0.52 × 9 = 4.68	(false positives) 0.04 × 991 = 39.64
Negative test	(false negatives) 0.48 × 9 = 4.32	(true negatives) 0.96 × 991 = 951.36

$$\text{Predictive value positive} = \frac{4.68}{4.68 + 39.64} = 10.56\%$$

Note that the predictive value is considerably enhanced by screening a higher-risk group.

13–9.   Yes, because we cannot assume the same rate of risk with sigmoidoscopy plus polypectomy or colonoscopy plus polypectomy as we did for simple observational sigmoidoscopy. The risk of bleeding accompanies the removal of polyps, and the risk of perforation increases with the increasing depth of examination by colonoscopy (approximately 1 per 1000 in the latter case alone). On the other hand, this aggressive follow-up might essentially eliminate the further development of colorectal cancer in populations so closely monitored.

13–10.   Fifty-percent survival of 30 cancers equals 15 patients, times 5 years equals 75 patient-years. Ninety percent of 30 patients equals 27 patients, times 5 years equals 135 patient-years. Ten thousand screenings times $50 per screening equals $500,000. Difference in lives saved equals 60 years. A cost of $500,000 over 60 years equals $8333 per additional year of life saved.

14–1.   The best test for initial screening is one that detects all or most cases of disease. It should also be a test that is easily available, fairly easy to perform, and acceptable to the population. Both the VDRL and the FTA-ABS tests partially meet these qualifications. However, the VDRL test is most often selected for screening since it is easier to perform than the FTA-ABS test. Another reason for not selecting the FTA-ABS test is that it remains positive after treatment so that it is difficult to interpret a positive test in a person who had syphilis and was appropriately treated for it in the past.

14–2.

$$\text{Sensitivity} = \frac{\text{TP}}{\text{TP} + \text{FN}} = \frac{57}{57 + 11} = \frac{57}{68} = 84\%$$

$$\text{Specificity} = \frac{\text{TN}}{\text{TN} + \text{FP}} = \frac{904}{904 + 31} = \frac{904}{935} = 97\%$$

These results underestimate sensitivity and overestimate specificity since the study does not consider borderline positive findings as positive tests.

14–3.   Construct a 2 × 2 table:

	Syphilis present (N = 100)	Syphilis absent (N = 900)
Negative FTA-ABS test	True-positive	False-positive
Positive FTA-ABS test	False-negative	True-negative

With a 10-percent prevalence, 100 individuals in a population of 1000 have the disease. Assuming a sensitivity of 99 percent, 99 of 100 individuals will have a negative FTA-ABS test. Assuming a specificity of 99 percent, 891 of 900 individuals will have a negative FTA-ABS test. Thus, one can construct the following table:

	Syphilis present (N = 900)	Syphilis absent (N = 900)
Positive FTA-ABS test	(true positives) 99	(false positives) 9
Negative FTA-ABS test	(false negative) 1	(true negatives) 891

From these values, one can calculate the predictive value of a positive and negative test.

$$\text{Predictive value} = \frac{\text{TP}}{\text{TP} + \text{FP}} = \frac{99}{99 + 9} = \frac{99}{108} = 92\%$$

$$\text{Predictive value negative} = \frac{FN}{FN + TN} = \frac{1}{1 + 891} = \frac{1}{892} = 0.11\%$$

14–4.   As the prevalence increases, the chances that a patient with a positive test has the disease greatly increases. Simultaneously, the chances that a patient with a negative test has the disease greatly decreases. Another way of saying this is that the higher the prevalence or probability of disease before obtaining the test, the more likely a positive test result actually indicates the presence of disease.

14–5.   If John has both a positive VDRL test and a positive FTA-ABS test, we need to estimate his pretest probability of having syphilis. Using Table 14-4, one can see that even if John has a relatively low pretest probability of syphilis (1 percent), his chance of having the disease if both tests are positive is 96.5 percent. This is a high enough probability to make most clinicians treat for the disease and follow John clinically and serologically thereafter.

14–6.   (a) There is evidence in epidemiologic studies that case and contact identification (and subsequent testing or treatment of these contacts) is crucial in the eradication of sexually transmitted diseases. Mandatory reporting of cases and potential contracts allows departments of public health to take responsibility for the costly and sometimes difficult task of tracking down all potential cases and ensuring proper follow-up and treatment. This task is much too cumbersome for the individual physician.

   (b) In the case of John and Mary, since you are the family physician, a meeting with the parties (perhaps individually and together) might be in order both to answer their questions and to identify other potential contacts. You might want to assure them of confidentiality with respect to their friends and family and also discuss with the health department what treatment you intend. If there are no other disclosed contacts, the health department may forego a large-scale investigation.

14–7.   In general, all four criteria are met by syphilis screening. We have seen that there is substantial morbidity or mortality associated with the untreated disease. Risk factors include sexual promiscuity and single contacts among high-risk groups. Treatment is possible and effective at the subclinical stage of latent syphilis, and serologic tests that are easy to perform are available for screening appropriate groups.

14–8.   The advantages of maintaining premarital screening programs are that many women can be reached before they deliver a child and that a group of individuals at risk are assured of being tested. Among the disadvantages are that it may constitute an invasion of privacy, it fails to reach homosexuals who are at high risk, and it fails to reach many women who deliver children out of wedlock.

15–1. Intuitively, we might assume that prevention of spread through more expedient identification and isolation of infectious cases would have steepened the slope of the curve. However, it is clear that the decline in death rate began well before the introduction of preventive or curative therapy. Such factors as better standards of living might have played a role early on. From an epidemiologic viewpoint, more accurate case identification methods might have made a difference in the number of deaths attributed to tuberculosis. It is interesting to note that the slope of the line does not change over time, regardless of the effect of interventions designed to control the disease. Thus, it is theoretically possible that biologic selection against bacilli survival has been the predominant factor contributing to the decline in the death rate associated with tuberculosis.

15–2. An individual, once infected by the tuberculosis organism, can at any time thereafter develop active disease. This risk probably decreases over time from initial infection. As a result of the decline in the incidence of disease, most younger members of the population have not been exposed to the tubercle bacillus, whereas those members of the population reaching 65 years of age or older probably were exposed to the organism. Thus, the greatest potential reservoir for development of active disease is among the elderly, who comprise the segment of the population still infected.

15–3. The incidence of tuberculosis will probably decline as the baby boomers advance into old age because the majority of these individuals will never have been exposed to the infecting organism.

15–4. Test sensitivity is 95 percent. The sensitivity of a test is the true positives divided by the true positives plus the false positives; therefore:

$$\frac{95}{95 + 5} = \frac{95}{100} = .95 = 95\%$$

15–5. (a) At a cutoff point of 10 mm, few individuals with *M. tuberculosis* will be missed by PPD testing, but infections with atypical organisms will be picked up also, constituting less than 1 percent of those tested. (b)

At a cutoff point of 12 mm, most individuals who test positively will be infected with *M. tuberculosis,* and a small number (approximately 8 percent or less) will be infected with atypical organisms. (c) At a cutoff point of 20 mm, most individuals who test positively will be infected with *M. tuberculosis,* and no atypical infections will be identified.

15–6. A PPD reaction of 10 mm in a population with a high incidence of tuberculosis would most likely signify infection with *M. tuberculosis,* as would a PPD reaction of 5 mm. A positive PPD of any size is less likely to signify a reaction to infection with atypical mycobacteria in this population.

15–7.

$$\text{Relative risk} = \frac{\text{risk of active } M.\ tuberculosis \text{ if placebo is taken}}{\text{risk of active } M.\ tuberculosis \text{ if isoniazid is taken}}$$

$$= \frac{62/(62\ +\ 11{,}977)}{14/(14\ +\ 12{,}439)} = 4.6$$

$$\text{Attributable risk} = \frac{\text{relative risk}\ -\ 1}{\text{relative risk}} = \frac{4.6\ -\ 1}{4.6} = \frac{3.6}{4.6} = 78\%$$

15–8.

$$\text{Relative risk} = \frac{\text{risk of active } M.\ tuberculosis \text{ if no treatment is given}}{\text{risk of active } M.\ tuberculosis \text{ if isoniazid is taken}}$$

$$= \frac{45/(45\ +\ 712)}{1/(1\ +\ 604)} = 36.0$$

$$\text{Attributable risk} = \frac{\text{relative risk}\ -\ 1}{\text{relative risk}} = \frac{36\ -\ 1}{36} = 97\%$$

15–9.

$$\text{Relative risk} = \frac{\text{risk of hepatitis if isoniazid is taken}}{\text{risk of hepatitis if no isoniazid is taken}}$$

$$= \frac{19/(19\ +\ 2302)}{1/(1\ +\ 2153)} = 17.6$$

$$\text{Attributable risk} = \frac{\text{relative risk}\ -\ 1}{\text{relative risk}} = \frac{17.6\ -\ 1}{17.6} = 94\%$$

15–10. One would need to consider the indication for use of isoniazid along with the following: the relative risk of developing active tuberculosis, the risk of spreading the disease if it became active, and the risk for a given individual of developing isoniazid-related hepatitis, such as age and history of or current use of alcohol.

15–11.   Persons in whom you should consider using chemoprophylaxis include: any household contact of an active case; an individual who is a recent converter, of any age; an individual with a positive PPD test of unknown duration who is younger than 35 years; a child younger than 5 years with exposure to active tuberculosis; an individual with fibrotic lesions on a chest roentgenogram that are suggestive of an old tuberculosis infection; an individual of any age with a positive PPD test who has any of the special conditions listed in the text.

Even though all of the aforementioned individuals are candidates for chemoprophylaxis, the decision to use isoniazid must be individualized. If an individual is noncompliant, the decision to use chemoprophylaxis might depend not only on his or her having an indication for its use but the relative potential for developing active disease, considered either separately or in conjunction with the relative public health risk, should the individual develop active disease.

If the person has a history of alcohol abuse, there is probably reason to suspect that he or she might be noncompliant. Depending on his or her nutritional status, or the possibility that he or she might use other drugs, this individual could be at increased risk for developing active disease. These factors must be weighed and discussed with the patient to arrive at a decision concerning isoniazid use. Perhaps most importantly, the possibility of developing irreversible hepatic damage, especially if the individual is older than 35 must be considered and compared with the risk of developing and also of spreading active tuberculosis.

15–12.   The patient in case A could be considered a recent converter. Therefore, simply because he is at increased risk for developing tuberculosis, he could be considered for chemoprophylaxis with isoniazid once active tuberculosis is ruled out with a chest roentgenogram. However, if isoniazid is used, he should also be closely monitored for signs of hepatotoxicity since, owing to his age, he is probably at high risk for developing isoniazid-related hepatitis.

Another possibly more prudent management approach might be first to rule out active tuberculosis and then, since he is in a closely monitored situation, to observe him for signs of active tuberculosis and treat accordingly if necessary.

One other consideration is to question whether this positive PPD test is actually owing to recent conversion. Even though records indicate he had a negative PPD test each of the 2 preceding years, these could have been falsely negative, perhaps owing to improper placement or reading. Obtaining old records might clarify the situation. This consideration might lend more weight to choosing observation.

15–13.   The child in case B is at an age associated with a very high risk for developing active tuberculosis, even though he has a negative PPD test, because he has been exposed to an active case of disease. According to official recommendations, he should be treated with isoniazid for a total of 12 months. A new PPD test should then be placed. If it is negative and exposure to the active case has ended, prophylactic therapy can be stopped.

15–14.   The patient in case C is not a known recent converter; nor is he in one of the age groups that would place him at high risk for developing active disease. However, he is in the age group at which the risk of isoniazid-related hepatitis begins to increase. Therefore, following him clinically and assessing for the presence of active disease would be prudent. In this situation, however, a question can be raised regarding whether this PPD result could represent a recent conversion. The decision to use prophylaxis would then depend on the patient's and your confidence that he will comply with the medication regimen and restrict his use of alcohol during the course of therapy.

Much of the patient's decision about what he wants, if he is regarded as a recent converter, will probably depend on his perception of the risk of developing active disease, of which you can apprise him. You would probably especially need to consider the potential risk for him to develop irreversible, substantial isoniazid-related hepatitis should he drink excessively while taking isoniazid versus the possibility of successfully treating and curing an active case of tuberculosis should it occur. The potential for him to spread active disease, should it develop, must also be considered.

In addition, if this patient has a history of being noncompliant with medications, the chance of successful prophylaxis is lessened. An alternative would be to rely on him to contact you in the event of upper respiratory symptoms. You might also want to schedule regular follow-up appointments.

16–1.   Although most physicians do not deal with questions such as this on a regular basis, not knowing the answer is in itself no problem. The only things you can remember about rabies are bad. You remember that the disease is virtually invariably fatal (there have been only 3 survivors documented in the past 20 years). Once clinical symptoms appear, the process is irreversible. You also remember that there is a highly effective preventive measure—postexposure vaccination—that can be undertaken. Nonetheless, this is not enough information to help you decide whether to treat the patient and how to go about it. Resources that might be of assistance in this decision-making process include standard texts and information available by direct consultation with the county or state health department.

16–2.   In Chapter 5, the concepts of primary, secondary, and tertiary prevention were introduced. Primary prevention seeks to eliminate acquisition of a disease. This usually is done by altering social, cultural, genetic, or environmental factors that serve to increase the risk of developing a particular illness.

Secondary prevention is the early detection of established illness in an asymptomatic individual. Its goal is the identification of a problem and its early treatment. Secondary prevention can be aimed at risk factor alleviation, but these risk factors are subclinical disease states rather than alterable social, cultural, or environmental conditions.

Tertiary prevention is the attempt to prevent either the occurrence of further complications or worsening of an established and usually symptomatic illness. Clinical medicine traditionally takes the form of tertiary prevention. This is true of palliative as well as curative interventions.

Postexposure vaccination is a form of secondary prevention.

16–3.   Any time a form of secondary prevention is effective, it does two things. First, it makes usage of the therapy far less discriminating: If there is a chance that exposure has occurred, vaccinations are readily prescribed, often without thought being given to their cost or inconvenience. Second, such a successful form of secondary prevention limits the desire to use other preventive measures, such as primary prevention.

16–4.   Each 70-kg person will need 1400 IU of HRIG, or five vials at $65 each, for a total cost of $325. In addition, each person will require five doses of HDSRV at $63 each, for a total of $315. The cost of vaccinating 25,000 people is therefore 25,000 × $640 = $16,000,000.

16–5.   Approximately 1000 individuals may be saved each year, but this is most likely an overestimate if one considers the number of cases that would have occurred in the prevaccine era. Regardless, given a total cost of $16,000,000, this leaves us with a crude estimate of $16,000 per case prevented.

16–6. In our case example, although Elisa was not bitten (bites are automatically considered an exposure), there was ample opportunity for saliva from the infected raccoon to come in contact with microscopic breaks in the skin barrier or to have been transmitted to a mucous membrane while Elisa handled the animal. If this is what is assumed to have happened, then the path to follow is obvious: Provide postexposure prophylaxis.

17–1. When Mary Sager was 36, during her first pregnancy, her risk of having a Down's syndrome child was 1 chance in 287. When she was 39, during her second pregnancy, the odds were 1 : 139, approximately a 2-fold increase. It is interesting to note that most major studies indicate that paternal age is not a risk factor for Down's syndrome.*

17–2. Practically, it would probably have been difficult to convince people to agree to randomization. In addition, there are moral questions raised about exposing not only the mother but also the fetus to an unknown level of risk unless both also stood to benefit in some way. Thus, random assignment to the treatment (amniocentesis) or nontreatment group would have been ethically problematic.

17–3. It would be important for the counseling physician, before advising a couple, to review how the fetal loss figures were calculated and consider whether any of the study's biases or limitations distorted the calculations. One would look at the fetal loss figures to determine whether any of the study's limitations could have resulted in a possible underestimate or overestimate of the difference between subjects and controls.

17–4. It is possible that the comparison between subjects and controls is unfair because, as was noted, the subject group is comprised of older patients, and older patients have a higher spontaneous abortion rate than younger ones. Thus, age must be considered a selection bias. To compensate for this potential selection bias, the investigators in the NICHD study calculated age-adjusted rates for the subject group and the control group and got 3.3 and 3.4 percent, respectively. It is possible, then, that the age bias did slightly distort the true difference between the subject group and the control group.

*Milunsky A. Genetic disorders and the fetus. 2nd ed. New York: Plenum, 1986.

17–5.   The study planners enlisted approximately 1000 subjects and 1000 controls so that a statistically significant difference could be demonstrated if there were a true doubling of the frequency of an adverse effect. Therefore, a small observed difference (0.3% percent, in this case) in spontaneous abortions, if true, between controls and subjects may indeed reflect a real increased risk for amniocentesis patients; however, the study may not have enough resolving power (numbers are too small) to demonstrate statistical significance. Statisticians refer to this as a type II error.

A number of authors state or imply that the spontaneous abortions they have seen in close proximity to amniocentesis are probably a result of the procedure and that the overall incidence of spontaneous abortions is slightly higher in amniocentesis subjects than in controls. In one paper, Pauker and Pauker* state that they have used the observed difference in the NICHD study† (0.3 percent) as the maximum likelihood estimate of the true difference. Other experts‡ estimate that the true risk of the procedure for causing fetal loss is probably less than 0.5 percent.

17–6.   This woman, because of the difficulty of conceiving, may not want to take even the slightest risk of losing the child. For this reason and because the risk of Down's syndrome is relatively small (1 : 175), she may elect not to have amniocentesis. The 0.3% difference in risk of spontaneous abortion between subjects and controls—although not statistically significant—may be very important for this individual.

17–7.   (a) There probably is only a slight increase in abortion rate with amniocentesis. The NICHD data should be very reassuring for the understandably worried couples we talked about previously. (b) One final caveat is necessary. Remembering the distinction made in Chapter 4, there is a difference between the *efficacy* shown in the somewhat artificial confines of a study and the *effectiveness* as translated into real-world situations. The excellent safety record demonstrated in the NICHD study, if it is to be applicable to our future patients, presumes that our patients will have access to physicians as skillful in performing amniocentesis as those in the study.

---

*Pauker SP, Pauker SG. The amniocentesis decision: an explicit guide for parents. Birth defects: original article series, 1979 (The National Foundation);15(5c):289–324.
†NICHD National Registry for Amniocentesis Study Group. Midtrimester amniocentesis for prenatal diagnosis. JAMA 1976;236(13):1471–1476.
‡Milunsky A. Genetic disorders and the fetus. 2nd ed. New York: Plenum, 1986.

17–8.   Considering her beliefs, she would probably rate not undergoing amniocentesis and having a Down's syndrome child as a low utility outcome, perhaps a 20. However, considering that she has very much wanted a child and tried for 11 years without success, she may rate the utility of spontaneous abortion after amniocentesis even lower, perhaps a 10. When her 1 : 175 age-related risk (and other risks) are integrated into the decision tree, the decision analysis may suggest that the choice most consistent with her beliefs and the risk data is for her not to have amniocentesis and take the relatively small risk 1 : 175 of having a Down's syndrome baby.

17–9.   Here is such an altered decision tree.

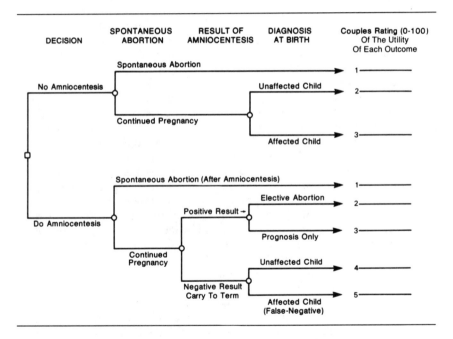

17–10.   The first frame presents the data in terms of mortality and the second in terms of survival. Surgery seemed much more attractive to the study population when presented in terms of probability of survival. The authors explained this difference by noting that "the risk of perioperative death looms larger when presented in terms of mortality." The way data are presented, then, introduces a bias into the decision-making process. This particular phenomenon is called the framing effect.

17–11. (a) Nondirective presentation of the data would be essential. However, in addition, decision analysis techniques might prove especially useful. They will help the patient deal with a complex body of mathematic information while at the same time incorporating her values into the decision-making process.

(b) In this case, you are confronted by a patient whose judgment may be distorted by an oversimplified concept of the facts. What sort of risk does she have in mind when she says that there is a "high risk of a Down's syndrome baby once you get to be older than 35?" Is it close to the actual risk for a 36-year-old woman (1 : 294)? Where did she hear about this high risk? You will want to know whether her thinking is influenced by availability bias: Did she have a friend who had a Down's syndrome baby at age 37, and did this event make her think that the risk was much higher than it really is? You will want to learn what information she does have and what fears she harbors about the nature of Down's syndrome itself? In such a case, where judgment may be distorted, the physician must first review the patient's understanding of the data (nondirective model) to ensure that it is accurate. The physician can then use judgment analysis; exploring with the patient in a supportive way the thought processes she used in making her judgment. Thus, the physician can uncover biases and misconceptions that interfere with the patient's ability to make decisions in accord with her beliefs. After reviewing the data, the physician could make this 36-year-old woman aware that her odds of having a Down's syndrome baby are only 1 : 294. If her perception of the risk of having a Down's syndrome baby was based simply on inaccurate information, presentation of the data by the physician will help her a great deal. If, after being given age-related risk information about Down's syndrome, she still seems unduly fearful, she might be reacting emotionally to her friend's experience. Judgment analysis could help uncover this and help her deal with it. Whether this woman merely has inaccurate information or has hidden fears (or both), helping her to think more realistically about the problem could ultimately bring her decision in line with her beliefs. She might opt not to have amniocentesis because, realistically, the odds against her having a Down's syndrome child are very good and her religious beliefs incline her away from abortion.

18–1. The first goal could be accomplished since, if a person were effectively vaccinated prior to any primary genital herpes infection, he or she would be protected from infection even if in contact with an actively infected individual. The seventh goal would also be attainable if there were an effective vaccine, as it would provide protection from herpes simplex virus whether it were shed from a recurrent or primary attack or were the result of asymptomatic shedding.

18–2. The first goal would be achieved since those under therapy during a primary episode of genital herpes would not be shedding virus and thus would not infect those who came into contact with them.

If the drug were safe, which is especially difficult to establish, the herpes simplex virus could be suppressed in terms of shedding and, therefore, newborns delivered vaginally would not be exposed to viral shedding. Thus, goal 2 could be accomplished.

By limiting the number of new lesions, such a drug would shorten the local manifestations during a primary episode, thus satisfying goal 3.

If the drug were able to suppress formation of new lesions in primary infections as well as successfully prevent viral shedding, a possible benefit would be the reduction of acute systemic complications of initial herpes simplex virus infection. Hence, goal 4 *might* be accomplished.

Finally, if we agree that the drug prevents recurrence as well as viral shedding, it would necessarily reduce transmission from those with established latent disease. Goal 7 would be met.

Only goals 5, 6, and 8 could not be satisfied by a drug that prevents additional lesions and stops viral shedding.

18–3. The first goal would be partially accomplished by such a drug, as those who come into contact with individuals with recurrent disease would not contract the herpes simplex virus if they were on appropriate treatment. Goal 2 might also be accomplished effectively but issues of safety for a fetus would be difficult to establish. Such a drug would be able to prevent subsequent clinical recurrence among those with established latent infection, thus satisfying goal 6. Finally, to the extent that all individuals with recurrent disease receive treatment with this drug, there would be a commensurate reduction in transmission from those with established latent disease (goal 7).

Since this drug is for recurrent disease, it would have no impact on primary episodes. Thus, goals 3 and 4 would not be satisfied. Since it does not eradicate the virus, it would also have no effect on latent infection, and therefore goals 5 and 8 could not be met.

18–4.

Acyclovir-5: Relative risk $= \dfrac{44/47}{13/45} = 3.2$

$$\text{Attributable risk} = \frac{2.2}{3.2} = 69\%$$

$$\text{Acyclovir-2:} \quad \text{Relative risk} = \frac{44/47}{18/5} = 2.65$$

$$\text{Attributable risk} = \frac{1.65}{2.65} = 62\%$$

18–5. Concerns of long-term therapy should be the development of resistant herpes simplex strains, which may occur by selection of strains that produce little or no thymidine kinase. In addition, for those patients on subjectively successful long-term suppression of genital herpes, newfound psychologic comfort may permit more promiscuous behavior. If the disease is spread in the absence of lesions, long-term suppression may, ironically, promote the spread of genital herpes.

18–6. Clinically small or unimpressive differences may be statistically significant.

18–7. In the self-initiated therapy patients, the 5.7 days ($\pm$ 0.3) needed for healing the lesions present at the first clinic visit is a shorter time than the 6.3 days for the same parameter in the physician-initiated therapy group. Although this appears to be a substantial improvement, the placebo patients in the self-initiated therapy group also healed more quickly than those in the physician-initiated therapy group.

A comparison of the difference in time between acyclovir users and placebo users in the other areas considered in this study reveals a small but statistically significant improvement in the duration of viral shedding with acyclovir use.

Self-initiated therapy produced especially impressive results in the percentage of patients who developed new lesions during the treatment period. The 7.3 percent who developed new lesions compare favorably with the 21.7 percent of controls and the 16 percent in the physician-initiated therapy group who developed new lesions.

18–8. Pregnancy potential and patient compliance need to be considered in individual patient selection.

18–9. You have the data. How you apply your professional values (e.g., how therapeutically conservative or aggressive you are) as well as your patient's concerns will determine the answer.

18–10. Longer-term therapy may lead to side effects not observed in short-term therapy. The efficacy may be affected by the development of resistant strains during treatment. Issues of informal consent and legal burden of proof arise when approved duration is exceeded.

19–1.

$$\text{Relative risk} = \frac{\text{observed/expected strokes with atrial fibrillation}}{\text{observed/expected strokes without atrial fibrillation}}$$

$$= \frac{5.60}{0.92}$$

$$= 6.09$$

$$\text{Attributable risk} = \frac{\text{relative risk} - 1}{\text{relative risk}} = \frac{5.09}{6.09} = 0.836 = 83.6\%$$

This means that in persons with atrial fibrillation, 83.6 percent of their strokes were attributable to atrial fibrillation.

19–2. The initial study included only persons who had atrial fibrillation on a prior examination. As can be seen from Table 19-2, in approximately 25 percent of persons who have a stroke and atrial fibrillation, the atrial fibrillation is noted for the first time at the time the stroke occurs. Thus, the initial Framingham data may underestimate the true risk of stroke from atrial fibrillation. (However, some people may develop atrial fibrillation because of a stroke.)

19–3. The risk we want is the population attributable risk. In other words, what percentage of all strokes in the population are caused by the presence of atrial fibrillation? We cannot simply use the raw data (i.e., the number of strokes in each group) since the raw data are not adjusted for the higher age, male predominance, and higher incidence of hypertension in the group with atrial fibrillation.

$$\begin{matrix}\text{Population} \\ \text{attributable} \\ \text{risk}\end{matrix} = \frac{b\,(RR - 1)}{b\,(RR - 1) + 1} = \frac{0.0044\,(5.1)}{0.0044\,(5.1) + 1} = 0.022$$

where b = prevalence of atrial fibrillation in total population

RR = relative risk

$$b = \frac{481 \text{ person-years in atrial fibrillation}}{109,532 \text{ total person-years}} = 0.0044$$

Thus, 2.2 percent of all strokes could be prevented if all strokes owing to atrial fibrillation (as detected in the initial Framingham study) were eliminated. Remember that by age 75, approximately 4 percent of the population (versus 0.4 percent in the Framingham group) have atrial fibrillation. Thus, the population attributable risk is probably much higher in those individuals aged 75 or older.

19–4.   Using the data of Svanborg and colleagues, we know that approximately 3 of every 100 individuals aged 70 years (4 percent males, 2 percent females) have atrial fibrillation. If 30 percent of them volunteered for the study, we would need to screen approximately 100 persons for each study subject obtained, or 273,400 to get our full complement of subjects. This would be a major task and, as noted, represents a *minimum* estimate. It is more likely that only new-onset, untreated cases could be used, which would increase the number we need to screen by 10-fold or more.

19–5.   Short-term anticoagulation is nearly always done with intravenous heparin, usually in the hospital. Long-term anticoagulation uses oral anticoagulants (usually of the coumarin type). The mechanism of action, efficacy, and side effects are different with these two drugs.

19–6.   Some likely events are survival with a major disability, complications, survival or death from a complication, and death owing to causes other than a stroke.

19–7.   See Figure 19-2.

19–8.   We will need to know (1) the probability of stroke in the 85-year-old person, given recent-onset atrial fibrillation, both with and without anticoagulation; (2) the probability of a complication, and of death from a complication, given anticoagulation; (3) the probability of death from causes other than stroke; (4) the probability of survival of major disability but death from a stroke with and without anticoagulation; and (5) the relative utility that the various outcomes (survival, stroke, stroke with a major disability, complication from anticoagulation, and death) have for our patient.

19–9.   One of the things that we can do when faced with a toss-up situation is to go back and reexamine the clinical situation to see whether minor losses or low-probability events that we omitted from the tree might sway us one way or the other. We often agonize over toss-up situations. However, it is important to recognize that a toss-up means that there is no clearly better or best option. Faced with these toss-ups, either option is acceptable.

19–10.   Consider that a 95-year-old with atrial fibrillation has a life expectancy of approximately 2 years, while a 55-year-old man with end-stage pulmonary disease and atrial fibrillation might have a life expectancy of less than 6 months. Clearly, the relative benefit in terms of gain in years of survival with anticoagulation would be greater with the 95-year-old man if other factors were the same in both patients.

19–11.   Do not institute anticoagulant therapy (result is below the curve).

19–12.   Anticoagulate (result is above the curve).

19–13.   This is a toss-up (result falls on the curve).

20.   Answers to questions in the section titled Testing Your Mastery of Important Concepts:
1. a
2. d
3. b
4. c
5. a
6. c
7. d
8. a
9. b
10. a

Index